HANDBOOK OF
MATERIALS FOR MEDICAL DEVICES

Edited by
J.R. Davis
Davis & Associates

ASM International
Materials Park, OH 44073-0002
www.asminternational.org

First printing, December 2003
Second Printing, March 2004
Third Printing, October 2004
Fourth Printing, October 2006

ASM International staff who worked on this project include Scott Henry, Assistant Director of Reference Publications; Bonnie Sanders, Manager of Production; and Nancy Hrivnak, Jill Kinson, and Carol Polakowski, Production Editors.

Library of Congress Cataloging-in-Publication Data

Handbook of materials for medical devices / edited by J.R. Davis.
   p. ; cm.
   Includes bibliographical references and index.
   1. Biomedical materials—Handbooks, manuals, etc. I. Davis, J. R. (Joseph R.) II. ASM International.
   [DNLM: 1. Biomedical and Dental Materials. QT 37 H2366 2003]
R857.M3H355 2003
610'.284 —dc22

2003057730

ISBN 13: 978-0-87170-790-1
ISBN 10: 0-87170-790-X
SAN:204-7586

ASM International®
Materials Park, OH 44073-0002
www.asminternational.org

Printed in the United States of America

Contents

Preface

In January of 2000, the National Institutes of Health (NIH) estimated that 8 to 10% of Americans, or about 20 to 25 million people, had some sort of medical device implanted in their bodies (refer to the NIH Technology Assessment Conference on Implants, held 10–12 Jan 2000 in Bethesda, MD). In the United States, the market for orthopedic implant devices such as total knee and hip replacements, spinal implants, and bone fixation devices, exceeds two billion dollars per year. Worldwide, this market exceeds $4.3 billion per year. These numbers, which clearly demonstrate the economic impact of the medical device industry, should continue to rise due to the combination of advances in the medical and materials science fields and an aging population (particularly in the United States, where some "baby boomers" are now in their sixties).

Humans have sought to restore function to the human body stricken by trauma or disease for thousands of years. For example, ancient civilizations such as the Phoenicians, Etruscans, Greeks, Romans, Chinese, and Aztecs used gold in dentistry as far back as 2700 BC. The use of sutures made from linen can be traced back to the Egyptians in circa 2000 BC. However, it has only been during the past 100 years that man-made materials and devices have been developed to the point where they can be used extensively to replace parts of living systems in the human body. These special materials—able to function in intimate contact with living tissue, with minimal adverse reaction or rejection by the body—are called *biomaterials*. Today, biomaterials play a major role in replacing or improving the function of every major body system (skeletal, circulatory, nervous, etc.). Some common implants include the orthopedic devices mentioned earlier; cardiac implants such as artificial heart valves and pacemakers; soft tissue implants such as breast implants and injectable collagen for soft tissue augmentation; and dental implants to replace teeth/root systems and bony tissue in the oral cavity.

Recognizing the growing importance of biomaterials and bioengineering, ASM International has published a number of reviews during the past 20 years that document the properties and failure mechanisms of metallic implant materials. The majority of these reviews can be found in various volumes of the *Metals/ASM Handbook* series. Until now, however, there was no single definitive source published by ASM that described the many important topics associated with the use of various implant materials (including metals, ceramics, polymers, composites, and coatings). These materials include:

- Implant material selection and applications
- The body/oral environment and its impact on implant material performance
- The basic concepts of biocompatibility
- Tissue attachment mechanisms
- Biophysical and biomechanical requirements of implant materials
- Corrosion and wear behavior, including degradation of polymeric materials

- Coatings technology, including the use of coatings to facilitate implant fixation and bone ingrowth, wear-resistant coatings, coatings to enhance blood clot resistance, antimicrobial action, and lubricity, and coatings for delivery of drugs
- Design considerations, particularly failures related to inadequate design

Each of these subjects is addressed in the *Handbook of Materials for Medical Devices.*

The genesis of this handbook can be attributed to the input of the ASM Handbook and Technical Books Committees, the ASM editorial staff (most notably, Scott Henry and Don Baxter), and the ASM Materials and Processes for Medical Devices Task Force. In particular, thanks are due to the following Task Force members for their thorough critique of the outline of the handbook at the outset of the project: Farrokh Farzin-Nia (Ormco Corporation), Darel E. Hodgson (Shape Memory Applications, Johnson Mathey), Terry C. Lowe (Los Alamos National Laboratory), and Sanjay Shrivastava (Edwards Lifesciences LLC). Their combined efforts led to the successful completion of this handbook.

Joseph R. Davis
Davis & Associates
Chagrin Falls, Ohio

CHAPTER 1

Overview of Biomaterials and Their Use in Medical Devices

A BIOMATERIAL, as defined in this handbook, is any *synthetic* material that is used to replace or restore function to a body tissue and is continuously or intermittently in contact with body fluids (Ref 1). This definition is somewhat restrictive, because it excludes materials used for devices such as surgical or dental instruments. Although these instruments are exposed to body fluids, they do not replace or augment the function of human tissue. It should be noted, however, that materials for surgical instruments, particularly stainless steels, are reviewed briefly in Chapter 3, "Metallic Materials," in this handbook. Similarly, stainless steels and shape memory alloys used for dental/endodontic instruments are discussed in Chapter 10, "Biomaterials for Dental Applications."

Also excluded from the aforementioned definition are materials that are used for external prostheses, such as artificial limbs or devices such as hearing aids. These materials are not exposed to body fluids.

Exposure to body fluids usually implies that the biomaterial is placed within the interior of the body, and this places several strict restrictions on materials that can be used as a biomaterial (Ref 1). First and foremost, a biomaterial must be biocompatible—it should not elicit an adverse response from the body, and vice versa. Additionally, it should be nontoxic and noncarcinogenic. These requirements eliminate many engineering materials that are available. Next, the biomaterial should possess adequate physical and mechanical properties to serve as augmentation or replacement of body tissues. For practical use, a biomaterial should be amenable to being formed or machined into different shapes, have relatively low cost, and be readily available.

Figure 1 lists the various material requirements that must be met for successful total joint replacement. The ideal material or material combination should exhibit the following properties:

- A biocompatible chemical composition to avoid adverse tissue reactions
- Excellent resistance to degradation (e.g., corrosion resistance for metals or resistance to biological degradation in polymers)
- Acceptable strength to sustain cyclic loading endured by the joint
- A low modulus to minimize bone resorption
- High wear resistance to minimize wear-debris generation

Uses for Biomaterials (Ref 3)

One of the primary reasons that biomaterials are used is to physically replace hard or soft tissues that have become damaged or destroyed through some pathological process (Ref 3). Although the tissues and structures of the body perform for an extended period of time in most people, they do suffer from a variety of destructive processes, including fracture, infection, and cancer that cause pain, disfigurement, or loss of function. Under these circumstances, it may be possible to remove the diseased tissue and replace it with some suitable synthetic material.

Orthopedics. One of the most prominent application areas for biomaterials is for orthopedic implant devices. Both osteoarthritis and rheumatoid arthritis affect the structure of freely movable (synovial) joints, such as the hip, knee, shoulder, ankle, and elbow (Fig. 2). The pain in such joints, particularly weight-bearing joints such as the hip and knee, can be considerable, and the effects on ambulatory function quite devastating. It has been possible to replace these joints with prostheses since the advent of anesthesia, antisepsis, and antibiotics, and the relief of pain and restoration of mobility is well known to hundreds of thousands of patients.

The use of biomaterials for orthopedic implant devices is one of the major focal points of this handbook. In fact, Chapters 2 through 7 and Chapter 9 (refer to Table of Contents) all deal with the materials and performance associated with orthopedic implants. As shown in Table 1, a variety of metals, polymers, and ceramics are used for such applications.

Cardiovascular Applications. In the cardiovascular, or circulatory, system (the heart and blood vessels involved in circulating blood throughout the body), problems can arise with heart valves and arteries, both of which can be successfully treated with implants. The heart valves suffer from structural changes that prevent the valve from either fully opening or fully closing, and the diseased valve can be replaced with a variety of substitutes. As with orthopedic implants, ceramics (carbons, as described in Chapter 6, "Ceramic Materials," in this handbook), metals, and polymers are used as materials of construction (Table 1).

Arteries, particularly the coronary arteries and the vessels of the lower limbs, become blocked by fatty deposits (atherosclerosis), and it is possible in some cases to replace segments with artificial arteries. As shown in Table 1, polymers are the material of choice for vascular prostheses (see Chapter 7, "Polymeric Materials," in this handbook for further details).

Ophthalmics. The tissues of the eye can suffer from several diseases, leading to reduced vision and eventually, blindness. Cataracts, for example, cause cloudiness of the lens. This may be replaced with a synthetic (polymer) intraocular lens (Table 1). Materials for contact lenses, because they are in intimate contact with the tissues of the eye, are also considered biomaterials. As with intraocular lenses, they too are used to preserve and restore vision (see Chapter 7, "Polymeric Materials," in this handbook for details).

Dental Applications. Within the mouth, both the tooth and supporting gum tissues can be readily destroyed by bacterially controlled diseases. Dental caries (cavities), the demineralization and dissolution of teeth associated with the metabolic activity in plaque (a film of mucus that traps bacteria on the surface of the teeth), can cause extensive tooth loss. Teeth in their entirety and segments of teeth both can be replaced or restored by a variety of materials (Table 1). A thorough review of these materials can be found in Chapter 10, "Biomaterials for Dental Applications," in this handbook.

Wound Healing. One of the oldest uses of implantable biomaterials can be traced back to the introduction of sutures for wound closure. The ancient Egyptians used linen as a suture as far back as 2000 B.C. Synthetic suture materials include both polymers (the most widely synthetic suture material) and some metals (e.g.,

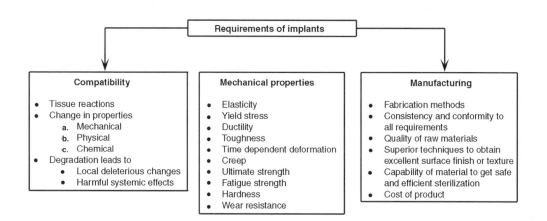

Fig. 1 Implant material requirements in orthopedic applications. Source: Ref 2

stainless steels and tantalum). Chapter 7, "Polymeric Materials," in this handbook discusses the characteristics and properties of synthetic suture materials.

Table 1 Examples of medical and dental materials and their applications

Material	Principal applications
Metals and alloys	
316L stainless steel	Fracture fixation, stents, surgical instruments
CP-Ti, Ti-Al-V, Ti-Al-Nb, Ti-13Nb-13Zr, Ti-Mo-Zr-Fe	Bone and joint replacement, fracture fixation, dental implants, pacemaker encapsulation
Co-Cr-Mo, Cr-Ni-Cr-Mo	Bone and joint replacement, dental implants, dental restorations, heart valves
Ni-Ti	Bone plates, stents, orthodontic wires
Gold alloys	Dental restorations
Silver products	Antibacterial agents
Platinum and Pt-Ir	Electrodes
Hg-Ag-Sn amalgam	Dental restorations
Ceramics and glasses	
Alumina	Joint replacement, dental implants
Zirconia	Joint replacement
Calcium phosphates	Bone repair and augmentation, surface coatings on metals
Bioactive glasses	Bone replacement
Porcelain	Dental restorations
Carbons	Heart valves, percutaneous devices, dental implants
Polymers	
Polyethylene	Joint replacement
Polypropylene	Sutures
PET	Sutures, vascular prosthesis
Polyamides	Sutures
PTFE	Soft-tissue augmentation, vascular prostheses
Polyesters	Vascular prostheses, drug-delivery systems
Polyurethanes	Blood-contacting devices
PVC	Tubing
PMMA	Dental restorations, intraocular lenses, joint replacement (bone cements)
Silicones	Soft-tissue replacement, ophthalmology
Hydrogels	Ophthalmology, drug-delivery systems
Composites	
BIS-GMA-quartz/silica filler	Dental restorations
PMMA-glass fillers	Dental restorations (dental cements)

Abbreviations: CP-Ti, commercially pure titanium; PET, polyethylene terephthalates (Dacron, E.I. DuPont de Nemours & Co.); PTFE, polytetra fluoroethylenes (Teflon, E.I. DuPont de Nemours & Co.); PVC, polyvinyl chlorides; PMMA, polymethyl methacrylate; BIS-GMA, bisphenol A-glycidyl. Source: Adapted from Ref 3

Another important wound-healing category is that of fracture fixation devices. These include bone plates, screws, nails, rods, wires, and other devices used for fracture treatment. Although some nonmetallic materials (e.g., carbon-carbon composite bone plates) have been investigated, almost all fracture fixation devices used for orthopedic applications are made from metals, most notably stainless steels (see Chapter 3, "Metallic Materials," in this handbook for details).

Drug-Delivery Systems. One of the fastest growing areas for implant applications is for devices for controlled and targeted delivery of drugs. Many attempts have been made to incorporate drug reservoirs into implantable devices for a sustained and preferably controlled release. Some of these technologies use new polymeric materials as vehicles for drug delivery. Chapters 7, "Polymeric Materials," and 9, "Coatings," in this handbook describe these materials.

Types of Biomaterials (Ref 1)

Most synthetic biomaterials used for implants are common materials familiar to the average materials engineer or scientist (Table 1). In general, these materials can be divided into the following categories: metals, polymers, ceramics, and composites.

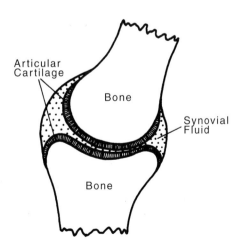

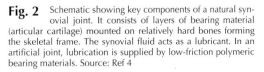

Fig. 2 Schematic showing key components of a natural synovial joint. It consists of layers of bearing material (articular cartilage) mounted on relatively hard bones forming the skeletal frame. The synovial fluid acts as a lubricant. In an artificial joint, lubrication is supplied by low-friction polymeric bearing materials. Source: Ref 4

Metals. As a class of materials, metals are the most widely used for load-bearing implants. For instance, some of the most common orthopedic surgeries involve the implantation of metallic implants. These range from simple wires and screws to fracture fixation plates and total joint prostheses (artificial joints) for hips, knees, shoulders, ankles, and so on. In addition to orthopedics, metallic implants are used in maxillofacial surgery, cardiovascular surgery, and as dental materials. Although many metals and alloys are used for medical device applications, the most commonly employed are stainless steels, commercially pure titanium and titanium alloys, and cobalt-base alloys (Table 1). The use of metals for implants is reviewed in Chapter 3, "Metallic Materials," in this handbook. Dental alloys are discussed in Chapters 10, "Biomaterials for Dental Applications," and 11, "Tarnish and Corrosion of Dental Alloys."

Polymers. A wide variety of polymers are used in medicine as biomaterials. Their applications range from facial prostheses to tracheal tubes, from kidney and liver parts to heart components, and from dentures to hip and knee joints (Tables 1, 2). Chapters 7, "Polymeric Materials," and 10, "Biomaterials for Dental Applications," in this handbook review the use of polymers for these applications.

Polymeric materials are also used for medical adhesives and sealants and for coatings that serve a variety of functions (see Chapters 8, "Adhesives," and 9, "Coatings," in this handbook for details).

Ceramics. Traditionally, ceramics have seen widescale use as restorative materials in dentistry. These include materials for crowns, cements, and dentures (see Chapter 10, "Biomaterials for Dental Applications," in this handbook for details). However, their use in other fields of biomedicine has not been as extensive, compared to metals and polymers. For example, the poor fracture toughness of ceramics severely limits their use for load-bearing applications. As shown in Table 1, some ceramic materials are used for joint replacement and bone repair and augmentation. Chapters 6, "Ceramic Materials," and 9, "Coatings," in this handbook review the uses of ceramics for nondental biomedical applications.

Composites. As shown in Table 1, the most successful composite biomaterials are used in the field of dentistry as restorative materials or dental cements (see Chapter 10, "Biomaterials for Dental Applications," in this handbook for details). Although carbon-carbon and carbon-reinforced polymer composites are of great interest for bone repair and joint replacement because of their low elastic modulus levels, these materials have not displayed a combination of mechanical and biological properties appropriate to these applications. Composite materials are, however, used extensively for prosthetic limbs, where their combination of low density/weight and high strength make them ideal materials for such applications.

Natural Biomaterials. Although the biomaterials discussed in this handbook are synthetic materials, there are several materials derived from the animal or plant world being considered for use as biomaterials that deserve brief mention. One of the advantages of using natural materials for implants is that they are similar to materials familiar to the body. In this regard, the field of biomimetics (or mimicking nature) is growing. Natural materials do not usually offer the problems of toxicity often faced by synthetic materials. Also, they may carry specific protein binding sites and other biochemical signals that may assist in tissue healing or integration. However, natural materials can be subject to problems of immunogenicity. Another problem faced by these materials, especially natural polymers, is their tendency to denature or decompose at temperatures below their melting points. This severely limits their fabrication into implants of different sizes and shapes.

An example of a natural material is collagen, which exists mostly in fibril form, has a characteristic triple-helix structure, and is the most

Table 2 Examples of polymers used as biomaterials

Application	Polymer
Knee, hip, shoulder joints	Ultrahigh molecular weight polyethylene
Finger joints	Silicone
Sutures	Polylactic and polyglycolic acid, nylon
Tracheal tubes	Silicone, acrylic, nylon
Heart pacemaker	Acetal, polyethylene, polyurethane
Blood vessels	Polyester, polytetrafluoroethylene, PVC
Gastrointestinal segments	Nylon, PVC, silicones
Facial prostheses	Polydimethyl siloxane, polyurethane, PVC
Bone cement	Polymethyl methacrylate

PVC, polyvinyl chloride. Source: Ref 1

prevalent protein in the animal world. For example, almost 50% of the protein in cowhide is collagen. It forms a significant component of connective tissue such as bone, tendons, ligaments, and skin. There are at least ten different types of collagen in the body. Among these, type I is found predominantly in skin, bone, and tendons; type II is found in articular cartilage in joints; and type III is a major constituent of blood vessels.

Collagen is being studied extensively for use as a biomaterial. It is usually implanted in a sponge form that does not have significant mechanical strength or stiffness. It has shown good promise as a scaffold for neotissue growth and is commercially available as a product for wound healing. Injectable collagen is widely used for the augmentation or buildup of dermal tissue for cosmetic reasons. Other natural materials under consideration include coral, chitin (from insects and crustaceans), keratin (from hair), and cellulose (from plants).

Examples of Biomaterials Applications

Biomedical devices range the gamut of design and materials selection considerations from relatively simple devices requiring one material, such as commercially pure titanium dental implants, to highly complex assemblies, such as the cardiac pacemaker described subsequently or the ventricular-assist device (VAD) discussed in Chapter 7, "Polymeric Materials" in this handbook (see, for example, Fig. 4 and Table 6 in Chapter 7, which illustrate the components and list the materials of construction, respectively, for a VAD).

Total Hip Replacement

Total joint replacement is widely regarded as the major achievement in orthopedic surgery in the 20th century. Arthroplasty, or the creation of a new joint, is the name given to the surgical treatment of degenerate joints aimed at the relief of pain and the restoration of movement. This has been achieved by excision, interposition, and replacement arthroplasty and by techniques that have been developed over approximately 180 years (Ref 2).

Design and Materials Selection. Hip arthroplasty generally requires that the upper femur (thigh bone) be replaced and the mating pelvis (hip bone) area be replaced or resurfaced.

As shown in Fig. 3, a typical hip prosthesis consists of the femoral stem, a femoral ball, and a polymeric (ultrahigh molecular weight polyethylene, or UHMWPE) socket (cup) with or without a metallic backing. Femoral components usually are manufactured from Co-Cr-Mo or Co-Ni-Cr-Mo alloys or titanium alloys (see Chapter 3, "Metallic Materials," in this handbook for details). The ball (articulating portion of the femoral component) is made either of highly polished Co-Cr alloys or of a ceramic (e.g., alumina). Modular designs, where the stem and ball are of two different materials, are common. For example, hip replacement implants featuring a titanium alloy femoral stem will have a Co-Cr femoral head. Similarly, the UHMWPE socket of the common acetabulum replacement can be implanted directly in the pelvis or be part of a modular arrangement wherein the cup is placed into a metallic shell

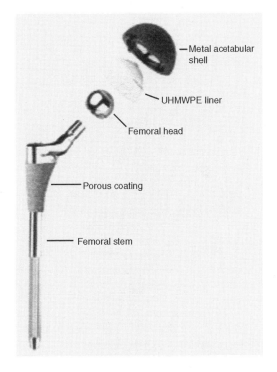

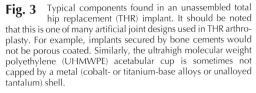

Fig. 3 Typical components found in an unassembled total hip replacement (THR) implant. It should be noted that this is one of many artificial joint designs used in THR arthroplasty. For example, implants secured by bone cements would not be porous coated. Similarly, the ultrahigh molecular weight polyethylene (UHMWPE) acetabular cup is sometimes not capped by a metal (cobalt- or titanium-base alloys or unalloyed tantalum) shell.

(Fig. 4). Design variations include the modular approach, straight stems, curved stems, platforms and no platforms, holes and holes in the femoral stem, and so on.

Table 3 lists some of the femoral head-to-socket combinations that have been used for total hip replacement arthroplasty. Cobalt-base alloys are the most commonly used metals for current metal-on-polymer implants. As indicated in Table 3 and elaborated in Chapter 3, "Metallic Materials," in this handbook, the oxide surface layer on titanium alloy femoral heads results in excessive wear to the UHMWPE acetabular cups. Figure 5 compares the wear behavior of various femoral head/cup combinations.

Knee Implants

In a total knee arthroplasty (TKA), the diseased cartilage surfaces of the lower femur

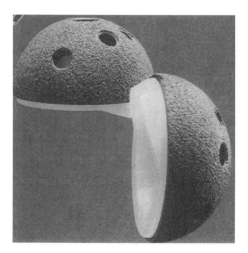

Fig. 4 Acetabular cup components, which are fitted over the the femoral head, featuring plasma-sprayed shell with anatomic screw hole placement

(thighbone), the tibia (shinbone), and the patella (kneecap) are replaced by a prosthesis made of metal alloys and polymeric materials. Most of the other structures of the knee, such as the connecting ligaments, remain intact.

Design. For simplicity, the knee is considered a hinge joint because of its ability to bend and straighten like a hinged door. In reality, the knee is much more complex, because the surfaces actually roll and glide, and the knee bends. The first implant designs used the hinge concept and literally included a connecting hinge between the components. Newer implant designs, recognizing the complexity of the joint, attempt to replicate the more complicated motions and to take advantage of the posterior cruciate ligament (PCL) and collateral ligaments for support.

Up to three bone surfaces may be replaced during a TKA: the lower ends (condyles) of the thighbone, the top surface of the shinbone, and the back surface of the kneecap. Components are designed so that metal always articulates against a low-friction plastic, which provides smooth movement and results in minimal wear.

The metal femoral component curves around the end of the thighbone (Fig. 6) and has an interior groove so the knee cap can move up and down smoothly against the bone as the knee bends and straightens.

The tibial component is a flat metal platform with a polymeric cushion (Fig. 6). The cushion may be part of the platform (fixed) or separate (mobile), with either a flat surface (PCL-retaining) or a raised, sloping surface (PCL-substituting).

The patellar component is a dome-shaped piece of polyethylene that duplicates the shape of the kneecap, anchored to a flat metal plate (Fig. 6).

Materials of Construction. The metal parts of the implant are made of titanium alloys (Ti-6Al-4V) or cobalt-chromium alloys. The plastic

Table 3 Materials combinations in total hip replacement (THR) prostheses

Femoral component	Socket component	Results
Co-Cr-Mo	Co-Cr-Mo	Early high loosening rate and limited use; new developments show lowest wear rate (THR only—in clinical use in Europe)
Co-Cr-Mo	UHMWPE	Widely employed; low wear
Alumina/zirconia	UHMWPE	Very low wear rate; zirconia more impact resistant
Alumina	Alumina	Minimum wear rate (components matched); pain—not in clinical use in the United States
Ti-6Al-4V	UHMWPE	Reports of high UHMWPE wear due to breakdown of titanium surface
Surface-coated Ti-6Al-4V	UHMWPE	Enhanced wear resistance to abrasion; only thin treated layer achieved

UHMWPE, ultrahigh molecular weight polyethylene. Source: Ref 2

parts are made of UHMWPE. All together, the components weigh between 425 and 565 g (15 and 20 oz), depending on the size selected.

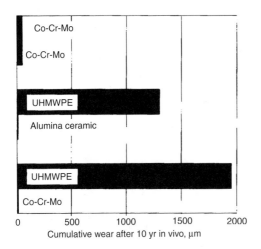

Fig. 5 Wear behavior of various femoral head/cup combinations. Even higher ultrahigh molecular weight polyethylene (UHMWPE) wear rates are encountered with titanium-base femoral heads. Source: Ref 2

Cardiac Pacemakers

Function. Cardiac pacemakers are generally used to manage a slow or irregular heart rate. The pacemaker system applies precisely timed electrical signals to induce heart muscle contraction and cause the heart to beat in a manner very similar to a naturally occurring heart rhythm. A pacemaker consists of a pulse generator, at least one electrode, and one or two pacing leads connecting the pacemaker to the heart. Figure 7 shows various types of pulse generators and pacing leads.

Components and Materials of Construction. The casing of the pulse generator functions as housing for the battery and circuits, which provide power. It is usually implanted between the skin and pectoral muscle. The sealed lithium iodine battery provides electrical energy to the pacemaker. This battery replaced the mercury-zinc battery in 1975, extending the life of some pacemaker models by over 10 yr. The circuitry converts the electrical energy to small electrical signals. The circuitry also con-

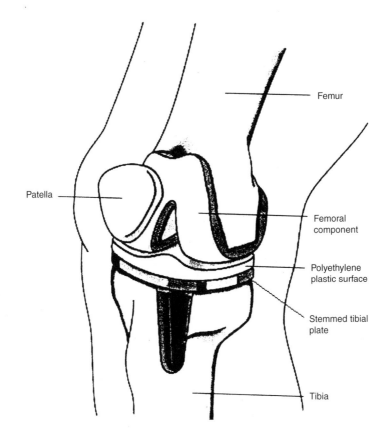

Fig. 6 Components of a total knee replacement arthroplasty. See text for details.

trols the timing of the electrical signals delivered to the heart. A connector block, made of polyurethane, is located at the top of the pacemaker (Fig. 7). It serves to attach the pacemaker to the pacemaker lead. Formerly, glass materials were used to comprise the connector block. The pulse generator is encased in ASTM grade 1 titanium. Titanium replaced ceramics and epoxy resin, which were used for encapsulation of some pacemakers in the past, with silicone rubber. This upgrade to titanium allowed patients to safely use appliances such as microwave ovens, because titanium helps to shield the internal components and reduce the external electromagnetic interference.

A pacing lead is vital to the pacemaker system, because it transmits the electrical signal from the pacemaker to the heart and information on the heart activity back to the pacemaker. One or two leads may be used, depending on the type

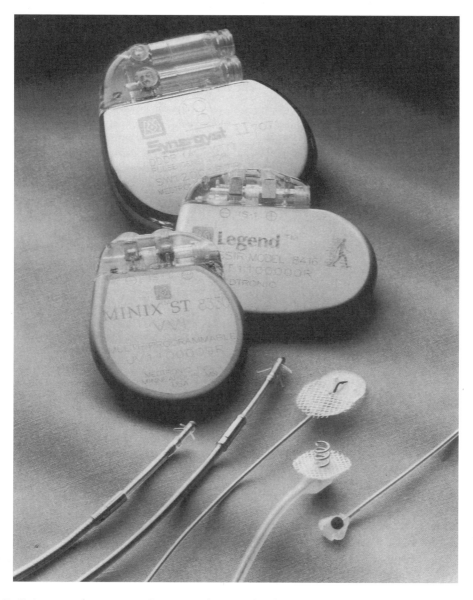

Fig. 7 Various pacemaker component designs. Top: Three examples of titanium-encased pulse generators. Connector blocks, which serve to attach the pacemaker to the pacemaker lead, are shown at the top of each pulse generator. Bottom: Various types of insulated endocardial and myocardial leads. Note that the lead shown at the center of the figure has a silicone sewing pad and Dacram mesh disk for implant fixation. Source: Ref 5

of pacemaker. One end of the lead is attached to the connector block of the pacemaker. The other end is inserted through a vein and placed in the right ventricle or right atrium of the heart. The lead is an insulated wire consisting of a connector pin, lead body, fixation mechanism (Fig. 7), and at least one electrode. The connector pin is the portion of the lead that is inserted into the connector block. The lead body is the insulated metal wire that carries electrical energy from the pacemaker to the heart.

The lead must be able to withstand the flexing induced by the cardiac contractions in the warm and corrosive environment in the body. Thus, the materials used must be inert, nontoxic, and durable. The lead body must be flexible, noncorrosive, and durable. It must also be a good electrical conductor. The early lead body was insulated with polyethylene. Currently, the lead body is insulated with a more resilient material such as silicone rubber tubing or polyurethanes. Polyurethanes are generally stronger than silicone rubbers, which are easily damaged. The strength of polyurethanes enables a thinner lead to be used in the pacemaker and offers greater lead flexibility. Another advantage of polyurethanes is their very low coefficient of friction when wet. However, metal-ion-induced oxidation may degrade polyurethanes, while silicones are not affected by this mechanism of degradation. The fixation mechanism serves to hold the tip of the lead in place in the heart. Currently, either a nickel-cobalt alloy with a silver core helix or an electrically active platinum-iridium helix may be used to anchor the electrode of the lead to the surface of the heart. The electrode is located at the tip of the lead. It serves to deliver the electrical energy from the pacemaker to the heart and information about the natural activity of the heart back to the pacemaker. Electrodes may be composed of platinum, titanium, stainless steel, silver, or cobalt alloys. Titanium has been used because it forms a nonconducting oxide layer at the surface. This surface prevents the exchange of charge carriers across the boundary. Titanium also exhibits a high modulus of elasticity, high resistance to corrosion, and high durability. Electrodes may be coated with iridium oxide to prevent nonconductive layers from forming. The coated electrodes may also provide lower acute and chronic thresholds due to the reduced local inflammation.

Drug-Eluting Leads. Leads have developed immensely since they were first introduced. The earliest leads were attached to the outer surface of the heart. In the mid-1960s, transverse leads were introduced. They could be inserted through a vein leading to the heart, thus eliminating the need to open the chest cavity during implantation. In the 1970s, tined and active fixation leads were developed to replace smooth tip leads. The prongs on the tined leads and the titanium alloy screws in the active fixation leads provide a more secure attachment to the heart and are still used today. In the early 1980s, steroid-eluting leads were developed. These leads emit a steroid drug from the tip of the electrode on the lead to suppress inflammatory response of the heart wall, thus reducing the energy requirements of the pacemaker. The steroid also results in low chronic thresholds. Ceramic collars surrounding the electrode tip were first used to contain and emit the steroid. This technique is still used, where dexamethasone sodium phosphate is the eluted steroid. A silicone rubber matrix contains the steroid, and this matrix is contained in a platinum-iridium porous tip electrode. The combination of platinum and iridium results in a material stronger than most steels. The porous tip electrode provides an efficient pacing and sensing surface by promoting fibrotic tissue growth and physically stabilizing the tissue interface. In order to facilitate passage of the fixation mechanism to the heart, either a soluble polyethylene glycol capsule or a mannitol capsule is placed on the electrode tip. When the electrode tip is exposed to body fluids, the steroid is released. The polyethylene glycol capsule dissolves within 2 to 4 min after the electrode tip is inserted into the vein. The mannitol capsule dissolves within 3 to 5 min after the insertion.

ACKNOWLEDGMENTS

The application examples describing knee implants and cardiac pacemakers were adapted from the following web sites:

- American Academy of Orthopaedic Surgeons, www.orthoinfo.aaos.org
- T. Reilly, "Structure and Materials of Cardiac Pacemakers," University of Wisconsin-Madison, www.pharmacy.wisc.edu/courses/718-430/2000presentation/Reilly.pdf

REFERENCES

1. C.M. Agrawal, Reconstructing the Human Body Using Biomaterials, *JOM,* Jan 1998, p 31–35
2. M. Long and H.J. Rack, Titanium Alloys

in Total Joint Replacement—A Materials Science Perspective, *Biomaterials,* Vol 19, 1998, p 1621–1639

3. D. Williams, An Introduction to Medical and Dental Materials, *Concise Encyclopedia of Medical & Dental Materials,* D. Williams, Ed., Pergamon Press and The MIT Press, 1990, p xvii–xx

4. D. Dowson, Friction and Wear of Medical Implants and Prosthetic Devices, *Friction, Lubrication, and Wear Technology,* Vol 18, *ASM Handbook,* ASM International, 1992, p 656–664

5. P. Didisheim and J.T. Watson, Cardiovascular Applications, *Biomaterials Science: An Introduction to Materials in Medicine,* B.D. Ratner, A.S. Hoffman, F.J. Schoen, and J.E. Lemons, Ed., Academic Press, 1996, p 283–297

SELECTED REFERENCES

General

- C.M. Agrawal, Reconstructing the Human Body Using Biomaterials. *J. Met.,* Vol 50 (No. 1). 1998, p 31–35
- S.A. Barenberg, Abridged Report of the Committee to Survey the Needs and Opportunities for the Biomaterials Industry, *J. Biomed. Mater. Res.,* Vol 22, 1988, p 1267–1291
- J.S. Benson and J.W. Boretos, Biomaterials and the Future of Medical Devices. *Med. Device Diag. Ind.,* Vol 17 (No. 4). 1995, p 32–37
- *Biomaterials Science: An Introduction to Materials in Medicine,* B.D. Ratner, A.S. Hoffman, F.J. Schoen, and J.E. Lemons, Ed., Academic Press, 1996
- M.M. Black et al., Medical Applications of Biomaterials, *Phys. Technol.,* Vol 13, 1982, p 50–65
- *Concise Encyclopedia of Medical Devices & Dental Materials,* D. Williams, Ed., Pergamon Press and The MIT Press, 1990
- Directory to Medical Materials, *Med. Device Diag. Ind.,* published annually in the April issue
- M. Donachie, Biomaterials, *Metals Handbook Desk Edition,* 2nd ed., J.R. Davis, Ed., ASM International, 1998, p 702–709
- E. Duncan, Biomaterials: Looking for Information, *Med. Device Diag. Ind.,* Vol 13 (No. 1), 1991, p 140–143
- P.M. Galletti. Artificial Organs: Learning to Live with Risk, *Tech. Rev.,* Nov/Dec 1988, p 34–40
- P.M. Galletti, Organ Replacement by Man-Made Devices. *J. Cardiothoracic Vascular Anesthesia,* Vol 7 (No. 5), Oct 1993, p 624–628
- J.S. Hanker and B.L. Giammara, Biomaterials and Biomedical Devices, *Science,* Vol 242, 11 Nov 1988, p 885–892
- R.D. Lambert and M.E. Anthony, Standardization in Orthopaedics, *ASTM Stand. News,* Aug 1995, p 22–29
- *Medical Devices and Services,* Section 13, *Annual Book of ASTM Standards,* ASTM
- J.B. Park and R.S. Lakes, *Biomaterials: An Introduction,* 2nd ed., Plenum Press, 1992

Biomaterials for Nondental or General Application

- J.M. Courtney and T. Gilchrist, Silicone Rubber and Natural Rubber as Biomaterials, *Med. Biol. Eng. Comput.,* Vol 18, 1980, p 538–540
- R.H. Doremus, Bioceramics. *J. Mater. Sci.,* Vol 27, 1992, p 285–297
- A.C. Fraker and A.W. Ruff, Metallic Surgical Implants: State of the Art. *J. Met.,* Vol 29 (No. 5), 1977, p 22–28
- R.A. Fuller and J.J. Rosen, Materials for Medicine, *Sci. Am.,* Vol 255 (No. 4), Oct 1986, p 119–125
- B.S. Gupta, Medical Testile Structures: An Overview, *Med. Plast. Biomater.,* Vol 5 (No. 1), 1998, p 16, 19–21, 24, 26, 28, 30
- G.H. Harth, "Metal Implants for Orthopedic and Dental Surgery," MCIC-74-18, Metals and Ceramics Information Center Report. Feb 1974
- G. Heimke and P. Griss, Ceramic Implant Materials, *Med. Biol. Eng. Comput.,* Vol 18, 1980, p 503–510
- D.S. Hotter, Band-Aids for Broken Bones, *Mach. Des.,* 4 April 1996, p 39–44
- M. Hunt, Get Hip with Medical Metals, *Mater. Eng.,* Vol 108 (No. 4), 1991, p 27–30
- A.J. Klein, Biomaterials Give New Life, *Adv. Mater. Process.,* May 1986, p 18–22
- F.G. Larson, Hydroxyapatite Coatings for Medical Implants. *Med. Device Diag. Ind.,* Vol 16 (No. 4). 1994, p 34–40
- M. Long and H.J. Rack, Titanium Alloys in Total Joint Replacement—A Materials Science Perspective, *Biomaterials,* Vol 19, 1998, p 1621–1639
- D.C. Mears, Metals in Medicine and Surgery, *Int. Met. Rev.,* Vol 22, June 1977, p 119–155

- D.S. Metsger and S.F. Lebowitz, Medical Applications of Ceramics. *Med. Device Diag. Ind.,* Vol 7, 1985, p 55–63
- M. Moukwa, The Development of Polymer-Based Biomaterials Since the 1920s, *J. Met.,* Vol 49 (No. 2) 1997, p 46–50
- S.J. Mraz, The Human Body Shop, *Mach. Des.,* 7 Nov 1991, p 90–94
- K. Neailey and R.C. Pond, Metal Implants, *Mater. Eng.,* Vol 3, June 1982, p 470–478
- D.E. Niesz and V.J. Tennery, "Ceramics for Prosthetic Applications—Orthopedic, Dental and Cardiovascular." MCIC-74-21, Metals and Ceramics Information Center Report, July 1974
- P.C. Noble, Special Materials for the Replacement of Human Joints, *Met. Forum,* Vol 6 (No. 2), 1983, p 59–80
- C.M. Rimnac et al., Failure of Orthopedic Implants: Three Case Histories, *Mater. Char.,* Vol 26, 1991, p 201–209
- W. Rostoker and J.O. Galante, Materials for Human Implantation, *Trans. ASME,* Vol 101, Feb 1979, p 2–14
- L.M. Sheppard, Building Teeth, Bones, and Other Body Parts with Ceramics, *Mater. Eng.,* April 1984, p 37–43
- L.M. Sheppard, Cure It with Ceramics. *Adv. Mater. Process.,* May 1986, p 26–31
- H. Shimizu, Metal/Ceramic Implants, *Med. Device Diag. Ind.,* Vol 8 (No. 7), 1986, p 30–35, 59–60
- E. Smethurst and R.B. Waterhouse. Causes of Failure in Total Hip Prostheses, *J. Mater. Sci.,* Vol 12, 1977, p 1781–1792
- T. Stevens, Prescription: Plastics. *Mater. Eng.,* Vol 108 (No. 4). 1991, p 23–26

Dental Materials

- S. Bandyopadhyay, Dental Cements. *Met. Forum,* Vol 3 (No. 4), 1980, p 228–235
- J.F. Bates and A.G. Knapton, Metals and Alloys in Dentistry. *Int. Met. Rev.,* Vol 22, March 1977, p 39–60
- M.P. Dariel et al., New Technology for Mercury Free Metallic Dental Restorative Alloys, *Powder Metall.,* Vol 37 (No. 2). 1994, p 88
- S. Espevik, Dental Amalgam, *Ann Rev. Mater. Sci.* Vol 7, 1977, p 55–72
- R.M. German, Precious-Metal Dental Casting Alloys. *Int. Met. Rev.,* Vol 27 (No. 5), 1982, p 260–288
- J.B. Moser, The Uses and Properties of Dental Materials, *Int. Adv. Nondestruct. Test.,* Vol 5, 1977, p 367–390
- J.M. Powers and S.C. Bayne, Friction and Wear of Dental Materials, *Friction, Lubrication, and Wear Technology,* Vol 18, *ASM Handbook,* ASM International, 1992, p 665–681
- *Restorative Dental Materials,* 11th ed., R.G. Craig and J.M. Powers, Ed., Mosby, Inc., An Affiliate of Elsevier Science, 2002
- D.E. Southan, Dental Porcelain, *Met. Forum,* Vol 3 (No. 4), 1980, p 222–227
- R.M. Waterstrat, Brushing up on the History of Intermetallics in Dentistry, *J. Met.,* Vol 42 (No. 3), 1990, p 8–14

Corrosion and Biocompatibility

- J. Black, *Biological Performance of Materials: Fundamentals of Biocompatibility,* Marcel Dekker, 1981
- A.C. Fraker, Corrosion of Metallic Implant and Prosthetic Devices. *Corrosion,* Vol 13, *ASM Handbook,* 1987, p 1324–1335
- K. Hayashi, Biodegradation of Implant Materials, *JSME Int. J.,* Vol 30 (No. 268), 1987, p 1517–1525
- H.J. Mueller, Tarnish and Corrosion of Dental Alloys. *Corrosion,* Vol 13, *ASM Handbook,* 1987, p 1336–1366
- K.R. St. John, Biocompatibility Testing for Medical Implant Materials, *ASTM Stand. News,* March 1994, p 46–49
- D.F. Williams, Corrosion of Implant Materials, *Ann Rev. Mater. Sci.,* Vol 6, 1976, p 237–266
- D.F. Williams, Tissue-Biomaterial Interactions, *J. Mater. Sci.,* Vol 22, 1987, p 3421–3445

CHAPTER 2

Physical and Mechanical Requirements for Medical Device Materials

BIOMATERIALS are the man-made metallic, ceramic, or polymeric materials used for intracorporeal applications in the human body. Intracorporeal uses may be for hard-tissue or soft-tissue augmentation or replacement. This chapter reviews some of the important requirements for biomaterials, including their response to the body environment (biocompatiblity), mechanical behavior, corrosion, and material response to sterilization.

Biomaterials: A Brief Overview (Ref 1)

As described in Chapter 1, "Overview of Biomaterials and Their Use in Medical Devices," in this handbook, metals frequently are used in the body for orthopedic purposes—such as hip stems and balls, knees, and so on—where hard tissue (bony structures) must be repaired or replaced. Metals also find application as stents (in angioplasty), leads and cases (in pacemakers), and surgical clips or staples. Dental applications of metals center around amalgam or gold to repair cavities or replace broken teeth, titanium alloys for posts on which to fix crowns or bridges, and nickel-chromium alloys and cobalt-chromium alloys for crowns and bridgework, partial dentures, or as the basis for porcelain-coated alloy teeth. Stainless steel and a few other alloys find use as wires and sheet in orthodontics.

Ceramics are used as the ball in the articulating region of a hip joint, as bioactive coatings on implants, and in certain aspects of dental use—for example, as fillers or for porcelain enameling (a ceramic process). Carbon finds use in heart valves and dental implants. As for polymeric materials, silicone has been used in joint replacement, polymethyl methacrylate as a cement (grout), and ultrahigh molecular weight polyethylene (UHMWPE) as the acetabular cup in hip joints. Polymers are also widely used in nonorthopedic applications, most notably as cardiovascular devices, ophthalmic devices, and drug-delivery systems. Composite materials, particularly polymeric material composites, are used in dental applications, but their use is limited elsewhere in the body. Composites or ceramics intended to resorb in the body have been shown to have potential application. Resorbable materials in the body are not new; resorbable sutures have been in use for many years.

Body Conditions (Ref 1)

Temperature conditions are not extreme for the materials used, body temperatures being a little less than 38 °C (100 °F). However, the chemical physiological environment and biomechanical environment can be extreme. For structural implants used to repair the hip, it is estimated that the average nonactive person may place 1 to 2.5×10^6 cycles of stress on his or her hip in a year. For a person 20 to 30 years of age, with a life expectancy of 70 to 80 years, that is the equivalent of approximately 10^8 cycles of loading in a lifetime. The actual loads and cycles are a function of the weight and activity level of the person, but the need for longtime cyclic capability in fatigue is obvious. Other applications in the body also impart many millions of fatigue cycles to the device or component implanted.

In considering the parameters of materials for intracorporeal applications, several factors are of major importance. It is generally agreed that the material must:

- Be nontoxic and noncarcinogenic, cause little or no foreign-body reaction, and be chemically stable and corrosion resistant. This is known as biocompatibility (see subsequent discussion).
- Be able to endure large and variable stresses in the highly corrosive environment of the human body
- Be able to be fabricated into intricate shapes and sizes

Many structural applications of materials in the body require that the replacement material fit into a space perhaps only one-fourth the area of the part being permanently or temporarily replaced or assisted. Consequently, the implant may have to withstand loads up to 16 or more times that which the human bone must withstand. In restorative dentistry, high compressive biting forces are combined with large temperature changes and acidity to produce a challenging environment. It is clear that there can be very great mechanical loading demands on biomaterials used for structural purposes.

The chemical structure of the body can cause corrosive attack, which may degrade the implant and/or cause release of ions that may adversely affect the body. This chemical interaction is described in terms of the biocompatibility of the biomaterial. Biocompatibility must consider the release of ions or molecules, the mobility of released species, and the interaction of released species or material surfaces with the body. Some ions or molecules are severely detrimental to the body. Among other things, a material might be carcinogenic, be thrombogenic (cause clotting), cause cell mutations, produce a fever, or cause sensitization. Ions released could cause tissue necrosis. The essence of developing a biomaterial has been to find a material with the necessary mechanical and/or physical properties that cause no damage, or a limited amount, to the human body.

Biocompatibility

Like other important scientific concepts that change over time, the definition of biocompatibility has evolved in conjunction with the continuing development of materials used in medical devices (Ref 2). Until recently, a biocompatible material was essentially thought of as one that would do no harm. The operative principle was that of inertness, as reflected, for example, in the definition of biocompatibility as "the quality of not having toxic or injurious effects on biological systems."

When more recently developed devices began to be designed with materials that were more responsive to local biological conditions, the salient principle became one of interactivity, with biocompatibility regarded as "the ability of a material to perform with an appropriate host response in a specific application" (Ref 3). There are four major points that should be elaborated on when using this definition (Ref 3):

- Biocompatibility is not a single event or a single phenomenon. It refers, instead, to a collection of processes involving different but interdependent mechanisms of interaction between the material and the tissue.
- Biocompatibility refers to the ability of the material to perform a function. This reflects the fact that all materials are intended to perform a specific function in the body rather than simply reside there. The ability to perform this function, and to continue to perform this function, depends not only on the intrinsic mechanical and physical properties of the material but also on its interaction with the tissues.
- The definition refers to the appropriate host responses. It does not stipulate that there should be no response, but rather that the response should be appropriate or acceptable in view of the function that has to be performed. It may be that the appropriate response is a minimal response. This is clearly allowed for in the definition but so are any more extensive reactions that are necessary for the continued safe and effective performance of the material or device.
- The definition also refers to the specific application. Biocompatibility of a material always should be described with reference to the situation in which it is used. While one type of interaction, or indeed one type of response of the tissue, may be seen with respect to one material in one situation, a different reaction or a different response may be seen in another situation. For example, the same material in two different physical forms (e.g., a solid

monolithic object and particulate matter) may elicit quite different responses. Thus, while it is perfectly satisfactory to deal with biocompatibility as a collection of phenomena with respect to defined conditions, there is no justification for using the adjectival counterpart *biocompatible* to describe a material. No material is unequivocally biocompatible; many materials may be biocompatible under one or more defined conditions but cannot be assumed to display biocompatibility under all conditions. Biocompatibility is not an intrinsic material property and cannot be considered as such.

Mechanical Behavior (Ref 1)

Metals generally are required to have both high static and cycle-dependent properties. Tensile yield and ultimate strength, modulus of elasticity, and fatigue endurance limit are the principal metallic strength attributes that must be determined. Temperature is not an issue. For dental materials, which experience very high point forces in the mouth, creep and compressive yield strengths are important. Ceramics offer excellent compressive yield, and thus are often used for such applications. Tension and bending or tension fatigue are not primary strength attributes for study in ceramics, because tensile loads cause relatively rapid nonductile crack propagation.

Important mechanical properties of polymeric materials include tensile strength, creep strength, modulus, and fatigue strength. Creep can be important, because the operating temperature of the body is a significant fraction of the melting or glass transition temperature for polymers. The first polymeric material (polytetrafluoroethylene, or Teflon, E.I. DuPont de Nemours & Co.) used for an acetabular cup in a hip implant failed because of extreme distortion due to creep.

Wear resistance is also an important criterion for all biomaterials. Excessive wear can lead to premature mechanical failure of the replacement component. More importantly, wear debris may not be biocompatible with the body.

Mechanical Property Tests

Under ideal conditions, mechanical property tests would be made in environments identical to that in the human body (i.e., in vivo). Practically, mechanical property tests are run either in normal air environments or, where the degrading effects of environment must be evaluated, in simulated human physiological solutions.

Fatigue Tests. Cyclic loading is applied to orthopedic implants during body motion, resulting in alternating plastic deformation of microscopically small zones of stress concentration produced by notches or microstructural inhomogeneities. The interdependency between factors such as implant shape, material, processing, and type of cyclic loading makes the determination of the fatigue resistance of a component an intricate but critical task. Because testing an actual implant under simulated implantation and load conditions is a difficult and expensive process, standardized fatigue tests have been selected for initial screening of orthopedic material candidates, joint simulator trials being generally reserved for a later stage in the implant development process. Fatigue tests include tension/compression, bending, torsion, and rotating bending fatigue testing, the latter, a relatively simple test, being widely used to evaluate orthopedic metallic materials. Standardized tests specific to implant materials include:

ASTM No.	Title
F 1160	Shear and Bending Fatigue Testing of Calcium Phosphate and Metallic Coatings
F 1440	Cyclic Fatigue Testing of Metallic Stemmed HIP Arthroplasty Femoral Components without Torsion
F 1539	Constant Amplitude Bending Fatigue Tests of Metallic Bone Staples
F 1659	Bending and Shear Fatigue Testing of Calcium Phosphate Coatings on Solid Metallic Substrates
F 1717	Static and Fatigue for Spinal Implant Constructs in a Corpectomy Model
F 1798	Evaluating the Static and Fatigue Properties of Interconnection Mechanisms and Subassemblies Used in Spinal Arthrodesis Implants
1800	Cyclic Fatigue Testing of Metal Tibial Tray Components of Total Knee Replacements
1801	Corrosion Fatigue Testing of Metallic Implant Materials

Wear Tests. The wear characteristics of implant materials, particularly UHMWPE mated against metal or ceramic materials, have been studied for approximately 40 years. There have been three major types of investigations during this period (Ref 4):

• Studies of the basic wear mechanisms on standard laboratory machines, such as pin-on-disk and pin-on-plate configurations (see, for example, ASTM F 732, "Test Method for Pin-on-Flat Wear Test for Polymeric Materials Used in Total Joint Prostheses which Experience Linear Reciprocating Wear Motion")

- Evaluations of complete implants in hip joint simulators and knee joint simulators. These evaluations involve weight-loss techniques such as gravimetric wear assessment (see, for example, ASTM F 1714 and F 1715, which describe laboratory methods for evaluating prosthetic hip and knee designs, respectively).
- Radiographic in vivo assessment of the performance of total replacement joints

Another area of great interest in implant material wear studies is the biological responses to wear debris. Standardized tests related to wear particles include:

ASTM No.	Title
F 1877	Characteristics of Particles
F 1903	Testing for Biological Responses to Particles in Vitro
F 1904	Testing the Biological Responses to Particles in Vivo

Elastic Modulus

Alloy design and thermomechanical processing have led to the development of implant materials, particulary cobalt-base alloys and titanium-base alloys, with enhanced properties. However, there has been, and still is, concern about the high elastic modulus of implant alloys compared to bone.

Long-term experience indicates that insufficient load transfer from the artificial implant to the adjacent remodeling bone may result in bone resorption and eventual loosening of the prosthetic device (Ref 5). Wolff's law ("The form being given, tissue adapts to best fulfill its mechanical function") suggests that coupling of an implant with a previously load-bearing natural structure may result in tissue loss. Indeed, it has been shown that when the tension/compression load or bending moment to which living bone is exposed is reduced, decreased bone thickness, bone mass loss, and increased osteoporosis ensue (Ref 5). This phenomenon, termed stress shielding, has been related to the difference in flexibility or stiffness, dependent in part on elastic moduli, between natural bone and the implant material. Dowson (Ref 6) appropriately pointed out that, as improvements in the combinations of total joint replacement slid-

ing material pairs have been recorded, the elastic modulus of the prosthetic materials has been moving further away from those of the natural joint they were intended to replace (Fig. 1). Any reduction in the stiffness of the implant, for example, through substitution of present orthopedic alloys with newer, lower-modulus materials, is expected to enhance stress redistribution to the adjacent bone tissues, therefore minimizing stress shielding and eventually prolonging device lifetime.

The problems related to implant stiffness-related stress shielding of bone have resulted in a number of proposed solutions for more flexible designs and low-modulus materials. For example, carbon-carbon and carbon-polymer composites, because of the ability to tailor their elastic modulus closer to bone than metals, have been investigated as candidates for a new generation of implants. However, they are far from being totally effective, due to potential environmental degradation and poor tribological behavior.

Alternatively, the first attempt at reducing the elastic modulus of orthopedic alloys was made by the introduction of α-β titanium alloys having elastic modulus values approximately half that of stainless steels or Co-Cr-Mo alloys (Fig. 1). However, the modulus of Ti-6Al-4V and related α-β alloys is still high (110 GPa, or 16×10^6 psi), approximately 4 to 10 times that of bone. Recent attempts at further minimizing orthopedic alloys moduli have led to the introduction of metastable β-titanium alloys with elastic modulus values as low as ~70 GPa (10×10^6 psi).

Corrosion (Ref 1)

Metals used as biomaterials must be either noble or corrosion resistant to the body environment. As described in Chapter 4, "Corrosion of Metallic Implants and Prosthetic Devices," in this handbook, many types of corrosion have been observed on biomaterials used in the body, including general corrosion, pitting and crevice corrosion, stress-corrosion cracking, corrosion fatigue, and intergranular corrosion. None of these forms, with the exception of general corrosion, can be tolerated in surgical implant materials. For a material to be considered resistant to corrosion in the body, its general corrosion rate usually must be less than 0.01 mil/yr (0.00025 mm/yr).

As with fatigue and wear, a number of standardized tests have been developed to evaluate the corrosion behavior of implant materials/devices. These include:

ASTM No.	Title
F 746	Pitting or Crevice Corrosion of Metallic Surgical Implant Materials
F 897	Fretting Corrosion of Osteosynthesis Plates and Screws
1801	Corrosion Fatigue Testing of Metallic Implant Materials
1814	Evaluating Modular Hip and Knee Joint Components
1875	Fretting Corrosion Testing of Modular Implant Interface: Hip Femoral Head-Bore and Cone Taper Interface

Ceramics. Corrosion testing of ceramic materials is not common practice, because the corrosion of oxide ceramics used for structural implants is very low. However, ceramics do show degradation of properties in vivo. Poly-crystalline ceramics of the alumina type show loss in static strength when exposed to body fluids. This strength loss is a form of environmental degradation. Generally, the greater the purity and the greater the density (lesser porosity) of a ceramic, the more resistant it is to strength loss in the body. Bioactive ceramics represent a different aspect of corrosion, because they are expected to transform into bony structures by gradually releasing their cations and anions to be incorporated in the growing bone or tissue structure. Corrosion testing is not implicitly required for bioactive ceramics.

Polymers. Although the physiological functions and biochemical reactions occuring in the body environment do not take place at high temperatures nor aggressive radiation conditions, the combination of an electrolyte with active biological species, including catalytic enzymes, intermediate oxygen species, and free radicals, constitutes a particularly reactive environment

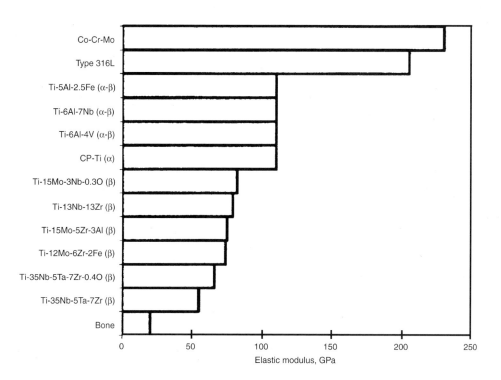

Fig. 1 The elastic modulus of various metallic implant materials compared to natural bone. The first implant alloys developed—stainless steels and cobalt-base alloys—have the highest elastic modulus values. The α-β titanium alloys have elastic modulus values approximately half of that of stainless steels and cobalt-base alloys. The newer-generation β-titanium alloys have the lowest elastic modulus values of any load-bearing implant alloy developed to date. Source: Ref 5

and leads to some degree of degradation of polymers. Among the individual mechanisms associated with polymer degradation are:

- Depolymerization
- Cross linking
- Oxidative degradation
- Leaching of additives
- Hydrolysis
- Crazing and stress cracking

An overview of polymer degradation can be found in Chapter 7, "Polymeric Materials," in this handbook.

Sterilization of Implants (Ref 7)

Sterilization is essential for all implanted materials/devices. In hospitals, economic considerations have also led to the repeated use of devices such as surgical instruments that are relatively expensive, thus necessitating repeated sterilization between use on different patients. Each sterilization method must accomplish the same goal: remove or destroy living organisms and viruses from the biomaterial. Sterility is generally quantified using the sterility assurance limit (SAL) and process conditions determined by performing fractional sterilization runs. The SAL is the probability that a given implant will remain nonsterile following a sterilization run, and the accepted minimum value for the SAL is 10^{-6}, or that one implant in one million will remain nonsterile. Three methods commonly employed include steam sterilization, ethylene oxide (EtO) gas sterilization, and gamma radiation sterilization. Selection of a specific sterilization method is based on economic considerations and implant material properties, for example, heat resistance and radiation sensitivity.

Steam Sterilization. The first sterilization method applied to biomedical implants was steam sterilization or autoclaving. With this method, sterilization is achieved by exposing the implant to saturated steam under pressure at 120 °C (250 °F). The main use of this method for implants occurs in hospitals, with the intraoperative steam sterilization of metallic devices. It is the method of choice for the sterilization of metallic surgical instruments and heat-resistant surgical supplies. A typical steam sterilization process lasts approximately 15 to 30 min after all surfaces of the implant reach 120 °C (250 °F).

The advantages of steam sterilization are efficacy, speed, process simplicity, and lack of toxic residues. The high temperature and pressure limit the range of implant and packaging compatibility, particularly for some polymers and adhesives that may undergo melting and softening during autoclaving.

Ethylene oxide sterilization has been exploited as a low-temperature process that is compatible with a wide range of implant and packaging materials. Components are vacuum processed in either pure EtO or a mixture of EtO and a diluent gas (e.g., CO_2 or a non-ozone-depleting chlorofluorocarbon-like compound) at 30 to 50 °C (85 to 120 °F). A typical EtO sterilization cycle ranges from 2 to 48 h.

Ethylene oxide is used to sterilize a wide range of medical implants, including surgical sutures, intraocular lenses, ligament and tendon repair devices, absorbable bone repair devices, heart valves, and vascular grafts.

The primary disadvantage associated with EtO processing is that EtO is toxic and a suspected human carcinogen. Contact with eyes and inhalation of vapors should be avoided.

Gamma Ray Sterilization. This method of sterilization uses ionizing radiation that involves gamma rays from a cobalt-60 isotope source. Gamma rays have a high penetrating ability, and the doses required to achieve sterilization (25 to 40 kGy) are readily delivered and measured. The devices to be sterilized are placed near the emitting source until they have been exposed to the required amount of radiation. Radiation-measuring devices called dosimeters are placed near the materials to be sterilized to document that the minimum dose required for sterilization was delivered and that the maximum dose for product integrity was not exceeded. No radiation is absorbed by the devices (i.e., they are not radioactive after sterilization), so they can be used immediately after sterilization.

Cobalt-60 radiation sterilization is widely used for medical products, such as surgical sutures and drapes, metallic bone implants, knee and hip prostheses, syringes, and neurosurgery devices. A wide range of materials is compatible with gamma radiation sterilization, and it has been widely accepted as the sterilization method of choice for polymeric materials that include polyethylene, polyesters, polystyrene, polysulfones, and polycarbonate. One exception is the fluoropolymer, polytetrafluoroethylene, which is not compatible with this sterilization method because of its extreme radiation sensitivity.

Cobalt-60 radiation sterilization is a simple process that is rapid and reliable, and it is readily controlled through straightforward dosimetry methods. Both large and small product volumes can be accommodated in a cost-effective manner.

Gamma radiation sterilization is not, however, without its drawbacks. Tests have shown that gamma radiation provides an environment conducive to the oxidation of UHMWPE implants. Oxidative degradation leads to an increase in density and crystallinity and, more importantly, in a loss of mechanical properties associated with progressive embrittlement. The use of inert environments (argon, nitrogen, vacuum) instead of air as the medium for gamma radiation sterilization greatly reduces the presence of any strong oxidizing species and improves the properties and shelf life of UHMWPE devices.

The packaging of UHMWPE components also influences oxygen degradation. Starting in the 1960s, joint replacement components were stored in air-permeable packaging. During the mid 1990s, air-permeable packaging was replaced by barrier packaging. The "barrier" in the package consists of polymer laminates or metallic foils to block gas diffusion. The goal of barrier packaging is to minimize oxidative degradation during long-term shelf storage. The loss of mechanical properties during long-term shelf aging in air frequently manifests most severely in a subsurface band, located 1 to 2 mm (0.04 to 0.08 in.) below the articulating surface. The development of this subsurface embrittled region has been associated with fatigue and delamination of UHMWPE implant components, particularly in the case of tricompartmental and unicondylar knee replacement.

Recently Developed Sterilization Techniques. Low-temperature gas plasma is a relatively new, commercially available sterilization method that was applied to UHMWPE in the 1990s. Gas plasma is an attractive method because it does not leave toxic residues or involve environmentally hazardous by-products. Two gas plasma methods have been evaluated. One uses a low-temperature peracetic acid gas plasma, the other a low-temperature hydrogen peroxide gas plasma. Gas plasma sterilization is carried out at temperatures lower than 50 °C (120 °F). Cycle times range from 75 min to 3 to 4 h, depending on the type of plasma used.

Ionized gases such as argon, nitrogen, oxygen, and carbon dioxide have also been used to kill microorganisms on surfaces. Polylactic acid (PLA), polyglycolic acid (PGA), and copolymers of PLA and PGA (PLGA) have been sterilized using these ionized gases. Treatment times are only 15 to 30 min.

Supercritical carbon dioxide fluid has also been used for bacterial inactivation. Applications include PLA and PLGA biodegradable polymers for drug-delivery systems, synthetic anterior cruciate prostheses constructed from knitted polyester, and human bone allografts.

REFERENCES

1. M. Donachie, Biomaterials, *Metals Handbook Desk Edition,* 2nd ed., J.R. Davis, Ed., ASM International, 1998, p 702–709
2. J. Katz, Developments in Medical Polymers for Biomaterials Applications, *Med. Device Diagnostic Ind.,* Jan 2001, p 122
3. D.F. Williams, Biocompatibility: An Overview, *Concise Encyclopedia of Medical & Dental Materials,* D. Williams, Ed., Pergamon Press and The MIT Press, 1990, p 51–59
4. D. Dowson, Friction and Wear of Medical Implants and Prosthetic Devices, *Friction, Lubrication, and Wear Technology,* Vol 18, *ASM Handbook,* ASM International, 1992, p 656–664
5. M. Long and H.J. Rack, Titanium Alloys in Total Joint Replacement—A Materials Perspective, *Biomaterials,* Vol 19, 1998, p 1621–1639
6. D. Dowson, Bio-Tribology of Natural and Replacement Synovial Joints, *Biomechanics of Diarthrodial Joints,* Vol 11, V.C. Mow, A. Ratcliffe, and S.L.-Y. Woo, Ed., Springer Verlag, 1992, p 305–345
7. J.B. Kowalski and R.F. Morrissey, Sterilization of Implants, *Biomaterials Science: An Introduction to Materials in Medicine,* B.D. Ratner, A.S. Hoffman, F.J. Schoen, and J.E. Lemons, Ed., Academic Press, 1996, p 415–420

CHAPTER 3

Metallic Materials

METALS have been successfully used as biomaterials for many years. Figures 1 to 3 show typical implant applications for orthopedic purposes. Figure 4 shows intramedullary rods and illustrates their use for fracture fixation. Besides orthopedics, there are other markets for metallic implants and devices, including oral and maxillofacial surgery (e.g., dental implants, craniofacial plates and screws) and cardiovascular surgery (e.g., parts of pacemakers, defibrillators, and artificial hearts; balloon catheters; valve replacements; stents; and aneurysm clips). Surgical instruments, dental instruments, needles, staples, and implantable drug pump housings are also made from metallic materials.

Relatively few metals in industrial use are biocompatible and capable of long-term success as an implant in the body. In developing a biomedical alloy, nontoxic elements must be selected as alloying elements. The biocompatibility of pure metals and some metallic biomedical alloys are compared in Fig. 5. For structural applications in the body (e.g., implants for hip, knee, ankle, shoulder, wrist, finger, or toe joints), the principal metals are stainless steels, cobalt-base alloys, and titanium-base alloys. These metals are popular primarily because of their ability to bear significant loads, withstand fatigue loading, and undergo plastic deformation prior to failure. Other metals and alloys employed in implantable devices include commercially pure titanium (CP-Ti), shape memory alloys (alloys based on the nickel-titanium binary system), zirconium alloys, tantalum (and, to a lesser extent, niobium), and precious metals and alloys.

Fatigue and yield strengths vary not only by alloy type (e.g., stainless steel versus titanium) but also with processing. The modulus, however, is more or less set by the alloy type (Table 1). The lowest moduli (105 to 125 GPa, or 15 to 18×10^6 psi) are for titanium alloys, while stainless steels have moduli near 205 GPa (30×10^6 psi), and cobalt-chromium alloys have moduli even higher, approximately 240 GPa (35×10^6 psi). The modulus is an important concern in the orthopedic application of biomaterials. Bone has a modulus on the order of 17 GPa (2.5×10^6 psi). The discrepancy between the modulus of bone and that of the alloys used to support structural loads means that the metallic devices implanted in the body take a disproportionate share of the load (stress). Bone adapts to the magnitude of the load it experiences. If the normal load experienced by a bone is shared between the bone and an implant, the portion of the load imposed on bone will be a function of the ratio of the elastic moduli of the bone and the implant material. Consequently, if the modulus of the implant material is significantly higher than bone, the actual load experienced by the bone will be proportionally lower due to the phenomenon known as stress shielding (Ref 3). Consequently, the bone will remodel itself to lower its load-bearing ability. This phenomenon, which leads to a deterioration of bone quality, along with the fact that significant differences in elastic moduli of the bone and the implant may lead to stress concentrations at their interface, behooves designers to try and match the stiffness of the implant and bone. The ideal alloy would have the modulus of magnesium, the strength of cobalt-chromium alloys, the corrosion resistance and biocompatibility of titanium, and the fabricability of stainless steel.

Alloys used in articulating prosthesis applications are often used in conjunction with other biomaterials, such as ultrahigh molecular weight polyethylene (UHMWPE), polyoxymethylene (Delrin-150, E.I. DuPont de Nemours & Co.), or aluminum oxide ceramics. A typical hip prosthesis consists of the stem, a ball, and a socket with a metallic backing.

The chemistry and manufacturing processes for metallic biomaterials are not necessarily unique to the biomedical device industry. Control of undesired elements is an important aspect of the successful application of metallic biomaterials. The principal requirement for each alloy is that it be corrosion resistant when inserted in the body and that it have optimal mechanical properties.

One of the unique aspects of the biomaterials and biomedical device industry is that, despite the general adherence to the ASTM International or other standards, materials are marketed and discussed in trade names. Thus, an alloy that has chemical origins that can be traced to a common cobalt-chromium alloy might have the following names: Vitallium, Plusmet, Endocast, Orthochrome, Protasul, and Zimaloy. It is necessary for each trade-marketed alloy to be reviewed to determine its underlying composition—that is, to which ASTM or other specification it is being made and sold.

Stainless steels and cobalt-chromium alloys depend for their general corrosion resistance on the presence of chromium and its ability to render the alloys passive. Additions of other alloy elements enhance resistance to nonuniform types of corrosion (e.g., pitting). Titanium and titanium alloys develop passivity without chromium. Surface passivity is the most important criteria, but surface finish also can affect performance. Highly polished surfaces perform better in terms of corrosion and wear.

Stainless Steels

Stainless steels are iron-base alloys that contain a minimum of 10.5% Cr, the amount needed to prevent the formation of rust in unpolluted atmospheres (hence the designation stainless). Few stainless steels contain more than 30% Cr or less than 50% Fe. They achieve their stainless characteristics through the formation of an invisible and adherent chromium-rich oxide surface film (~2 nm thick). This oxide forms and heals itself in the presence of oxygen.

Increasing the chromium content beyond the minimum of 10.5% confers still greater corrosion resistance. Further improvement in corrosion resistance and a wide range of properties may be achieved by the addition of nickel. The addition of other alloying elements may be used to enhance resistance to specific corrosion mechanisms or to develop desired mechanical and physical properties. For example, molybdenum further increases resistance to pitting corrosion, while nitrogen increases mechanical strength as well as enhances resistance to pitting. Carbon is normally present in amounts ranging from less than 0.03% to over 1.0% in certain martensitic grades.

Approximately 1% of the total tonnage of stainless steels is used for biomedical applications. Most nonimplant medical devices (e.g., surgical and dental instruments) are manufactured from commercial-grade stainless steels. These stainless steels adequately meet clinical requirements where contact with human tissue is transient.

Stainless steels used for implants must be suitable for close and prolonged contact with human

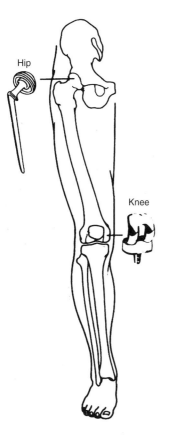

Fig. 1   Diagram of total hip and knee replacements showing component shape and location of implantation

tissue (i.e., warm, saline conditions). Specific requirements for resistance to pitting and crevice corrosion and the quantity and size of nonmetallic inclusions apply to implant-grade stainless steels. Hence, special production routes such as vacuum melting (VM), vacuum arc remelting (VAR), or electroslag refining (ESR) are required to produce implant steels. Table 2 lists various nonimplantable and implantable device applications for stainless steels.

Designations for Stainless Steels

In the United States, wrought grades of stainless steels are generally designated by the American Iron and Steel Institute (AISI) numbering system, the Unified Numbering System (UNS), or the proprietary name of the alloy. In addition, designation systems have been established by most of the major industrial nations. Of the two institutional numbering systems used in the United States, AISI is the older and more widely used. Most of the grades have a three-digit designation; the 200 and 300 series are generally austenitic stainless steels, whereas the 400 series are either ferritic or martensitic.

Some of the grades have a one- or two-letter suffix that indicates a particular modification of the composition.

The UNS system includes a considerably greater number of stainless steels than AISI, because it incorporates all of the more recently developed stainless steels. The UNS designation for a stainless steel consists of the letter S, followed by a five-digit number. For those alloys that have an AISI designation, the first three digits of the UNS designation usually correspond to an AISI number. When the last two digits are 00, the number designates a basic AISI grade. Modifications of the basic grades use two digits other than zeroes.

Classification of Stainless Steels

Stainless steels can be divided into five families. Four are based on the characteristic crystallographic structure/microstructure of the alloys in the family: martensitic, ferritic, austenitic, or duplex (austenitic plus ferritic). The fifth family, the precipitation-hardenable alloys, is based on the type of heat treatment used, rather than microstructure.

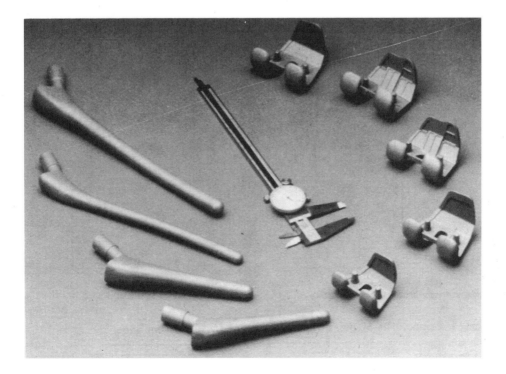

Fig. 2   Investment-cast titanium alloy knee and hip implant prostheses

Martensitic stainless steels are essentially Fe-Cr-C alloys that possess body-centered tetragonal crystal structure (martensitic) in the hardened condition. They are ferromagnetic, hardenable by heat treatments, and generally resistant to corrosion only in relatively mild environments. Chromium content is generally in the range of 10.5 to 18%, and carbon content can exceed 1.2%. The chromium and carbon contents are balanced to ensure a martensitic structure. Elements such as niobium, silicon, tungsten, and vanadium can be added to modify the tempering response after hardening. Small amounts of nickel can be added to improve corrosion resistance in some media and to improve toughness. Sulfur or selenium is added to some grades to improve machinability.

The high hardness of martensitic stainless steels (up to 97 HRB) makes them ideally suited for dental and surgical instruments. Examples include bone curettes, chisels and gouges, dental burs, dental chisels, curettes, explorers, root elevators and scalers, forceps, hemostats, retractors, orthodontic pliers, and scalpels. Chemical compositions of martensitic stainless steels used for dental and surgical instruments are given in Table 3.

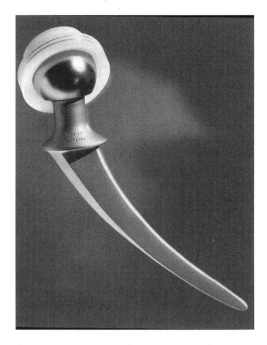

Fig. 3 Hip joint made of a Co-Ni-Cr-Mo alloy MP35N (ASTM F 562). Source: Timken Co.

Ferritic stainless steels are essentially iron-chromium alloys with body-centered cubic (bcc) crystal structures. Chromium content is usually in the range of 11 to 30%. Some grades may contain molybdenum, silicon, aluminum, titanium, and niobium to confer particular characteristics. Sulfur or selenium can be added to improve machinability.

Unlike the martensitic stainless steels, the ferritic stainless steels cannot be strengthened by heat treatment. Also, because the strain-hardening rates of ferrite are relatively low, and cold work significantly lowers ductility, the ferritic stainless steels are not often strengthened by cold work.

Ferritic stainless steels find few applications in medical devices. Examples are solid handles for instruments, guide pins, and fasteners.

Austenitic stainless steels constitute the largest stainless family in terms of number of alloys and use. Like the ferritic alloys, they cannot be hardened by heat treatment. However, their similarity ends there. The austenitic stainless steels are essentially nonmagnetic in the annealed condition and can be hardened only by cold working. They usually possess excellent cryogenic properties and good high-temperature strength and oxidation resistance. Chromium content generally varies from 16 to 26%; nickel content is less than or equal to approximately 35%; and manganese content is less than or equal to 15%. The 200-series steels contain nitrogen, 4 to 23% Mn, and lower nickel contents (up to 7% Ni). The 300-series steels contain larger amounts of nickel and up to 2% Mn. Molybdenum, copper, silicon, aluminum, titanium, and niobium can be added to confer certain characteristics, such as halide pitting resistance or oxidation resistance. Austenitic stainless steels offer excellent formability, and their response to deformation can be controlled by the nickel content (i.e., higher nickel contents result in improved formability).

Austenitic stainless steels find applications in nonimplantable medical devices where good corrosion resistance and moderate strength are required, for example, canulae, dental impression trays, guide pins, holloware, hypodermic needles, steam sterilizers, storage cabinets and work surfaces, thoracic retractors, and so on. These applications often require a material that is easily formed into complex shapes. Chemical compositions of stainless steels used for nonimplantable medical devices or dental appliances are given in Table 4.

Austenitic stainless steels are also widely used for implants. See the section "Implant-Grade Stainless Steels" in this chapter for details.

Duplex stainless steels are two-phase alloys based on the Fe-Cr-Ni system. These materials typically comprise approximately equal proportions of ferrite and austenite phases in their microstructure and are characterized by their low carbon contents (<0.03%) and additions of molybdenum, nitrogen, tungsten, and copper. Typical chromium and nickel contents are 20 to 30% and 5 to 8%, respectively. The specific advantages offered by duplex stainless steels over conventional 300-series stainless steels are strength (approximately twice that of austenitic stainless steels), improved toughness and ductility (compared to ferritic grades), and superior chloride stress-corrosion cracking resistance and pitting resistance.

Duplex stainless steels have yet to make an impact in the biomedical field. They are com-monly used in the oil and gas, petrochemical, and pulp and paper industries.

Precipitation-hardenable (PH) stainless steels are chromium-nickel grades that can be hardened by an aging treatment. These grades are classified as austenitic (e.g., A-286), semi-austenitic (e.g., 17-7PH), or martensitic (e.g., 17-4PH). The classification is determined by their solution-annealed microstructure. The semiaustenitic alloys are subsequently heat treated so that the austenite transforms to martensite. Cold work is sometimes used to facilitate the aging reaction. Various alloying elements, such as aluminum, titanium, niobium, or copper, are used to achieve aging.

Both semiaustenitic and martensitic PH steels are used for medical applications. Examples include neurosurgical aneurysm and microvascular clips (Table 2) and various types of surgical and dental instruments. Austenitic grades are not currently being used for medical devices. Chemical compositions of semi-

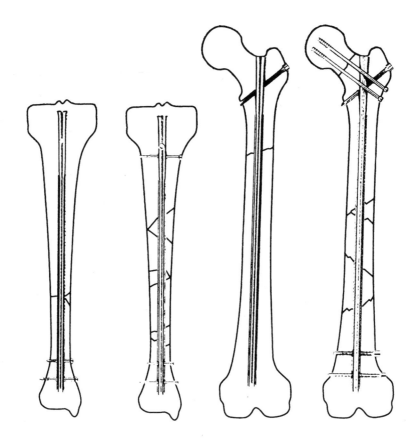

Fig. 4   Intramedullary rods and locking nails applied to tibia or femur

austenitic and martensitic PH steels used in the medical industry are listed in Table 5.

Implant-Grade Stainless Steels

Austenitic stainless steels are popular for implant applications because they are relatively inexpensive, they can be formed with common techniques, and their mechanical properties can be controlled over a wide range for optimal strength and ductility. Stainless steels for implants are wrought alloys (i.e., they are fabricated by forging and machining). Passivity of stainless steel implants is enhanced by nitric acid passivation before the implant is sterilized and packaged for delivery to a medical facility.

Austenitic stainless steels are not sufficiently corrosion resistant for long-term use as an implant material. They find use as bone screws, bone plates, intramedullary nails and rods, and other temporary fixation devices with a number of applicable ASTM standards, including:

ASTM No.	Stainless steel implant material
F 138/139(a)	Low-carbon stainless steels (type 316L or UNS S31673)
F 1314	Nitrogen-strengthened 22Cr-12.5Ni-5Mn-2.5Mo (UNS S20910)
F 1586	Nitrogen-strengthened 21Cr-10Ni-3Mn-2.5Mo (UNS S31675)
F 2229	Nitrogen-strengthened 23Mn-21Cr-1Mo (UNS S29108)

(a) F 138 covers bar and wire; F 139 covers sheet and strip.

Type 316L (18Cr-14Ni-2.5Mo) is a vacuum-melted low-carbon variant of the standard type 316 composition. Table 6 lists chemistries for type 316L and three comparative stainless steel implant alloys. The vacuum melting step imparts improved cleanliness, and the chemistry is designed to maximize the pitting corrosion resistance and provide a ferrite-free microstructure. The pitting resistance equivalent (PRE) meets the following requirement:

$$\%Cr + 3.3 \times \%Mo \geq 26$$

The recommended grain size for type 316L is ASTM No. 5 or finer when tested in accordance with ASTM test method E 112 for determining average grain size. The grain size should be relatively uniform throughout the specimen/device.

Type 316L is ordinarily used in the 30% cold-worked state (Ref 5), because cold-worked metal has a markedly increased yield, ultimate tensile, and fatigue strength relative to the annealed state. The trade-off is decreased ductility, but ordinarily, this is not a major concern in implant products. A summary of representative mechanical properties of 316L stainless steel is provided in Table 7 and Fig. 6.

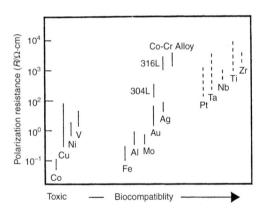

Fig. 5 The relationship between polarization resistance and biocompatibility of pure metals, cobalt-chromium alloy, and stainless steels. Source: Ref 1

Table 1 Comparison of mechanical properties of metallic implant materials with those of cortical bone

Material	Young's modulus		Ultimate tensile strength		Fracture toughness	
	GPa	10⁶ psi	MPa	ksi	MPa √m	ksi √in.
Cobalt-chromium alloys	230	35	900–1540	130–225	~100	~90
Austenic stainless steel	200	30	540–1000	80–145	~100	~90
Ti-6Al-4V	106	15	900	130	~80	~70
Cortical bone	7–30	1–4	50–150	7–20	2–12	2–11

Source: Ref 2

Table 2   Medical device applications for stainless steels

Application	Description(a)
Bone screws and pins	Internal fixation of diaphyseal fractures of cortical bone, and metaphyseal and epiphyseal fractures of cancellous bone: screw comprised of hexagonal or Phillips recess driving head, threaded shaft, and self-tapping or non-self-tapping tip; type 316L stainless steel
Onlay bone plates	Internal fixation of shaft and mandibular fractures: thin, narrow plate with slots or holes for retaining screws; type 316L stainless steel
Blade and nail bone plates	Internal fixation of fracture near the ends of weight-bearing bones: plate and nail, either single unit or multicomponent; type 316L stainless steel
Intramedullar bone nails	Internal fixation of long bones: tube or solid nail; type 316L stainless steel
Percutaneous pin bone fixation	External clamp fixation for fusion of joints and open fractures of infected nonunions: external frame supporting transfixing pins; stainless steel
Total joint prostheses	Replacement of total joints with metal and plastic components (shoulder, hip, knee, ankle, and great toe): humeral, femoral (hip and knee), talus, and metatarsal components; type 316L stainless steel
Wires	Internal tension band wiring of bone fragments or circumferential cerclage for comminuted or unstable shaft fractures; type 316L stainless steel
Harrington spine instrumentation	Treatment of scoliosis by application of correction forces and stabilization of treated segments: rod and hooks; type 316L stainless steel
Mandibular wire mesh prostheses	Primary reconstruction of partially resected mandible; types 316 and 316L stainless steel
Fixed orthodontic appliances	Correction of malocclusion by movement of teeth: components include bands, brackets, archwires, and springs; types 302, 303, 304, and 305 stainless steel
Preformed dental crowns	Restoration for extensive loss of tooth structure in primary and young permanent teeth: preformed shell; type 304 stainless steel
Preformed endodontic post and core	Restoration of endodontically treated teeth: post fixed within root canal preparation, with exposed core providing a crown foundation; types 304 and 316 stainless steel
Retention pins for dental amalgam	Retention of large dental amalgam restorations: cemented, friction lock, and self-threading pins, placed approximately 2 mm (0.08 in.) within dentin with approximately 2 mm (0.08 in.) exposed; types 304 and 316 stainless steel
Wire mesh	Inguinal hernia repair, cranioplasty (with acrylic), orthopedic bone cement restrictor; types 316 and 316L stainless steel
Sutures	Wound closure, repair of cleft lip and palate, securing of wire mesh in cranioplasty, mandibular and hernia repair and realignment, tendon and nerve repair; types 304, 316, and 316L stainless steel
Stapedial prostheses	Replacement of nonfunctioning stapes: various types comprised of wire and piston or wire and cup piston (synthetic fluorine-containing resin/stainless steel piston, platinum and stainless steel cup piston, and all stainless steel prostheses); types 316 and 316L stainless steel
Neurosurgical aneurysm and microvascular clips	Temporary or permanent occlusion of intracranial blood vessels; tension clips of various configurations, approximately 2 cm (0.8 in.) or less in length and constructed of one piece or jaw, pivot, and spring components (similar and dissimilar compositions); 17-7PH, 17-7PH (Nb), PH-15-7Mo, and types 301, 304, 316, 316L, 420, and 431 stainless steel
Self-expanding stent	Treatment of tracheobronchial stenosis, tracheomalacia, and air collapse following tracheal reconstruction: 0.457 mm (0.018 in.) stainless steel wire formed in a zigzag configuration of 5–10 bends
Balloon-expandable stent	Dilation and postdilation support of complicated vascular stenosis (experimental): stainless steel
Hydrocephalus drainage valve	Control of intercranial pressure: one-way valve; type 316 stainless steel
Trachea tube	Breathing tube following tracheotomy and laryngectomy: tube-within-a-tube construction; type 304 stainless steel
Electronic laryngeal prosthesis system	Electromagnetic voicing source following total laryngectomy: implanted unit comprised of subdermal transformer, rectifier pack, and transducer encased in type 316 stainless steel, with spring steel diaphragm
Electrodes and lead wires	Anodic, cathodic, and sensing electrodes and lead wires: intramuscular stimulation, bone growth stimulation, cardiac pacemaker (cathode), electromyography (EMG), electroencephalogram (EEG), and lead wires in a large number of devices; types 304, 316, and 316L stainless steel
Arzbaecher pill electrode	Atrial electrocardiograms: swallowed sensing electrode of short metal tubing segments forced over plastic tubing; stainless steel
Cardiac pacemaker housing	Hermetic packaging of electronics and power source: welded capsule; type 316L stainless steel
Variable capacitance transducer	Measurement of pressure on sound: metal diaphragm, mounted in tension; stainless steel
Variable resistance transducer	Measurement of respiratory flow: metal arms supporting wire strain gage; stainless steel
Intrauterine device (IUD)	Contraception: stainless steel (Majzlin spring, M-316, M device), stainless steel and silicone rubber (Comet, M-213, Ypsilon device), stainless steel and natural rubber (K S Wing IUD), stainless steel and polyether urethane (Web device)
Intrauterine pressure-sensor case	Protective shroud for transducer: stainless steel
Osmotic minipump	Continuous delivery of biologically active agents: implanted unit comprising elastomeric reservoir, osmotic agent, rate-controlling membrane, and stainless steel flow moderator and filling tube
Radiographic marker	Facilitation of postoperative angiography of bypass graft: open circle configuration of 25 gage suture wires; stainless steel
Butterfly cannula	Intravenous infusion: stainless steel
Cannula	Coronary perfusion: silicone rubber reinforced with an internal wire spiral; stainless steel
Acupuncture needle	Acupuncture: 0.26 mm (0.01 in.) diameter × 5–10 cm (2–4 in.) length needles; stainless steel
Limb prostheses, orthoses, and adaptive devices	Substitution, correction, support, or aided function of movable parts of the body, and technical aids not worn by the patient: components such as braces, struts, joints, and bearings of many items; steel and stainless steel

(a) Stainless steel types other than those listed for each application may also be used. Source: Ref 4

Table 3 Chemical compositions of martensitic stainless steels commonly used for surgical and dental instruments

UNS No.	Type/designation	Composition(a), %							
		C	Mn	Si	Cr	Ni	P	S	Other
S41000	410	0.15	1.00	1.00	11.5–13.5	. . .	0.04	0.03	. . .
S41600	416	0.15	1.25	1.00	12.0–14.0	. . .	0.06	0.15 min	0.6 Mo(b)
S42000	420	0.15 min	1.00	1.00	12.0–14.0	. . .	0.04	0.03	. . .
S42010	TrimRite	0.15–0.30	1.00	1.00	13.5–15.0	0.25–1.00	0.040	0.030	0.40–1.00 Mo
S42020	420F	0.15 min	1.25	1.00	12.0–14.0	. . .	0.06	0.15 min	0.6 Mo(b)
S43100	431	0.20	1.00	1.00	15.0–17.0	1.25–2.50	0.04	0.03	. . .
S44002	440A	0.60–0.75	1.00	1.00	16.0–18.0	. . .	0.04	0.03	0.75 Mo

(a) Single values are maximum values unless otherwise indicated. (b) Optional

Table 4 Chemical compositions of austenitic stainless steels commonly used for nonimplant medical devices and dental appliances

UNS No.	Type/designation	Composition(a), %							
		C	Mn	Si	Cr	Ni	P	S	Other
S30100	301	0.15	2.0	1.00	16.0–18.0	6.0–8.0	0.045	0.03	. . .
S30200	302	0.15	2.0	1.00	17.0–19.0	8.0–10.0	0.045	0.03	. . .
S30300	303	0.15	2.0	1.00	17.0–19.0	8.0–10.0	0.20	0.15 min	0.6 Mo(b)
S30400	304	0.08	2.0	1.00	18.0–20.0	8.0–10.5	0.045	0.03	. . .
S30500	305	0.12	2.0	1.00	17.0–19.0	10.5–13.0	0.045	0.03	. . .
S31600	316	0.08	2.0	1.00	16.0–18.0	10.0–14.0	0.045	0.03	2.0–3.0 Mo
S31700	317	0.08	2.0	1.00	18.0–20.0	11.0–15.0	0.045	0.03	3.0–4.0 Mo

(a) Single values are maximum values unless otherwise indicated. (b) Optional

Table 5 Chemical compositions of precipitation-hardenable stainless steels used for medical devices and surgical and dental instruments

UNS No.	Alloy	Composition(a), %								
		C	Mn	Si	Cr	Ni	Mo	P	S	Other
Martensitic types										
S13800	PH13-8 Mo	0.05	0.10	0.10	12.25–13.25	7.5–8.5	2.0–2.5	0.01	0.008	0.90–1.35 Al;0.01 N
S15500	15-5PH	0.07	1.00	1.00	14.0–15.5	3.5–5.5	. . .	0.04	0.03	2.5–4.5 Cu; 0.15–0.45 Nb
S17400	17-4PH	0.07	1.00	1.00	15.0–17.5	3.0–5.0	. . .	0.04	0.03	3.0–5.0 Cu; 0.15–0.45 Nb
S45000	Custom 450	0.05	1.00	1.00	14.0–16.0	5.0–7.0	0.5–1.0	0.03	0.03	1.25–1.75 Cu; 8 × %C min Nb
S45500	Custom 455	0.05	0.50	0.50	11.0–12.5	7.5–9.5	0.50	0.04	0.03	1.5–2.5 Cu; 0.8–1.4 Ti; 0.1–0.5 Nb
Semiaustenitic types										
S15700	PH15-7 Mo	0.09	1.00	1.00	14.0–16.0	6.50–7.75	2.0–3.0	0.04	0.04	0.75–1.50 Al
S17700	17-7 PH	0.09	1.00	1.00	16.0–18.0	6.50–7.75	. . .	0.04	0.04	0.75–1.50 Al
S35000	AM-350	0.07–0.11	0.50–1.25	0.50	16.0–17.0	4.0–5.0	2.50–3.25	0.04	0.03	0.07–0.13 N
S35500	AM-355	0.10–0.15	0.50–1.25	0.50	15.0–16.0	4.0–5.0	2.50–3.25	0.04	0.03	0.07–0.13 N

(a) Single values are maximum values unless otherwise indicated.

Type 316L can be welded, but care must be taken not to sensitize the component. Type 316L, as well as other austenitic grades, has been used as wire for limited-duration applications in the body. Welding and soldering are used to join one wire section to another or to form smooth tips on guide wires.

Vacuum melted 316L remains the most widely used stainless steel for implant devices. Table 2 reviews the many medical device applications for this alloy.

Nitrogen-Strengthened Stainless Steels. Recently, other stainless steels have been developed and standardized that have increased corrosion resistance and improved mechanical properties when compared to 316L (ASTM F 138/139). As listed earlier in the introduction to this section, these include ESR-processed nitrogen-strengthened alloys covered by ASTM F 1314, F 1586, and F 2229. Table 6 lists chemical composition requirements for these alloys. Nitrogen-strengthened alloys are being used for bone plates, bone screws, spinal fixation components, and other medical components.

ASTM F 1314, which has a nominal composition of 22Cr-12.5Ni-5Mn-2.5Mo plus 0.20 to 0.40% N, was one of the first nitrogen-strengthened stainless steels developed for fracture fixation devices (Ref 7). It falls in the 200-series classification of stainless steels (UNS S20910). This ferrite-free alloy is capable of being cold worked to ultimate tensile strengths exceeding 1380 MPa (200 ksi). Minimum mechanical requirements for S20910 wire and bar are listed in Table 8.

ASTM F 1586, like type 316L (UNS S31673), is another variant of the standard-grade type 316. It has a UNS designation of S31675 and a nominal composition of 21Cr-10Ni-3Mn-2.5Mo plus 0.25 to 0.50% N. This alloy exhibits improved tensile strength, impact strength, fatigue strength, and crevice and pitting corrosion when compared with type 316L. Minimal mechanical requirements for S31675 bars are listed in Table 9.

ASTM F 2229 is an essentially nickel-free (<0.05% Ni) 200-series austenitic stainless steel (UNS S29108) with a nominal composition of

Table 6   Chemical compositions of austenitic stainless steels used for implantable fracture fixation devices

ASTM designation	UNS No.	Composition(a), %										
		C	Mn	P	S	Si	Cr	Ni	Mo	N	Cu	Others
F 138	S31673	0.030	2.00	0.025	0.010	0.75	17.00–19.00	13.00–15.00	2.25–3.00	0.10	0.50	...
F 1314	S20910	0.030	4.00–6.00	0.025	0.010	0.75	20.50–23.50	11.50–13.50	2.00–3.00	0.20–0.40	0.50	0.10–0.30 Nb; 0.10–0.30 V
F 1586	S31675	0.08	2.00–4.25	0.025	0.010	0.75	19.50–22.00	9.00–11.00	2.00–3.00	0.25–0.50	0.25	0.25–0.80 Nb
F 2229	S29108	0.08	21.00–24.00	0.03	0.010	0.75	19.00–23.00	0.10	0.50–1.50	0.90 min	0.25	...

(a) Single values are maximum values unless otherwise indicated.

Table 7   Mechanical requirements for ASTM F 138 (UNS S31673) bar and wire

Condition	Diameter or thickness		Ultimate tensile strength, min		Yield strength (0.2% offset), min		Elongation in 4D or 4W, min(a), %	Brinell hardness, max(b), HB
	mm	in.	MPa	ksi	MPa	ksi		
Hot worked (c)	All		...	...	...	...	...	250
Annealed	1.60 and over	0.063 and over	490	71	190	27.5	40	...
Cold worked	1.60–38.1	0.063–1.500	860	125	690	100	12	...
Extra hard	1.60–6.35	0.063–0.250	1350	196	...	...	...	...

(a) 4D = 4 × diameter; 4W = 4 × width. Alternately, a gage length corresponding to ISO 6892 may be used when agreed on between supplier and purchaser. (b) 29 kN (3000 kgf) load. (c) Typically supplied as hot-rolled bar for forging applications

23Mn-21Cr-1Mo plus ~1.0% N. It was developed in response to nickel-allergy problems associated with nickel-containing stainless steels. In addition to providing austenitic stability (ferrite-free structure), the high nitrogen content contributes to high levels of corrosion resistance and strength. Typical mechanical properties for S29108 bars are listed in Table 10.

All of the nitrogen-strengthened stainless steels discussed previously have better crevice

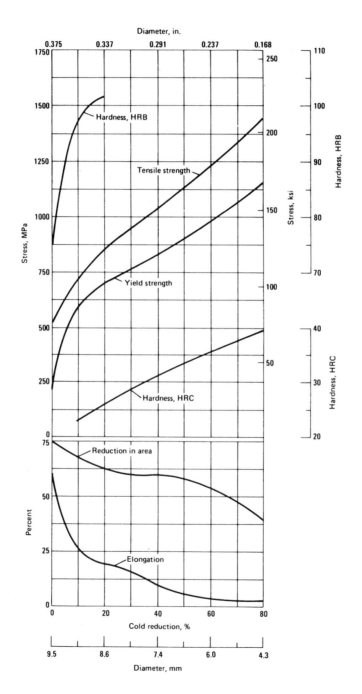

Fig. 6 Effect of cold reduction on the tensile properties of annealed type 316L stainless steel rods (9.53 mm, or 0.375 in. diam). Elongation was measured in 50 mm (2 in.); yield strength at 0.2% offset. Source: Ref 6

and pitting corrosion resistance when compared to type 316L. Figure 7 shows the critical crevice temperature (the critical temperature to initiate crevice corrosion in a 6% ferric chloride/1% hydrochloric acid solution accordance with ASTM G 48, method D) and the PRE for ASTM 138 (type 316L), 1314, 1586, and 2229, respectively. The nitrogen-strengthened grades have PRE values in excess of 30. Similarly, yield strength levels for cold-worked, nitrogen-strengthened stainless steels are higher than type 316L (Fig. 8).

Cobalt-Base Alloys

Cobalt-base alloys were first used in the 1930s. The Co-Cr-Mo alloy Vitallium was used as a cast dental alloy and then adopted to orthopedic applications starting in the 1940s. The corrosion of cobalt-chromium alloys is more than an order of magnitude greater than that of stainless steels, and they possess high mechanical property capability.

Although cobalt alloys were first used as cast components, wrought alloys later came into use. Although a number of specifications exist for cobalt-base alloys, the four main alloys used are:

- ASTM F 75, a Co-28Cr-6Mo casting alloy
- ASTM F 90, a Co-20Cr-15W-10Ni wrought alloy
- ASTM F 799, a Co-28Cr-6Mo thermomechanically processed alloy with a composition nearly identical to ASTM F 75 casting alloy

Table 8   Mechanical requirements for ASTM F 1314 (UNS S20910) bar and wire

| Condition | Diameter or thickness | | Ultimate tensile strength, min | | Yield strength (0.2% offset), min | | Elongation in 4D, min(a),% | Brinell hardness, max(b), HB |
	mm	in.	MPa	ksi	MPa	ksi		
Hot worked(c)	Up to 50.8	Up to 2	. . .	. . .	. . .	. . .	. . .	325
Annealed	All		690	100	380	55	35	. . .
Cold worked	1.59–19.1(d)	$^1/_{16}$–$^3/_4$(d)	1035	50	862	125	12	. . .

(a) $4D = 4 \times$ diameter. (b) 29,400 N (3000 kgf) load. (c) Typically supplied as hot-rolled bar for forging applications. (d) Other sizes may be furnished by agreement between the producer and the purchaser.

Table 9   Mechanical requirements for ASTM F 1586 (UNS S31675) bars

| Condition | Diameter or thickness | | Ultimate tensile strength, min | | Yield strength (0.2% offset), min | | Elongation in 4D, min(a),% |
	mm	in.	MPa	ksi	MPa	ksi	
Annealed(b)	All		740	107	430	62.4	35
Medium hard	1.59–19.1(c)	$^1/_{16}$–$^3/_4$(c)	1000	145	700	102	20
Hard	1.59–19.1(c)	$^1/_{16}$–$^3/_4$(c)	1100	160	1000	145	10

(a) $4D = 4 \times$ diameter. (b) Corresponds to ISO 5832-9. (c) Other sizes may be furnished by agreement between the producer and the purchaser.

Table 10   Tensile properties of ASTM F 2229 (UNS S29108) bars

| Cold work, % | Ultimate tensile strength | | Yield strength | | Elongation in 4D, % | Reduction in area, % |
	MPa	ksi	MPa	ksi		
(Annealed)	931	135	586	85	52	75
10	1062	154	786	114	37	73
20	1262	183	952	138	25	68
30	1496	217	1227	178	19	63
40	1731	251	1551	225	12	59

Note: Data represent bar cold drawn various amounts from a starting diameter of 25 mm (1.0 in.) Tests represent 12.8 mm (0.505 in.) diameter specimens machined from the bar center. Source: Carpenter Technology Corporation

- ASTM F 562, a Co-35Ni-20Cr-10Mo wrought alloy

Compositions for these and other alloys covered by ASTM specifications are listed in Table 11.

Strengthening in cobalt alloys is produced by solid-solution elements and the presence of carbides. In wrought alloys where working is possible, cold work enhances strength. In order to produce wrought cobalt-chromium alloys, carbon must be reduced compared to the level in cast alloys (0.05% versus approximately 0.25% or higher). Low carbon contents mean that less strengthening is produced by carbides. To

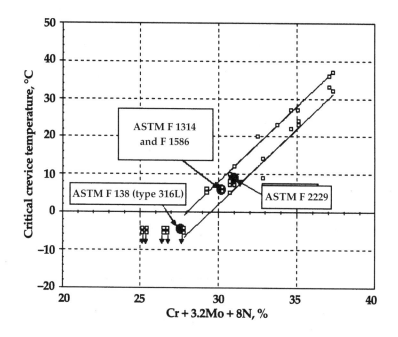

Fig. 7 Critical crevice temperature (CCT) for stainless steel implant alloys plotted versus the Cr + 3.2Mo + 8N pitting resistance equivalent. The CCT tests were conducted in accordance with ASTM G 48, method D. Source: Ref 8

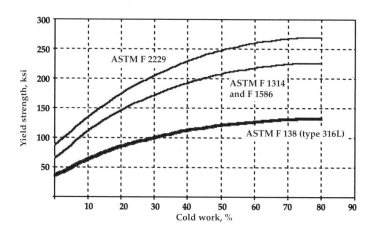

Fig. 8 Yield strength versus cold work levels for three nitrogen-strengthened implant alloys and type 316L. Source: Ref 8

enhance fabricability, chromium contents generally are reduced and nickel added. Wrought alloys can be hot worked, and some can be cold drawn. Yield strengths vary with grain size and the degree of cold work imparted from the wrought fabrication process.

Alloys produced for structural applications such as hip prostheses can be forged if optimal properties are desired. The forging process results in maximum strength and toughness for cobalt-chromium alloys but may not produce uniform grain sizes. Data have been reported on forging of a modified F 75 composition wherein finer grain size occurred in the distal end (tip of the femoral stem, farthest from the ball) than in the proximal end (Table 12). Strength (fatigue, yield) was correspondingly better in specimens taken from the distal end.

Cobalt-chromium alloys are difficult to machine. Closed-die forging can minimize machining requirements, but wrought processed

components still may require more machining than cast components. Consequently, investment casting often is used to produce cobalt-chromium implants at the lowest cost. The grain size of cast components is invariably greater than that of comparable wrought components, so strength properties of castings do not approach those of wrought cobalt-chromium alloys. Porosity can be a problem in castings but can be controlled by improved mold design and by application of hot isostatic pressing (HIP) in postcast treatment of vacuum investment-cast alloys. Powder metallurgy has been used to make some cobalt-chromium components. Hot isostatic pressing of powder is claimed to result in very fine grains and exceptional properties, but costs may be higher.

The preferred method of producing cobalt-base alloy implants will be a function of the trade-off between cost and properties. Where the properties of castings are sufficient, castings will

Table 11 Chemical compositions of cobalt-base alloys used for surgical implants

ASTM designation	UNS No.	Composition(a), wt%										
		Cr	Mo	Ni	Fe	C	Si	Mn	W	P	S	Others
F 75	R30075	27.0–30.0	5.0–7.0	1.00	0.75	0.35	1.00	1.00	0.20	0.020	0.010	0.25 N; 0.30 Al; 0.01 B
F 90	R30605	19.0–21.0	...	9.0–11.0	3.00	0.05–0.15	0.40	1.00–2.00	14.00–16.00	0.040	0.030	...
F 562	R30035	19.0–21.0	9.0–10.5	33.0–37.0	1.00	0.025	0.15	0.15	...	0.015	0.010	1.0 Ti
F 563	R30563	18.00–22.00	3.00–4.00	15.00–25.00	4.00–6.00	0.05	0.50	1.00	3.00–4.00	...	0.010	0.50–3.50 Ti
F 799	R31537	26.0–30.0	5.0–7.0	1.00	0.75	0.35	1.00	1.00	...	...	...	0.25 N
F 1058 grade 1	R30003	19.0–21.0	6.0–8.0	14.0–16.0	Bal(b)	0.15	1.20	1.5–2.5	...	0.015	0.015	0.10 Be; 39.0–41.0 Co
F 1058 grade 2	R30008	18.5–21.5	6.5–7.5	15.0–18.0	Bal(b)	0.15	1.20	1.00–2.00	...	0.015	0.015	0.001 Be; 39.0–42.0 Co

(a) Single values are maximum values unless otherwise indicated. (b) The iron content is approximately equal to the difference between 100% and the sum percentage of the other specified elements. ASTM F 1058 grade 1 contains between 39.0 and 41.0 wt% Co; ASTM F 1058 grade 2 contains between 39.0 and 42.0 wt% Co.

Table 12 Effect of forging on Vitallium alloy (Co-28Cr-6Mo) mechanical properties

Material condition	Tensile strength		0.2% yield strength		Elongation, %	Fatigue strength (10^6 cycles implied, $R = -1$)	
	MPa	ksi	MPa	ksi		MPa	ksi
Forged							
Proximal stem	1406.6	204.0	889.5	129.0	28.3	792.9	115.0
Distal stem	1506.6	218.5	1029.4	149.3	27.5	827.4–965.3	120.0–140.0
Cast (typical)	790	115	520	75	15	310	45

Source: Ref 2

dominate. When maximum strength is required, hot pressing and/or forging will rule. Table 13 shows that forged, cold-worked, and HIPed wrought cobalt alloys have substantial mechanical property advantages over the cast alloy.

ASTM F 75 is a cast Co-Cr-Mo alloy with a UNS No. of R30075 (Table 11). Commonly used commercial/proprietary names to describe this alloy include Vitallium and Haynes 21. The main attribute of this alloy is corrosion resistance in chloride environments, which is related to its bulk composition (particularly the high chromium content) and the surface oxide (nominally Cr_2O_3). This alloy has a long history in the aerospace and biomedical implant industries.

When F 75 is cast into shapes by investment casting, the alloy is melted at 1350 to 1450 °C (2460 to 2640 °F) and then poured into ceramic molds of the desired shape (e.g., femoral stems for artificial hips) (Ref 5). The molds are made by fabricating a wax pattern to near-final dimensions and then coating (or investing) the pattern with a special ceramic. A ceramic mold remains after the wax is melted out. Then, the molten metal is poured into the mold. Once the metal has solidified into the shape of the mold, the ceramic mold is cracked away, and processing continues toward the final device. More detailed information on the investment (or lost wax) casting process can be found in Ref 9.

As-cast F 75 alloy typically consists of a cobalt-rich matrix (alpha phase) plus interdendritic and grain-boundary carbides (primarily $M_{23}C_6$, where M represents cobalt, chromium, or molybdenum). There can also be interdendritic cobalt and molybdenum-rich sigma intermetallic, and cobalt-base gamma phases.

If nonequilibrium cooling occurs during casting solidification, a cored microstructure can develop (Ref 5). In this situation, the interdendritic regions become solute (chromium, molybdenum, carbon)-rich and contain carbides, while dendrites become chromium depleted and richer in cobalt. This is an unfavorable electrochemical situation, with the chromium-depleted regions being anodic with respect to the rest of the microstructure. This coring also results in small differences in the mechanical properties between the cobalt-rich dendrites and the chromium-rich interdendritic regions. Subsequent solution annealing heat treatments at 1225 °C (2235 °F) for 1 to 3 h can help alleviate the problems associated with coring.

A further feature of cast cobalt implant alloys is the extremely large grain size observed in the original castings. This problem is particularly severe in castings having a large cross section, because here any chilling effect from the mold wall is quickly lost, and the remaining liquid solidifies slowly, resulting in coarse grain size (Ref 10). As stated earlier, a finer grain size results in superior mechanical properties.

ASTM F 799. This is a modified F 75 alloy (Table 11) that has been mechanically processed by hot forging rough billets to final shape. In this process, it is common to use several steps, during which the alloy is successively brought closer to the required shape. The temperature at which these operations are carried out varies, because even though a higher temperature allows a greater deformation to be achieved, it results in less strengthening (Ref 10). Consequently, it is common for the early forging steps to be carried out at a comparatively high temperature, to allow easy deformation, and the later steps at a lower temperature, to induce as much cold working as possible. In this way, the finished product may exhibit

Table 13 Typical properties of cast and wrought cobalt-base alloys

ASTM designation	Condition	Young's modulus		Yield strength		Tensile strength		Fatigue endurance limit (at 10^7 cycles, $R = -1$)	
		GPa	10^6 psi	MPa	ksi	MPa	ksi	MPa	ksi
F 75	As-cast/annealed	210	30	448–517	65–75	655–889	95–129	207–310	30–45
	P/M HIP(a)	253	37	841	122	1277	185	725–950	105–138
F 799	Hot forged	210	30	896–1200	130–174	1399–1586	203–230	600–896	87–130
F 90	Annealed	210	30	448–648	65–94	951–1220	138–177	Not available	
	44% cold worked	210	30	1606	233	1896	275	586	85
F 562	Hot forged	232	34	965–1000	140–145	1206	175	500	73
	Cold worked, aged	232	34	1500	218	1795	260	689–793(b)	100–115(b)

(a) P/M, powder metallurgy; HIP, hot isostatic pressing. (b) Axial tension, $R = 0.05$, 30 Hz. Source: Ref 5

extremely high strength levels, while there are minimal quantities of metal to be subsequently removed by machining.

The microstructure of hot-forged F 799 reveals a more worked grain structure than as-cast F 75 and a hexagonal close-packed (hcp) phase that forms via a shear-induced transformation of face-centered cubic (fcc) matrix to hcp platelets. The fatigue, yield, and ultimate tensile strengths of this alloy are approximately twice those for as-cast F 75 (Table 13).

As an alternative to conventional casting and forging practices, powder metallurgy techniques have been used successfully to achieve extremely good mechanical properties. In this process, inert-gas-atomized spherical powders (Fig. 9) are compacted to final shapes by HIP (Fig. 10). Hot isostatic pressing of prealloyed

powders produces a much finer microstructure than cast products (Fig. 11). The very fine, uniformly distributed carbides give HIPed cobalt alloys superior wear properties when mating with UHMWPE or when mating to itself in a metal-to-metal joint. As shown in Table 13, significant improvements in mechanical properties are also achieved. More detailed information on HIP can be found in Ref 11.

ASTM F 90 is a wrought Co-Cr-W-Ni alloy with a UNS No. of R30605 (Table 11). Commonly used commercial/proprietary names to describe this alloy include Haynes 25 and L-605. Tungsten and nickel are added to improve machinability and fabrication characteristics (Ref 5). In the annealed state, its mechanical properties approximate those of cast F 75, but when cold worked to 44%, the properties more than double (Table 13). This difference in properties between F 90 in the annealed and work-hardened condition means that great care must be taken to ensure even and thorough deformation of the component (Ref 10). Without this, the variation in properties may allow unexpected failure to occur.

ASTM F 562 is a wrought Co-Ni-Cr-Mo alloy with a UNS No. of R30035 (Table 11). Known as MP35N, this material was originally developed as a high-performance aerospace fastener alloy that combines strength, high ductility, and corrosion resistance, including resistance to stress-corrosion cracking in the high-strength condition (Ref 12). The prime strengthening mechanism in F 562 is the solid-state

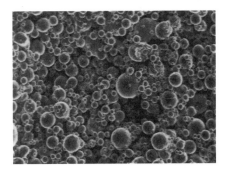

Fig. 9 Scanning electron micrograph of inert-gas-atomized prealloyed Co-Cr-Mo powder used to produce fully dense implants. 180×

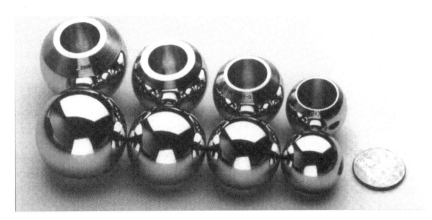

Fig. 10 Femoral bearing caps made from hot isostatic pressed Co-Cr-Mo alloy (ASTM F 799). Source: Carpenter Technology Corporation

phase transformation of part of the matrix from a fcc crystal structure to a hcp structure by cold working. This transformation occurs because of the high cobalt content in the alloy and has been termed the multiphase reaction. The presence of two distinct crystal structures poses a barrier to the motion of dislocations and leads to pronounced strengthening. Subsequent age hardening in the 425 to 650 °C (800 to 1200 °F) range acts to stabilize these two phases through the process of solute partitioning (Ref 12). Cold-worked and aged F 562 can exceed tensile strength levels in excess of 1795 MPa (260 ksi), which is the highest strength of any of the surgical implant alloys (Table 13). Figure 12 shows the effects of cold work and cold work plus aging on the tensile properties of the alloy. It is interesting to note that even at high yield strength levels of 1600 MPa (230 ksi), F 562 is still capable of exhibiting elongations in excess of 8%.

Other Cobalt-Base Surgical Implant Alloys. Although the four cobalt-chromium

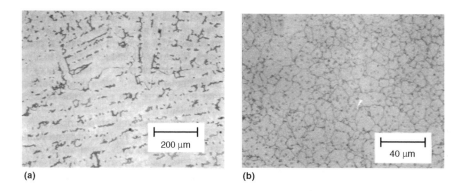

(a)   (b)

Fig. 11   Comparison of microstructures of investment-cast and hot isostatic pressed Co-Cr-Mo alloys. (a) Cast structure consisting of a Co-Cr-Mo solid solution with large carbides. Macrograin size is ASTM 7.5. (b) Hot isostatic pressed structure featuring fine carbides and significant reduction in grain size compared to the cast structure. Micrograin size is ASTM 12–14.

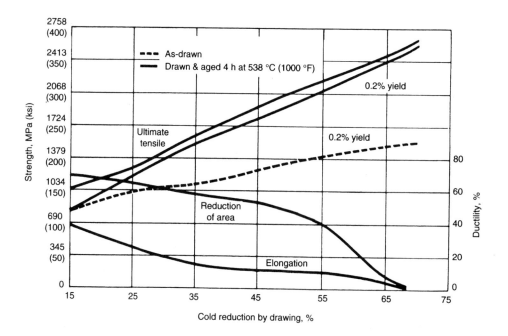

Fig. 12   Tensile properties of cold-drawn and aged ASTM F 562 (MP35N) alloy. Source: Ref 12

and cobalt-nickel-chromium alloys discussed previously are the most widely used cobalt alloys for implant applications, there are other alloys that have been rigorously tested and standardized for medical devices. Each of the alloys discussed subsequently has been shown to be innocuous for cytotoxicity, systemic toxicity, intracutaneous irritation, intramuscular implantation, skin sensitization, blood hemolysis, and pyrogenicity.

ASTM F 563 is a wrought Co-Ni-Cr-Mo-W-Fe alloy with a UNS No. of R30563 (see Table 11 for composition requirements). It is available in the form of bars, wires, and forgings. Like F 562, this alloy can be strengthened by cold working and cold working plus aging. Table 14 lists mechanical requirements for F 563.

ASTM F 1058 is a wrought Co-Cr-Ni-Mo-Fe alloy that is available in two grades, both of which are strengthened by cold working and cold working plus aging. Both grades are available in wire and strip forms. F 1058 grade 1 has a UNS No. of R30003 (see Table 11 for composition requirements). Commonly known as Elgiloy, this alloy has an elastic modulus of 190 GPa (27.5×10^6 psi), which is slightly lower

than the moduli of the cobalt implant alloys listed in Table 13. Elgiloy has been used for artificial heart springs. F 1058 grade 2 has a UNS No. of R30008 (see Table 11 for composition requirements). The chemical composition of grade 2 is in agreement with the composition limits specified in ISO 5832-7. This alloy has been used in devices for neurosurgery and vascular surgery (e.g., cartoid artery clamps). Table 15 lists mechanical requirements for cold-worked and aged F 1058 wire.

UNS R30004, commonly known as Havar, is another cobalt alloy being considered for medical implants. Available in foil and strip forms, the alloy has a nominal composition of:

Element	Content, wt%
Cobalt	42
Chromium	19.5
Nickel	12.7
Tungsten	2.7
Molybdenum	2.2
Manganese	1.6
Carbon	0.2
Iron	Bal

Havar is also strengthened by cold working and cold working and age hardening. Typical mechanical properties for this alloy are given in Table 16. There is no current ASTM standard for UNS R30004 alloy.

Table 14 Mechanical requirements for ASTM F 563 (UNS R30563) wrought products

Conditions	Ultimate tensile strength, min		Yield strength (0.2% offset), min		Elongation in 4D or 4W, min(a), %	Reduction of area, min, %
	MPa	ksi	MPa	ksi		
Fully annealed	600	87	276	40	50	65
Cold worked or cold worked and aged(b)						
Medium hard	1000	145	827	120	18	50
Hard	1310	190	1172	170	12	45
Cold worked and aged (for special purposes), extra hard	1586	230	1310	190	. . .	. . .

(a) $4D = 4 \times$ diameter; $4W = 4 \times$ width. (b) Aging in the temperature range from 400 to 550 °C (750 to 1020 °F)

Table 15 Mechanical requirements for cold-worked and aged ASTM F 1058 wire

Diameter		Ultimate tensile strength, min psi		Yield strength (0.2% offset), min	
mm	in.	MPa	ksi	MPa	ksi
0.02 to 0.12, incl	0.001 to 0.005, incl	2275	330	. . .	
Over 0.12 to 1.00, incl	Over 0.005 to 0.040, incl	2000	290	1450	210
Over 1.00 to 1.50, incl	Over 0.040 to 0.060, incl	1965	285	1380	200
Over 1.50 to 2.00, incl	Over 0.060 to 0.080, incl	1895	275	1380	200
Over 2.00 to 2.50, incl	Over 0.080 to 0.100, incl	1895	275	1345	195
Over 2.50 to 3.00, incl	Over 0.100 to 0.120, incl	1860	270	1275	185
Over 3.00 to 3.50, incl	Over 0.120 to 0.140, incl	1860	270	1240	180

Note: Wire thermally aged by heating to a temperature within the range of 480 to 540 °C (900 to 1000 °F), holding at the selected temperature within ±15 °C (±25 °F) for 5 to 5^1/$_2$ h, and cooling in air to room temperature

Titanium and Titanium-Base Alloys

Titanium is a low-density element (approximately 60% of the density of iron) that can be highly strengthened by alloying and deformation processing. Titanium and its alloys used for implant devices have been designed to have excellent biocompatibility, with little or no reaction with tissue surrounding the implant. Titanium derives it corrosion resistance from the stable oxide film that forms on its surface, which can reform at body temperatures and in physiological fluids if damaged. Increased use of titanium alloys as biomaterials is occurring due to their lower modulus (see, for example, Table 1), superior biocompatibility, and enhanced corrosion resistance when compared to more conventional stainless steels and cobalt-base alloys. These attractive properties were a driving force for the early introduction of commercially pure titanium (CP-Ti) and $\alpha + \beta$ (Ti-6Al-4V) alloys as well as for the more recent development of new titanium alloy compositions and orthopedic metastable β alloys.

Physical Metallurgy (Ref 13)

Titanium undergoes an allotropic transformation at approximately 885 °C (1625 °F), changing from a hcp crystal structure (α phase) to a bcc crystal structure (β phase). The transformation temperature (β transus—completion of transformation to β on heating) is strongly influenced by the interstitial elements oxygen, nitrogen, and carbon (α stabilizers), which raise the transformation temperature; by hydrogen (β stabilizer), which lowers the transformation temperature; and by metallic impurity or alloying elements, which may either raise or lower the transformation temperature.

Depending on their microstructure, titanium alloys fall into one of four classes: α, near-α, α-β, or β. These classes denote the general type of microstructure after processing. Most α alloys will have a minimal amount of β phase, sometimes as a result of tramp iron, as in CP-Ti, and sometimes due to minor β stabilizer additions to enhance workability (e.g., the molybdenum and vanadium additions in Ti-8Al-1Mo-1V). A near-α or super-α alloy may appear microstructurally similar to an α alloy. An α-β alloy consists of α and retained or transformed β, and commercial β alloys tend to retain the β phase on initial cooling to room temperature but precipitates secondary phases during heat treatment.

Effects of Alloying Elements. The role of the interstitial elements oxygen, nitrogen, and carbon was described previously. The substitutional alloying elements also play an important role in controlling the microstructure and properties of titanium alloys.

Tantalum, vanadium, molybdenum, and niobium are β isomorphous (i.e., have similar phase relations) with bcc titanium. Titanium does not form intermetallic compounds with the β isomorphous elements. Eutectoid systems are formed with chromium, iron, copper, nickel, palladium, cobalt, manganese, and certain other transition metals. These elements have low solubility in α titanium and decrease the transformation temperature. They usually are added to alloys in combination with one or more of the β isomorphous elements to stabilize the β phase and prevent or minimize formation of intermetallic compounds, which could occur during thermomechanical processing, heat treatment, or service at elevated temperature.

Zirconium and hafnium are unique in that they are isomorphous with both the α and β phases of titanium. Tin and aluminum have significant solubility in both α and β phases. Aluminum increases the transformation temperature significantly, whereas tin lowers it slightly. Aluminum, tin, and zirconium commonly are used together in α and near-α alloys. In α-β

Table 16   Typical mechanical and physical properties for UNS R30004 (Havar) wrought products

Condition	Ultimate tensile strength		0.2% offset yield strength		Elongation in 50 mm (2 in.), %	Hardness, HRC	Modulus of elasticity in tension	
	MPa	ksi	MPa	ksi			GPa	10⁶ psi
Annealed	965	140	483	70	40	25	203	29.5
Cold rolled	1862	270	1724	250	1	50	. . .	. . .
Cold rolled and aged	2275	330	2069	300	1	60	. . .	. . .

Source: Hamilton Precision Metals

alloys, these elements are distributed approximately equally between the α and β phases. Almost all commercial titanium alloys contain one or more of these three elements because they are soluble in both α and β phases, and particularly because they improve creep strength in the α phase.

Many more elements are soluble in β titanium than in α. Beta isomorphous alloying elements are preferred as additions because they do not form intermetallic compounds. However, iron, chromium, and other compound formers sometimes are used in β-rich α-β alloys or in β alloys, because they are strong β stabilizers and improve hardenability and response to heat treatment. Nickel, molybdenum, palladium, and ruthenium improve corrosion resistance of unalloyed titanium in certain media.

Alloy Systems (Ref 13)

There are several grades of unalloyed titanium. The primary difference between grades is oxygen and iron content. Grades of higher purity (lower interstitial content) are lower in strength, hardness, and transformation temperature than those higher in interstitial content, and have greater formability. The high solubility of the interstitial elements oxygen and nitrogen makes titanium unique among metals and also creates problems not of concern in most other metals. For example, heating titanium in air at high temperature results not only in oxidation but also in solid-solution hardening of the surface as a result of inward diffusion of oxygen (and nitrogen). A surface-hardened zone of α-case (or air contamination layer) is formed. Normally, this layer is removed by machining, chemical milling, or other mechanical means prior to placing a part in service, because the presence of α-case reduces fatigue strength and ductility.

Commercial and semicommercial titanium grades and alloys are subdivided into four groups: unalloyed (CP-Ti) grades, α and near-α alloys, α-β alloys, and β alloys. The α-β alloy Ti-6Al-4V is the most widely used titanium alloy, accounting for approximately 45% of total titanium production. Unalloyed grades comprise approximately 30% of production, and all other alloys combined comprise the remaining 25%. In terms of biomedical applications, Ti-6Al-4V and its extra-low interstitial variant (Ti-6Al-4V ELI) and CP-Ti grades are also the most widely used, although the past

decade has seen increased use of β-titanium alloys for surgical implant applications. Table 17 lists applicable ASTM standards for titanium and titanium alloys used for medical implants.

Selection of an unalloyed grade of titanium, an α or near-α alloy, an α-β alloy, or a β alloy depends on desired mechanical properties, service requirements, cost considerations, and the other factors that enter into any materials selection process.

Commercially pure titanium (98.9 to 99.6% Ti) is essentially all α titanium (hcp crystal structure), with relatively low strength and high ductility. Unalloyed titanium is selected for its excellent corrosion resistance, especially in applications where high strength is not required. Yield strengths of CP-Ti grades (Table 18) vary from 170 to 480 MPa (25 to 70 ksi) simply as a result of variations in the interstitial and impurity levels. Oxygen and iron are primary variants in these grades; strength increases with increasing oxygen and iron contents. Similarly, fatigue strengths are also increased with higher levels of oxygen (Ref 5). At 0.085% O (slightly purer than grade 1), the fatigue limit (10^7 cycles) is approximately 88.2 MPa (12.9 ksi), while at 0.27% O (close to grade 2 oxygen level), the fatigue limit is approximately 216 MPa (31 ksi).

Examples of biomedical applications for CP-Ti grades include pacemaker cases, housings for ventricular-assist devices and implantable infu-

Table 17 ASTM specifications, nominal compositions, and UNS designations for titanium and titanium alloys used for biomedical applications

ASTM specification	Alloy	UNS No.
Alpha microstructures		
F 67	CP-Ti grade 1	R50250
	CP-Ti grade 2	R50400
	CP-Ti grade 3	R50550
	CP-Ti grade 4	R50700
Alpha-beta microstructures		
F 136	Ti-6Al-4V ELI	R56401
F 1472	Ti-6Al-4V	R56400
F 1295	Ti-6Al-7Nb	R56700
F 2146	Ti-3Al-2.5V	R56320
Beta microstructures		
F 1713	Ti-13Nb-13Zr	. . .
F 1813	Ti-12Mo-6Zr-2Fe	R58120
F 2066	Ti-15Mo	R58150

sion drug pumps, dental implants, maxillofacial and craniofacial implants, and screws and staples for spinal surgery.

Alpha and Near-α Alloys. Alpha alloys that contain aluminum, tin, and/or zirconium are preferred for high-temperature as well as cryogenic applications. Alpha-rich alloys generally are more resistant to creep at high temperature than α-β or β alloys. The extra-low interstitial α alloys (ELI grades) retain ductility and toughness at cryogenic temperatures, and Ti-5Al-2.5Sn-ELI has been used extensively in such applications.

Unlike α-β and β alloys, α alloys cannot be significantly strengthened by heat treatment. Generally, α alloys are annealed or recrystallized to remove residual stresses induced by cold working. Alpha alloys have good weldability because they are insensitive to heat treatment. They generally have poorer forgeability and narrower forging temperature ranges than α-β or β alloys, particularly at temperatures below the β transus. This poorer forgeability is manifested by a greater tendency for strain-induced porosity or surface cracks to occur, which means that small reduction steps and frequent reheats must be incorporated in forging schedules.

Alpha alloys that contain small additions of β stabilizers (Ti-8Al-1Mo-1V or Ti-6Al-2Nb-1Ta-0.8Mo, for example) sometimes have been classed as super-α or near-α alloys. Although they contain some retained β phase, these alloys consist primarily of α and behave more like conventional α alloys than α-β alloys

To date, α and near-α alloys have not been used for biomedical applications. Their utility for medical devices has been limited by their low ambient temperature strength when compared to α-β or β alloys. For non-load-bearing corrosion-resistant applications, CP-Ti grades are preferred.

Alpha-beta alloys contain one or more α stabilizers or α-soluble elements plus one or more β stabilizers. These alloys retain more β phase after solution treatment than do near-α alloys, the specific amount depending on the quantity of β stabilizers present and on heat treatment.

Alpha-beta alloys can be strengthened by solution treating and aging. Solution treating usually is done at a temperature high in the two-phase α-β field and is followed by quenching in water, oil, or other suitable quenchant. As a result of quenching, the β phase present at the solution-treating temperature may be retained or may be partly, or fully, transformed during cooling by either martensitic transformation or nucleation and growth. The specific response depends on alloy composition, solution-treating temperature (β-phase composition at the solution temperature), cooling rate, and section size. Solution treatment is followed by aging, normally at 480 to 650 °C (900 to 1200 °F), to precipitate α and produce a fine mixture of α and β in the retained or transformed β phase. Transformation kinetics, transformation products, and specific response of a given alloy can be quite complex; a detailed review of the subject is beyond the scope of this chapter.

Solution treating and aging can increase the strength of α-β alloys 30 to 50%, or more, over the annealed or overaged condition. Response to solution treating and aging depends on section size; alloys relatively low in β stabilizers (Ti-6Al-4V, for example) have poor hardenability and must be quenched rapidly to achieve significant strengthening. For Ti-6Al-4V, the cooling rate of a water quench is not rapid enough to significantly harden sections thicker than approximately 25 mm (1 in.). As the content of β stabilizers increases, hardenability increases; Ti-5Al-2Sn-2Zr-4Mo-4Cr, for example, can be through hardened with relatively uniform

Table 18 Tensile properties and impurity limits for ASTM F 67 unalloyed titanium

Designation	Tensile strength (min)		0.2% yield strength (min)		Elongation, %	Impurity limits (max), wt%				
	MPa	ksi	MPa	ksi		N	C	H	Fe	O
ASTM grade 1	240	35	170	25	24	0.03	0.08	0.015	0.20	0.18
ASTM grade 2	340	50	280	40	20	0.03	0.08	0.015	0.30	0.25
ASTM grade 3	450	65	380	55	18	0.05	0.08	0.015	0.30	0.35
ASTM grade 4	550	80	480	70	15	0.05	0.08	0.015	0.50	0.40

response throughout sections up to 150 mm (6 in.) thick. For some alloys of intermediate β-stabilizer content, the surface of a relatively thick section can be strengthened, but the core may be 10 to 20% lower in hardness and strength. The strength that can be achieved by heat treatment is also a function of the volume fraction of β phase present at the solution-treating temperature. Alloy composition, solution temperature, and aging conditions must be carefully selected and balanced to produce the desired mechanical properties in the final product.

Although the ability of α-β alloys to be precipitation hardened has been studied in laboratory programs since the early days of the titanium industry, there have been relatively few production applications of solution-treated and precipitation-(age)-hardened alloys. This situation appears to be changing, because alloys such as Ti-6Al-2Sn-4Zr-6Mo, Ti-5Al-2Sn-2Zr-4Mo-4Cr, and certain high-hardenability β alloys have been developed specifically to be age hardened for improved strength—approximately 30 to 40% above that of annealed alloys.

As shown in Table 17, there are four ASTM standardized α-β alloys currently used for medical devices. Ti-6Al-4V and Ti-6Al-4V ELI are the most commonly employed alloys. They are widely used for total joint replacement arthroplasty (primarily hips and knees, as shown in Fig. 2). Ti-6Al-7Nb and Ti-5Al-2.5Fe (not currently standardized by ASTM) are metallurgically quite similar to Ti-6Al-4V, except for the absence of vanadium. As shown in Fig. 5, vanadium is considered a toxic element in terms of its biocompatibility. Ti-6Al-7Nb has been used for femoral hip stems, fracture fixation plates, spinal components, fasteners, nails, rods, screws, and wire. Ti-3Al-2.5V is known for its excellent cold formability. Its tensile properties are 20 to 50% higher than CP-Ti grades. It is used for tubing and intramedullary nails. Table 19 lists the elastic moduli and tensile properties of α-β alloys used for medical devices.

Beta alloys are richer in β stabilizers and leaner in α stabilizers than α-β alloys. They are characterized by high hardenability, with β phase completely retained on air cooling of thin sections or water quenching of thick sections. Beta alloys have excellent forgeability, cold-rolling capabilities, and in sheet form can be cold brake-formed more readily than high-strength α-β or α alloys. It is more difficult to perform more complex triaxial-strain-type forming operations with β alloys because they exhibit almost no work hardening, and necking occurs early. After solution treating, β alloys are aged at temperatures of 450 to 650 °C (850 to 1200 °F) to partially transform the β phase to α. The α forms as finely dispersed particles in the retained β, and strength levels comparable or superior to those of aged α-β alloys can be attained. The chief disadvantages of β alloys in comparison with α-β alloys are higher density, lower creep strength, and lower tensile ductility in the aged condition. Although tensile ductility

Table 19 Properties of titanium alloys developed for orthopedic implants

Alloy designation	Elastic modulus		0.2% yield strength		Ultimate tensile strength (min)		Elongation, %
	GPa	10⁶ psi	MPa	ksi	MPa	ksi	
Alpha-beta alloys							
Ti-6Al-4V	110	16	860	125	930	135	10–15
Ti-6Al-7Nb	105	15.2	795	115	860	125	10
Ti-5Al-2.5Fe	110	16	820	119	900	130	6
Ti-3Al-2.5V	100	14.5	585	85	690	100	15
Beta alloys							
Ti-13Nb-13Zr	79–84	11.5–12.2	836–908	121–132	973–1037	141–150	10–16
Ti-12Mo-6Zr-2Fe (TMZF)	74–85	10.7–12.3	1000–1060	145–154	1060–1100	154–160	18–22
Ti-15Mo	78	11.3	655	95	795	115	22
Ti-15Mo-5Zr-3Al	75–88	10.9–12.8	870–968	126–140	882–975	128–141	17–20
Ti-15Mo-2.8Nb-0.2Si-0.260 (21SRx)	83	12.0	945–987	137–143	979–999	142–145	16–18
Ti-16Nb-10Hf	81	11.7	736	107	851	123	10
Ti-35.5Nb-7.3Zr-5.7Ta (TNZT)	55–66	7.9–9.6	793	115	827	120	20

Source: Ref 14 and product literature from Stryker Howmedica Osteonics and Allvac, an Allegheny Technologies Company

is lower, the fracture toughness of an aged β alloy generally is higher than that of an aged α-β alloy of comparable yield strength.

In the solution-treated condition (100% retained β), β alloys have good ductility and toughness, relatively low strength, and excellent formability. Solution-treated β alloys begin to precipitate α phase at slightly elevated temperatures and thus are unsuitable for elevated-temperature service without prior stabilization or overaging treatment.

Beta alloys (at least commercial β alloys), despite the name, actually are metastable, because cold work at ambient temperature can induce a martensitic transformation, or heating to a slightly elevated temperature can cause partial transformation to α or other transformation products. The principal advantages of β alloys are that they have high hardenability, excellent forgeability, and good cold formability in the solution-treated condition.

The 1990s witnessed considerable advances in the development of β alloys for orthopedic implant applications similar to those listed previously for α-β alloys. The β alloys offer lower elastic moduli and enhanced biocompatibility when compared to Ti-6Al-4V and other α-β alloys. The principal alloying elements in these alloys are niobium, zirconium, molybdenum, tantalum, and iron, all of which exhibit good-to-excellent biocompatibility (Fig. 5). In addition, they are vanadium-free alloys (vanadium has been reported to be toxic and to show adverse tissue effects). Table 19 lists the elastic moduli and tensile properties of various β alloys used for medical devices. The most recently synthesized alloys are based on the Ti-Nb-Zr-Ta system (TNZT alloys). These alloys offer the lowest elastic moduli of any metallic implant alloy developed to date. Table 20 compares the elastic modulus values for a variety of natural and synthetic joint materials.

Fatigue Properties (Ref 14). Ti-6Al-4V is generally considered as a standard material when evaluating the fatigue resistance of orthopedic titanium alloys. The mechanical response of Ti-6Al-4V is extremely sensitive to prior thermomechanical processing history (Ref 14). The prior-β grain size, the ratio of primary α to transformed β, the α grain size, and the α-β morphologies all impact performance, particularly high-cycle fatigue. Another important consideration is the sensitivity of titanium alloy fatigue properties to surface condition, which is

associated with their high notch sensitivity. Rotating bending fatigue (RBF) strength is reduced by 40% with notched samples (Ref 14). For biomedical applications, the notch sensitivity of Ti-6Al-4V is a critical factor in the performance of porous coated implants. Porous coated hip stems show a large reduction in the fatigue limit as compared to the smooth condition (see Chapter 9, "Coatings," in this handbook for a discussion on the effects of porous coatings on fatigue properties).

Table 21 compares the smooth fatigue strength of CP-Ti, α-β, and β-titanium alloys as well as Co-Cr-Mo alloys and type 316L stainless steel. The smooth fatigue resistance of β-titanium alloys is generally lower when compared to α-β alloys on an equivalent yield strength basis. However, the lower stress-controlled smooth fatigue limit of β alloys may not be an appropriate characterization for orthopedic applications, where notch fatigue behavior, more closely associated with strain-controlled fatigue, may be more representative of in vivo conditions. For example, hip stems rarely have a smooth surface but are typically structured with wedges and coatings, creating stress-concentration sites. When considering the fatigue strain, that is, the ratio between fatigue stress and elastic modulus (Fig. 13), the strain-controlled fatigue behavior of certain β alloys is comparable to that of α-β Ti-6Al-4V alloy. In fact, a smaller reduction in fatigue limit occasioned by the introduction of notches is typi-

Table 20 Elastic modulus values for natural and synthetic joint materials

Joint material	Elastic modulus	
	GPa	10^6 psi
Articular cartilage	0.001–0.17	0.000145–0.0247
PTFE	0.5	0.07
UHMWPE	0.5	0.07
Bone cement (PMMA)	3.0	0.44
Bone	10–30	1.45–4.35
TNZT alloys	55–66	7.9–9.6
"New generation" β-Ti alloys	74–85	10.7–12.3
Ti-6Al-4V alloy	110	16
Zirconia	200	29
Stainless steel	205	30
Co-Cr-Mo alloy	230	33
Alumina	350	51

PTFE, polytetrafluoroethylene; UHMWPE, ultrahigh molecular weight polyethylene; PMMA, polymethyl methacrylate; TNZT, titanium-niobium-zirconium-tantalum. Source: Ref 14

cally observed in Ti-13Nb-13Zr and TMZF β alloys when compared to Ti-6Al-4V (Table 22).

The friction and wear properties of titanium are quite different from those of most other metals (Ref 2). This is the result of its tenacious oxide (passive) film. The film will remain intact under low loads and slow sliding speeds in articulating conditions. However, if the film is worn away and not regenerated promptly, galling will cause metal-to-metal contact and cold welding. This process leads to very high friction and wear rates; consequently, titanium-to-titanium (or to other metal) articulating joints are not used. Methods such as physical vapor deposition coating (TiN, TiC), ion implantation (N^+), thermal treatments (nitriding and oxygen diffusion hardening), and laser alloying with TiC have been examined for improving wear (Ref 14). Ion implantation has been the most common treatment employed (see Chapter 9, "Coatings," in this handbook for further details).

Table 21 Smooth (unnotched) fatigue strength of orthopedic implant alloys

Alloy designation	Test conditions(a)	Fatigue limit(b)		Fatigue limit/yield strength
		MPa	ksi	
CP-Ti	RBF($R = -1$/100 Hz)	430	62	0.6
Ti-6Al-4V	Axial ($R = -1$/292 Hz)	500	73	0.6
	Axial ($R = 0.1$/292 Hz)	330	48	0.4
	RBF ($R = -1$/60 Hz)	610	88	0.7
Ti-6Al-7Nb	RBF ($R = -1$)	500–600	73–87	0.7
Ti-5Al-2.5Fe	RBF ($R = -1$)	580	84	0.8
Ti-15Mo-5Zr-3Al (aged β + α condition)	RBF ($R = -1$/100 Hz)	560–640	81–93	0.5
Ti-13Nb-13Zr	Axial ($R = 0.1$/60 Hz)	500	73	0.6
Ti-12Mo-6Zr-2Fe (TMZF)	RBF ($R = -1$/167 Hz)	525	76	0.5
Ti-15Mo-3Nb-0.3O (21SRx)	RBF ($R = -1$/60 Hz)	490	71	0.5
TNZT	RBF ($R = -1$/60 Hz)	265	38	0.5
TNZT-0.4O	RBF ($R = -1$/60 Hz)	450	65	0.5
SS 316L	RBF ($R = -1$/100 Hz)	440	64	0.6
Co-Cr-Mo	RBF ($R = -1$)	400–500	58–73	0.4–0.5
	RBF ($R = -1$/100 Hz)	500–580	73–84	. . .

(a) RBF, rotating bending fatigue. (b) Fatigue limit at 10^7 cycles. Source: Ref 14

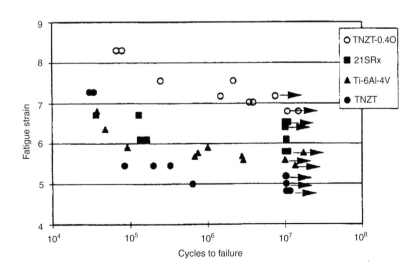

Fig. 13 Total strain-controlled (rotating bending fatigue, $R = -1$, 60 Hz) fatigue response for α-β (Ti-6Al-4V) and β alloys. Source: Ref 14

The wear properties of titanium probably prevent its more widespread use in orthopedic prostheses (Ref 2). For the most part, however, titanium is not articulated against other metallic materials or itself but is used for components of modular construction where a titanium femoral stem will be used with a cobalt-chromium or a ceramic ball to articulate against a UHMWPE liner (e.g., in a total hip replacement).

Hip simulator testing has shown that wear rates for UHMWPE mated against Ti-6Al-4V are 35% greater than that for Co-Cr-Mo alloy. Like the metal-to-metal wear described previously, the high UHMWPE wear rates associated with titanium alloy counterparts have been related to the mechanical instability of the metal oxide layer (Ref 14). It has been proposed that when normal or shear stresses are high enough to induce breakdown of the surface passive layer, the oxide will be disrupted. The exposed metal surface layer may then either reform a passive layer or adhesively bond (cold weld) to the polymer surface. The latter situation leads to continuous removal (material disruption) and reformation (oxidation) of the passivating layer and results in gradual consumption of alloy material. Concurrently, the surface roughness of the metal surface will increase, which results in yet higher UHMWPE wear. Ultimately, the breakdown of the oxide layer creates the potential for abrasive wear, where the hard oxide debris acts as third-body abrasive components (Fig. 14).

Wear of joint prosthesis materials unavoidably represents a long-term limitation to the lifetime of a total joint replacement, because the accumulation of UHMWPE and, to a lesser extent, metal or ceramic wear debris has been associated with incidence of nonspecific pain and prosthesis loosening (Ref 14). The former is a result of adverse tissue reaction, while the latter is a result of adverse reaction to wear debris of the implant/bone fixation. There is, therefore, an increasing concern over the long-term use of UHMWPE, underscored by recent recognition

Table 22 Notch fatigue strength of orthopedic titanium alloys

Alloy designation	Smooth fatigue limit(a) MPa	Smooth fatigue limit(a) ksi	Notch fatigue limit(a) MPa	Notch fatigue limit(a) ksi	K_f(b)	$K_{\text{Ti-6Al-4V}}$(c)
Ti-6Al-4V	500	73	290 ($K_f = 3.3$)	42 ($K_f = 33$)	0.6	. . .
Ti-5Al-2.5 Fe	580	84	300 ($K_f = 3.6$)	44 ($K_f = 3.6$)	0.5	. . .
Ti-15Mo-5Zr-3Al (aged)	560–640	81–93	190 ($K_f = 2.8$)	28 ($K_f = 2.8$)	0.3	1.0
Ti-13Nb-13Zr	500	73	335 ($K_f = 1.6$)	49 ($K_f = 1.6$)	0.7	1.0
			215 ($K_f = 3.0$)	31 ($K_f = 3.0$)	0.4	1.3
Ti-12Mo-6Zr-2Fe	525	76	410 ($K_f = 1.6$)	59 ($K_f = 1.6$)	0.8	1.4

(a) At 10^7 cycles. (b) K_f is a fatigue strength reduction factor defined as fatigue limit (notch)/fatigue limit (smooth control) under same test conditions. (c) $K_{\text{Ti-6Al-4V}}$ is a fatigue strength factor relative to Ti-6Al-4V defined as fatigue limit (alloy)/fatigue limit (Ti-6Al-4V) under same test conditions. Source: Ref 14

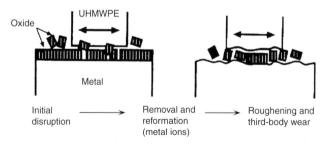

Fig. 14 Schematic illustration of the suggested oxidative/abrasive wear process during articulation of Ti-6Al-4V on ultrahigh molecular weight polyethylene (UHMWPE). Source: Ref 14

of the nonuniformity (variable molecular weight, or MW, and MW distribution, processing and fabrication history) of the material, reports of the possible harmful effects of UHMWPE sterilization, and the interaction of UHMWPE wear debris with the body fluids and tissues (Ref 14).

Comparison of Orthopedic Implant Materials

Thus far in this chapter, the three primary metallic material groups used for orthopedic implant devices have been reviewed—austenitic stainless steels, cobalt-base alloys, and titanium and titanium alloys. Each of these metallic alloys has distinct advantages and disadvantages. Table 23 compares some of the characteristics of these alloys. Additional comparative information pertaining to elastic moduli for these and other materials can be found in Tables 1 and 20.

Shape Memory Alloys (Ref 15)

The term *shape memory alloys* (SMA) is applied to that group of metallic materials that demonstrates the ability to return to some previously defined shape or size when subjected to the appropriate thermal procedure. Generally,

these materials can be plastically deformed at some relatively low temperature and, on exposure to some higher temperature, will return to their shape prior to the deformation. Materials that exhibit shape memory only on heating are referred to as having a one-way shape memory. Some materials also undergo a change in shape on recooling. These materials have a two-way shape memory.

Although a relatively wide variety of alloys is known to exhibit the shape memory effect, only those that can recover substantial amounts of strain or that generate significant force on changing shape are of commercial interest. To date, this has been the NiTi alloys and copper-base alloys such as Cu-Zn-Al and Cu-Al-Ni. Of these, only NiTi alloys have been used for biomedical devices.

A shape memory alloy is further defined as an alloy that yields a thermoelastic martensite. In this case, the alloy undergoes a martensitic transformation of a type that allows the alloy to be deformed by a twinning mechanism below the transformation temperature. The deformation is then reversed when the twinned structure reverts on heating to the parent phase.

General Characteristics

The martensitic transformation that occurs in the shape memory alloys yields a thermoelastic

Table 23 Comparison of some of the characteristics of orthopedic metallic implant materials

	Stainless steels	Cobalt-base alloys	Ti and Ti-base alloys
Designation	ASTM F 138 (type 316LVM)	ASTM F 75 ASTM F 799 ASTM F 562 (Cast and wrought)	ASTM F 67 ASTM F 136 ASTM F 1295 (Cast and wrought)
Principal alloying elements (wt%)	Fe (bal) Cr (17–20) Ni (12–14) Mo (2–4)	Co (bal) Cr (19–30) Mo (0–10) Ni (0–37)	Ti (bal) Al (6) V (4) Nb (7)
Advantages	Cost, availability, processing	Wear resistance, corrosion resistance, fatigue strength	Biocompatibility, corrosion, minimum modulus, fatigue strength
Disadvantages	Long-term behavior, high modulus	High modulus, biocompatibility	Lower wear resistance, low shear strength
Primary uses	Temporary devices (fracture plates, screws, hip nails); used for THR stems in United Kingdom (nitrogen-strengthened stainless steels)	Dentistry castings, prostheses stems, load-bearing components in TJR (wrought alloys)	Used in THRs with modular (Co-Cr-Mo or ceramic) femoral heads; long-term, permanent devices (nails, pacemakers)

THR, total hip replacement; TJR, total joint replacement. Source: Ref 14

martensite and develops from a high-temperature austenite phase with long-range order. The martensite typically occurs as alternately sheared platelets, which are seen as a herringbone structure when viewed metallographically. The transformation, although a first-order phase change, does not occur at a single temperature but over a range of temperatures that varies with each alloy system. The usual way of characterizing the transformation and naming each point in the cycle is shown in Fig. 15. Most of the transformation occurs over a relatively narrow temperature range, although the beginning and end of the transformation during heating or cooling actually extends over a much larger temperature range. The transformation also exhibits hysteresis in that the transformation on heating and on cooling does not overlap (Fig. 15). This transformation hysteresis (shown as T in Fig. 15) varies with the alloy system.

Nickel-Titanium Alloys

The basis of the nickel-titanium system of alloys is the binary, equiatomic (49 to 51 at. % Ni) intermetallic compound of NiTi. This intermetallic compound is extraordinary because it has a moderate solubility range for excess nickel or titanium, as well as most other metallic elements, and it also exhibits a ductility comparable to most ordinary alloys. This solubility allows alloying with many of the elements to modify both the mechanical properties and the transformation properties of the system. Excess nickel, in amounts up to approximately 1%, is the most common alloying addition. Excess nickel strongly depresses the transformation temperature and increases the yield strength of the austenite. Other frequently used elements are iron and chromium (to lower the transformation temperature) and copper (to decrease the hysteresis and lower the deformation stress of the martensite). Because common contaminants such as oxygen and carbon can also shift the transformation temperature and degrade the mechanical properties, it is also desirable to minimize the amount of these elements.

Properties. Table 24 shows the major physical properties of the basic binary nickel-titanium system and some of the mechanical properties of the alloy in the annealed condition. Note that this is for the equiatomic alloy with an A_f value of approximately 110 °C (230 °F). Selective work hardening, which can exceed 50% reduction in some cases, and proper heat treatment can greatly improve the ease with which the martensite is deformed, give an austenite with much greater strength, and create material that spontaneously moves itself both on heating and on cooling (two-way shape memory). One of the biggest challenges in using this family of alloys is in developing the proper processing procedures to yield the properties desired.

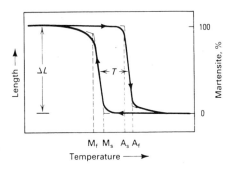

Fig. 15 Typical transformation versus temperature curve for a shape memory alloy specimen under constant load (stress) as it is cooled and heated. T transformation hysteresis. M_s, martensite start; M_f, martensite finish; A_s, austenite start; A_f, austenite finish

Table 24 Properties of binary nickel-titanium shape memory alloys

Properties	Property value
Melting temperatures, °C (°F)	1300 (2370)
Density, g/cm³ (lb/in.³)	6.45 (0.233)
Resistivity, Ω · cm	
Austenite	~100
Martensite	~70
Thermal conductivity, W/m · °C	
(Btu/ft · h · °F)	
Austenite	18 (10)
Martensite	8.5 (4.9)
Corrosion resistance	Similar to 300-series stainless steel or titanium alloys
Young's modulus, GPa (10^6 psi)	
Austenite	~83 (~12)
Martensite	~28–41 (~4–6)
Yield strength, MPa (ksi)	
Austenite	195–690 (28–100)
Martensite	70–140 (10–20)
Ultimate tensile strength, MPa (ksi)	895 (130)
Transformation temperatures, °C (°F)	–200 to 110 (–325 to 230)
Hysteresis, Δ°C (Δ°F)	~30(~55)
Latent heat of transformation, kJ/kg · atom (cal/g · atom)	167 (40)
Shape memory strain	8.5% max

Processing. Because of the reactivity of the titanium in these alloys, all melting of them must be done in a vacuum or an inert atmosphere. Methods such as plasma arc melting, electron beam melting, and vacuum induction melting are all used commercially. After ingots are melted, standard hot-forming processes such as forging, bar rolling, and extrusion can be used for initial breakdown. The alloys react slowly with air, so hot working in air is quite successful. Most cold-working processes can also be applied to these alloys, but they work harden extremely rapidly, and frequent annealing is required. Wire drawing is probably the most widely used of the techniques, and excellent surface properties and sizes as small as 0.05 mm (0.002 in.) are made routinely.

Heat treating to impart the desired memory shape is often done at 500 to 800 °C (950 to 1450 °F), but it can be done as low as 300 to 350 °C (600 to 650 °F) if sufficient time is allowed. The SMA component may need to be restrained in the desired memory shape during the heat treatment; otherwise, it may not remain there.

Applications. To illustrate the application of NiTi SMAs, consider osteosynthesis plates. These are attached to a bone to stabilize a fracture and promote healing. The plate is produced in its desired final geometry using a NiTi SMA, then is stretched 8% and cooled. Screw attachment holes are drilled without heating the plate. Then, the plate is attached to the patient's fractured bone. A local heat source (warm water or hot air) is applied to raise the temperature to above the transition temperature; the plate reverts to its original dimensions, contracting and pulling the fractured surfaces together.

Other current biomedical applications for NiTi alloys include:

- Medical staples. Like bone plates, compression staples are used to set broken bones and promote healing. They are implanted directly into the area of the break to compress the two parts of the bone.
- Blood-clot (Cava) filters (NiTi wire is shaped to anchor itself in a vein and catch passing clots.)
- Vascular stents to reinforce blood vessels
- Orthodontic wires (for braces) and endodontic instruments (see Chapter 10, "Biomaterials for Dental Applications," in this handbook for details)

Potential applications for NiTi alloys include hip prostheses, anterior cruciate ligament prostheses, and endoprotheses. More detailed information on these applications can be found in Ref 16.

Applicable standards for NiTi alloys include:

- ASTM F 2063, which covers processing and properties of wrought NiTi alloys (bar, wire, flat-rolled products, and tubing)
- ASTM F 2005, which covers standard terminology associated with shape memory alloys
- ASTM F 2082, which covers the determination of the transformation temperature of NiTi alloys by bend and free recovery
- ASTM F 2004, which covers the determination of the transformation temperature of NiTi alloys by thermal analysis

Other Metallic Materials Used for Medical Devices

Tantalum belongs to a group of metals commonly referred to as refractory metals. In addition to tantalum, the refractory metals consist of niobium, molybdenum, tungsten, and rhenium. With the exception of two of the platinum-group metals (osmium and iridium), the refractory metals have the highest melting temperatures (>2000 °C, or 3630 °F) and the lowest vapor pressures of all metals. The use of niobium, molybdenum, and tungsten for biomedical applications is largely confined to their use as an alloying element in stainless steels, cobalt-base alloys, and titanium alloys. There are no current applications for rhenium in the medical device field. Tantalum is also used as an alloying additive in titanium alloys, but commercially pure (unalloyed) tantalum (99.90% Ta, minimum) is also fabricated into a variety of medical devices.

Tantalum has excellent resistance to corrosion by a large number of acids, by most aqueous solutions of salts, by organic chemicals, and by various combinations and mixtures of these agents. The corrosion resistance of tantalum is approximately the same as glass, but offers the intrinsic fabrication advantages of a metal. As shown in Fig. 5, tantalum is among the most biocompatible metals used for implantable devices.

The chemical requirements for surgical implant applications of tantalum and the average impurity limits for commercially available tantalum are listed in Table 25. Elastic modulus ranges and tensile properties for annealed and cold-worked unalloyed tantalum are given in Table 26.

Tantalum implants have been used successfully in general surgery and neurosurgery as monofilament and braided suture wires for skin closure, tendon, and nerve repair; as foils and sheets for nerve anastomoses; clips for the ligation of vessels; staples for abdominal surgery; and as pliable sheets and plates for cranioplasty and reconstructive surgery. Sintered tantalum capacitor electrodes are also in electrical stimulation devices.

Tantalum is also used to coat carbon foam skeletons used as a biocompatible replacement for the vertebral bodies that make up the spinal column. These coatings, which are 70 to 80%

porous, have the appearance of cancellous bone. In addition to spinal implants, carbon-tantalum cellular materials are being considered for hip and knee construction and bone scaffold void-filling applications.

Zirconium Alloys. Zirconium is similar to titanium in that it is considered a reactive metal; that is, it has a high affinity for oxygen. When zirconium is exposed to an oxygen-containing environment, an adherent, protective oxide film forms on its surface. This film is formed spontaneously in air or water at ambient temperature and below. Moreover, this film is self-healing and protects the base metal from chemical attack at temperatures up to 300 °C (570 °F). As a result, zirconium is very resistant to corrosive attack in most mineral and organic acids, strong alkalies, and saline solutions. As shown in Fig. 5, zirconium exhibits the highest biocompatibility of all metals.

In terms of its use in biomedical applications, zirconium has largely been used as an alloying additive in β-titanium alloys (Table 19). Recently, however, a zirconium alloy knee implant with a hard ceramic (zirconium oxide) surface has been developed (Ref 17). The zirconium alloy is Zr-2.5Nb, with small additions of oxygen for increased strength. The ceramic coating is developed through heating at 500 °C (930 °F). At that temperature, the zirconium reacts with oxygen to produce zirconium oxide, or zirconia. The ceramic zone extends approximately 5 μm deep. Underneath the ceramic, the material gradually transitions from the ceramic into zirconium metal through another several micrometers. The Zr-2.5Nb alloy has a relatively low modulus of 100 GPa (14.5×10^6 psi).

Metals for Medical Electrodes. An important and challenging medical use of implanted electrodes is in prosthetic devices for neural control (Ref 18). These devices employ metal electrodes to transmit the current required for electrical stimulation of appropriate areas of the nervous system. Neural prostheses for direct control of peripheral organs include the cardiac pacemaker, the phrenic stimulator for respiratory control, and the spinal cord stimulators for bladder control. More complex neural-control devices are auditory prostheses for the sensory deaf, experimental visual prostheses for the blind, and neuromuscular prostheses for restoration of hand, arm, or leg function in paralyzed individuals.

Table 25 Chemical requirements for unalloyed tantalum in accordance with ASTM F 560

	Compositions, maximum weight percent allowed	
Element	UNS R05200(a)	UNS R05400(b)
Carbon	0.010	0.010
Oxygen	0.0150	0.030
Nitrogen	0.010	0.010
Hydrogen	0.0015	0.0015
Niobium	0.100	0.100
Iron	0.010	0.010
Titanium	0.010	0.010
Tungsten	0.05	0.05
Molybdenum	0.020	0.020
Silicon	0.0050	0.0050
Nickel	0.010	0.010
Tantalum	Bal	Bal

(a) Electron beam or vacuum arc cast tantalum. (b) Sintered tantalum

Table 26 Elastic modulus range and tensile properties for unalloyed tantalum

	Condition	
Property	Annealed	Cold worked
Hardness, HV	80–110	120–300
Elastic modulus, GPa (10^6 psi)	186–191 (27–28)	
Yield strength, MPa (ksi)	140 (20)	345 (50)
Tensile strength, MPa (ksi)	205 (30)	480 (70)
Elongation, %	20–30	1–25

The most frequently considered metals for electrical stimulation are the so-called noble or precious metals: platinum, iridium, rhodium, gold, and palladium. This is because of their resistance to chemical and electrochemical corrosion. However, all of these metals show corrosion effects during both in vitro and in vivo electrical stimulation. Corrosion effects include weight loss, formation of unstable surface films that tend to spall from the surface, and dissolution of metal (Ref 18). Of the noble metals mentioned previously, platinum and platinum-iridium alloys containing 10 to 30% Ir are the most widely used for electrical stimulation. Metal oxides such as iridium oxide have also shown promise.

Some nonnoble metals are candidates for electrode applications requiring high mechanical strength and fatigue resistance such as demanded of intramuscular electrodes. These include (Ref 18):

- Vacuum melted type 316L stainless steel
- Cobalt alloys Elgiloy and MP35N
- Pure metals zirconium, tungsten, tantalum, and titanium
- Tungsten bronzes made by powder metallurgy processing

Silver. Silver salts, complexes, and the metal itself have played an important part in the development of medicine. Interest in the use of silver is being renewed in a wide variety of biomedical applications, where it can prevent the growth of microorganisms responsible for disease (Ref 19).

Metallic silver is used in a number of surgical applications, both for structural devices (e.g., cranial support plates, suture wire, aneurysm clips, and tracheostomy tubes) and for prostheses (e.g., silicon-silver penile implants). The antimicrobial properties of silver are used in the form of silver salts and complexes that break down to release silver ions (Ag^+). As described in Chapter 9, "Coatings," in this handbook, antimicrobial silver ions can also be incorporated into polymeric coatings.

REFERENCES

1. N. Niinomi, Recent Titanium R&D for Biological Applications in Japan, *JOM,* June 1999, p 32–34

2. M. Donachie, Biomaterials, *Metals Handbook Desk Edition,* 2nd ed., J.R. Davis, Ed., ASM International, 1998, p 702–709

3. C.M. Agrawal, Reconstructing the Human Body Using Biomaterials, *JOM,* Jan 1998, p 31–35

4. E.J. Sutow, Iron-Based Alloys, *Concise Encyclopedia of Medical & Dental Materials,* D. Williams, Ed., Pergamon Press and The MIT Press, 1990, p 232–240

5. J.B. Brunski, Metals, *Biomaterials Science: An Introduction to Materials in Medicine,* B.D. Ratner, A.S. Hoffman, F.J. Schoen, and J.E. Lemons, Ed., Academic Press, 1996, p 37–50

6. P. Harvey, Ed., *Engineering Properties of Steel,* American Society for Metals, 1982, p 298

7. R.H. Shetty, L.N. Gilbertson, and C.H. Jacobs, The 22-13-5 Stainless Steel—An Alternative to Hot Forged 316L Stainless Steel in Fracture Fixation, *Trans. Ortho. Res. Soc.,* Vol 10, 1985, p 246

8. R.C. Gebeau and R.S. Brown, Tech Spotlight: Biomedical Implant Alloy, *Adv. Mater. Process.,* Sept 2001, p 46–48

9. R.A. Horton, Investment Casting, *Casting,* Vol 15, *Metals Handbook,* 9th ed., ASM International, 1988, p 253–269

10. A.M. Weinstein and A.J.T. Clemow, Cobalt-Based Alloys, *Concise Encyclopedia of Medical & Dental Materials,* D. Williams, Ed., Pergamon Press and The MIT Press, 1990, p 106–112

11. J.J. Conway and F.J. Rizzo, Hot Isostatic Pressing of Metal Powder, *Powder Metal Technologies and Applications,* Vol 7, *ASM Handbook,* ASM International, 1998, p 605–620

12. Cobalt-Base Alloys, *ASM Specialty Handbook: Nickel and Cobalt and Their Alloys,* J.R. Davis, Ed., ASM International, 2000, p 362–370

13. R. Boyer, Titanium and Titanium Alloys, *Metals Handbook Desk Edition,* 2nd ed., J.R. Davis, Ed., ASM International, 1998, p 575–588

14. M. Long and H.J. Rack, Titanium Alloys in Total Joint Replacement—A Materials Science Perspective, *Biomaterials,* Vol 19, 1998, p 1621–1639

15. Shape Memory Alloys, *Metals Handbook Desk Edition,* 2nd ed., J.R. Davis, Ed., ASM International, 1998, p 668–669

16. D. Mantovani, Shape Memory Alloys: Properties and Biomedical Applications, *JOM,* Oct 2000, p 36–44

17. Medical Materials, *Adv. Mater. Process.,* Sept 2002, p 24–27

18. L.S. Robblee and S.F. Cogan, Metals for Medical Electrodes, *Concise Encyclopedia of Medical & Dental Materials,* D. Williams, Ed., Pergamon Press and The MIT Press, 1990, p 245–251

19. G.J. Grashoff and R.O. King, Silver in Medical Applications, *Concise Encyclopedia of Medical & Dental Materials,* D. Williams, Ed., Pergamon Press and The MIT Press, 1990, p 321–326

SELECTED REFERENCES

- R. Boyer, G. Welsch, E.W. Collings, and S. Lampman, Ed., *Materials Properties Handbook: Titanium Alloys,* ASM International, 1994

- J.R. Davis Ed., *ASM Specialty Handbook: Nickel, Cobalt, and Their Alloys,* ASM International, 2000

- J.R. Davis, Ed., *ASM Specialty Handbook: Stainless Steels,* ASM International, 1994

- J.R. Davis, Ed., *Metals Handbook Desk Edition,* 2nd ed., ASM International, 1998

CHAPTER 4

Corrosion of Metallic Implants and Prosthetic Devices

THE NEED TO ENSURE MINIMAL COR-ROSION has been a major determining factor in the selection of materials for use in the body environment. The first requirement for any material—whether a metal/alloy, ceramic, or polymer—to be placed in the body is that it should be biocompatible and not cause any adverse reaction in the body. The material must withstand the body environment and not degrade to the point that it cannot function in the body as intended. For example, metals used in the cardiovascular system must be nonthrombogenic, and, in general, the more electronegative the metal with respect to blood, the less thrombogenic the metal will be. Cobalt-chromium alloys of the HS-21 and HS-25 compositions (ASTM F 75 and F 90, respectively) and titanium are used in heart valves. Design also is an important factor in preventing thrombus formation. Corrosion is included in the topic of biocompatibility because it is an important factor in the release of metal ions into the body environment and in the degradation of the implant metal. In vitro electrochemical measurements can be conducted in controlled environments, and these techniques provide methods of determining the basic corrosion reactions necessary for predicting the corrosion behavior of materials and for screening and characterizing materials intended for use in surgical applications.

This chapter discusses the corrosion of metallic materials. Historical background information is given on the metals used in prosthetic devices, biocompatibility, significance of corrosion, and standards. This is followed by discussions of electrochemistry and corrosion processes, the types of corrosion to be expected, and the test methods used to evaluate the corrosion behavior of surgical implant metals. Information on specific materials and on corrosion processes is provided in the references cited in this chapter.

Historical Background

The earliest attempts at repairing the human body probably went unrecorded. There are a number of historical accounts of the development of the use of metals in the human body (Ref 1–5). The first record of metal implantation discusses the repair of a cleft palate with a gold plate by Petronius in 1565 (Ref 1, 3). Approximately 100 years later, Hieronymus Fabricius described the use of gold, iron, and bronze wires for sutures. In 1775, arguments arose between Pujol, a surgeon opposing internal fixation, and Icart, a surgeon who favored internal fixation and used brass wires (Ref 1, 3, 6). Icart encountered problems with infection but cited the work of two French surgeons, Lapeyode and Sicre, who had successfully used wire to repair bone fractures. In 1886, Hansmann used metal plates for internal fixation (Ref 7). These plates, which were nickel-plated steel, had holes through which screws were inserted into the bone. Some had a bend at one end and protruded through the skin for ease of removal. X-rays were discovered by Roentgen in 1895. The use of x-rays to observe the healing of fractures revealed the advantages of internal fixation and stimulated its use.

It was difficult in early times to determine whether the infection and inflammation were due to the metal or to other factors. The development of aseptic techniques by Baron Joseph

Lister in the 1860s made it possible to determine the most suitable metals for use as implants (Ref 1, 8). As the success of surgery increased, it became clear that the metals were an important limiting factor. The metals tested for implant use included platinum, gold, silver, lead, zinc, aluminum, copper, and magnesium (Ref 1); all of these were found to be too malleable. Magnesium was found to be highly reactive in the body. Steel plates coated with gold or nickel came into use. The need for strong and corrosion-resistant metals became apparent. Stainless steels were introduced as implants in 1926, and Co-Cr-Mo-C alloys were first used in 1936 (Ref 2). Titanium was determined to be inert in the body (Ref 9, 10); titanium and titanium alloys were not introduced until the 1960s and came into increased use in the 1970s. Tantalum, which was studied in the early 1950s, does show some tissue reaction (Ref 11, 12).

Observations eventually led to the discovery of electrochemical reactions in the body in the 1930s. Steel screws in a magnesium plate produced the dramatic result of having the magnesium plate disappear before the fracture healed. The combination of copper with zinc was found to be highly reactive, as was the combination of brass screws with an aluminum plate. Surgeons and scientists began to believe that homogeneous metals should be used to prevent these reactions. At this time, many scientists were beginning to notice electrochemical reactions with surgical implants; one of the first actual measurements of an electrode potential difference between uncorroded and corroded areas of screws was made by F. Masmonteil (Ref 13). C.S. Venable, W.P. Stuck, and A. Beach are responsible for bringing electrolytic effects to the attention of surgeons and scientists in the United States (Ref 14). This interest in and discovery of electrochemical effects with surgical implants in the 1930s occurred more than 140 years after Italian physician Luigi Galvani published his electrochemical discoveries (Ref 15). Electrochemistry was already a well-established science. A. Volta showed that the electricity was generated by the contact of dissimilar metals, not from "animal electricity," as stated by Galvani (Ref 15). Galvani did later demonstrate the electrical nature of nerve action.

The latter half of the 20th century saw marked advances in the successful use of prosthetic devices. The success of the total hip prosthesis increased because of the addition of the acetabular component (hip socket) and the surgical procedures introduced by J. Charnley (Ref 16) and others, who used polymethyl methacrylate bone cement to affix the metal femoral component and ultrahigh molecular weight polyethylene acetabular cup. Biomaterials research was promoted by the founding of the Society for Biomaterials in 1974 and by increased interest among other medical and scientific societies. More emphasis was placed on standards and specifications, and ASTM International established Committee F-4 on Medical Materials and Devices in 1964 (Ref 17). Congress passed the Medical Device Amendments (Ref 18) and placed responsibility for the implementation of this legislation with the United States Food and Drug Administration.

J.S. Hirschhorn and J.T. Reynolds explored the use of a totally porous Co-Cr-Mo implant that had an elastic modulus closer to that of bone, but the porosity made the strength insufficient for the load (Ref 19). Metal porous coated implants were introduced, and they provided a porous coating for bony ingrowth attachment and maintained the strength of the solid substrate (Ref 20–24). Hydroxyapatite filler within the porous coating increases bone growth during the first 4 weeks (Ref 24). Electrical stimulation also increases the early stages of bone ingrowth (Ref 25, 26). Corrosion of porous coatings is a concern because of the increased surface area and the changed surface morphology. E.P. Lautenschlager (Ref 27) studied the corrosion of porous Ti-6Al-4V, and H.V. Cameron (Ref 28) studied porous cobalt-chromium. Corrosion studies of porous Ti-6Al-4V and Co-Cr-Mo indicated no changes in corrosion behavior except for increased current due to the increased surface area of the porous materials; however, caution should be exercised regarding possible contamination or crevice corrosion due to porous configurations (Ref 23, 29). More recent studies discuss the biocompatibility of some of the more recently developed beta-titanium alloys for implant applications. These materials are discussed in Chapter 3, "Metallic Materials," in this handbook.

Types of Metals Used

Metals and alloys used as implants undergo an active-passive transition; therefore, corrosion resistance results from the growth of a protective surface film. These metals are in the passive state with a protective surface oxide film when used as implants and are highly corrosion resistant in saline environments. The metals currently used for surgical implants include stainless steel (AISI type 316L), Co-Cr-Mo-C, Co-Cr-W-Ni, Co-Ni-Cr-Mo, titanium, Ti-6Al-4V, and tantalum. The compositions and mechanical properties of these metals and alloys as recommended by ASTM (Ref 17) are given in Tables 1 and 2.

The metals and alloys most frequently used as implant materials are discussed in terms of metallurgical factors to provide a better understanding of their effect on corrosion resistance. For example, small changes in alloying additions of certain elements can result in significant changes in corrosion behavior. Such microstructural changes as grain size, precipitates, location of precipitates, and the presence of impurities can be important. Additional infor-

mation on the metallurgical aspects is available in Chapter 5, "Failure Analysis of Metallic Orthopedic Implants," in this handbook, and Ref 5, 30, and 31.

Stainless Steels. Steels and coated steels were used in the early 1900s for surgical purposes (Ref 1–3). The Frenchman Berthier is credited with discovering in 1821 that adding chromium to iron greatly improves corrosion resistance (Ref 32). Stainless steel was introduced in 1912 (Ref 32). In 1926, type 302 and other stainless steels were used in orthopedic surgery, and type 316 stainless steel came into use during World War II (Ref 3).

Type 316L (18Cr-14Ni-2.5 Mo) is used most widely in applications in which the implant is temporary, although it is also used for some permanent implants. The composition and mechanical properties are given in Tables 1 and 2, respectively. Type 316L is the least corrosion resistant to body fluids of the implant metals

Table 1   Compositions of selected metals and alloys used for implant applications

Metal/alloy	Co	Cr	Ni	Mo	Fe	Ti	C	Other
Stainless steel, F 138	...	17.0–19.0	13.0–15.0	2.0–3.0	bal	...	0.030	Max 0.5 Cu, 2.0 Mn, 0.025 P, 0.75 Si, 0.20 S, 0.10 N
Co-Cr-Mo, cast, F 75	bal	27.0–30.0	1.0	5.0–7.0	0.75	...	0.35	1.0 Si, 1.0 Mn
Co-Cr-W-Ni, wrought, F 90	bal	19.0–21.0	9.0–11.0	...	3.0 max	...	0.05–0.15	14.0–16.0 W, 1.0–2.0 Mn; max 0.4 Si, 0.04 P, 0.03 S
Co-Ni-Cr-Mo, wrought, F 562	bal	19.0–21.0	33.0–37.0	9.0–10.5	1.0 max	1.0 max	0.025 max	Max 0.15 Mn, 0.15 Si, 0.015 P, 0.010 S
Titanium, F 67	...	...	...	...	0.20 max	bal	0.10 max	Max 0.03 N, 0.015 H, 0.18 O
Ti-6Al-4V, wrought, F 136	...	...	...	...	0.25 max	bal	0.08 max	5.5–6.5 Al, 3.5–4.5 V; max 0.05 N, 0.012 H, 0.13 O
Tantalum, F 560	...	...	0.010	0.020	0.010	0.010	0.010	0.015 O, 0.010 N, 0.0015 H, 0.10 Nb, 0.05 W, 0.005 Si

Values shown represent wt%.

Table 2   Mechanical properties of selected metals and alloys used for implant applications

Metal or alloy	Yield strength		Tensile strength		Modulus of elasticity		Elongation, %
	MPa	ksi	MPa	ksi	GPa	10^6 psi	
316L stainless steel, annealed	207	30	517	75	...	...	40
316L stainless steel, cold worked	689	100	862	125	200	29	12
Co-Cr-Mo, cast	450	65	655	95	248	36	8
Co-Cr-Mo, thermomechanically processed	827	120	1172	170	...	...	12
Co-Cr-W-Ni, wrought	379	55	896	130	242	35	...
Co-Ni-Cr-Mo, annealed	241–448	35–65	793–1000	115–145	228	33	50
Co-Ni-Cr-Mo, cold worked and aged	1586	230	1793	260	...	...	8
Titanium, grade 1	170–310	25–45	240	35	...	...	24
Titanium, grade 4	483–655	70–95	550	80	110	16	16
Ti-6Al-4V, ELI annealed	827	120	896	130	124	18	10
Tantalum, annealed	138	20	172	25	...	...	...
Tantalum, cold worked	345	50	480	70	...	...	...

ELI, extra-low interstitial

discussed, but its corrosion resistance is adequate for some purposes, and if the material is in the cold-worked condition, the mechanical properties are good. Figure 1 shows type 316L stainless steel in the cold-worked condition. Deformation lines are evident, indicating that the material is work hardened. This material is virtually free of inclusions. Inclusions often contain sulfur, which is detrimental to pitting corrosion resistance.

The effects of alloying are important when variations in steels are under consideration. Iron exists in two different crystal structures (Ref 34), but there are two structure transitions as the structure transforms from the high-temperature body-centered cubic (bcc) δ-ferrite at 1390 °C (2534 °F) to the face-centered cubic (fcc) γ-austenite, which in turn transforms to bcc α-ferrite at 910 °C (1670 °F):

$$\text{bcc } \delta\text{-iron} \xrightarrow{1390\,°C} \text{fcc } \gamma\text{-iron} \xrightarrow{910\,°C} \text{bcc } \alpha\text{-iron}$$

Details of the metallurgy of stainless steels used for surgical implants are available in Ref 32. Chromium, which is the key element in the corrosion resistance of stainless steel, is a ferrite former. Carbon is an austenite stabilizer. Nickel

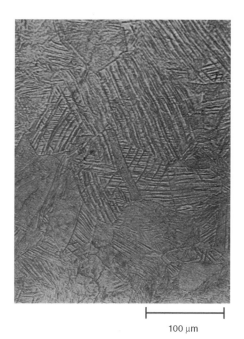

Fig. 1 Microstructure of cold-worked AISI type 316L stainless steel. Etchant: 20 mL HCl, 10 mL HNO₃, and 3 g FeCl₃ for 2 to 5 s

is added to steel to stabilize the austenite phase. Austenitic stainless steels, such as type 316L, contain chromium and nickel. The minimum combined content of these elements is 23%; the minimum chromium content is 16%, and the minimum nickel content is 7%. The type 316L stainless steel used for surgical implants contains 17 to 19% Cr and 12 to 14% Ni. Other austenitic stainless steels used for implant applications are nitrogen-strengthened 21Cr-10Ni-3Mn-2.5Mo and 22Cr-12.5Ni-5Mn-2.5Mo grades.

Molybdenum is added in amounts of 2 to 3% to strengthen the protective surface film in saline and acidic environments and to increase resistance to pitting. Molybdenum in amounts above 3% can reduce the corrosion resistance to strongly oxidizing environments and can result in the formation of some ferrite.

Carbon content in the type 316L surgical implant stainless steel should not exceed 0.08%. The greatest corrosion resistance is obtained when the carbon is in solid solution and when there is a homogeneous single-phase structure. A homogeneous austenitic structure can be produced by heat treating type 316L in the range of 1050 to 1100 °C (1920 to 2010 °F) and cooling rapidly. This rapid cooling (water quenching for large pieces) is essential for keeping the carbides in solution. Slower cooling allows chromium carbides to form at the grain boundaries and leaves the steel susceptible to intergranular corrosion. There is a depletion of chromium in areas adjacent to the grain-boundary carbides, and this further enhances corrosion in grain boundaries. The formation of these grain-boundary carbides in stainless steels is known as sensitization. The susceptibility of low-carbon stainless steels to sensitization is less than that of stainless steels with higher carbon contents.

When carbon is added to stainless steels containing little or no nickel and the stainless steel is heat treated, the result is the formation of tetragonal martensite, a nonequilibrium, hard, needlelike phase. Martensitic stainless steels are part of the type 400 series, which are not used for surgical implants.

Austenitic stainless steels are not ferromagnetic, they work harden easily, and corrosion resistance is acquired by the presence of a surface film. Magnetic alloys should not be used in the body, because they could become dislodged in a magnetic field. Ferrite should not be present in implants, not only from the standpoint of its corrosion resistance but also because it is magnetic. Magnetic-resonance imaging should not be used for an individual with any type of magnetic material in his body, and, if possible, it should be avoided for any patient who has a metallic implant. Two possible problems are the heating of the metal and the distortion of position produced by the metal even though it is not magnetic.

The corrosion resistance of stainless steel can be improved by electropolishing. Electropolishing provides a uniform surface, removes surface defects that could serve as pit sites, and leaves a protective surface film. Another method of improving corrosion resistance is the development of a protective film by passivating the steel in a 20 to 40 vol% nitric acid (HNO_3) solution at 60 °C (140 °F) for 30 min (Ref 35).

Cobalt Alloys. Cobalt-chromium alloys were first studied in 1895 by E. Haynes (Ref 36, 37), who received U.S. patents in 1907 for a cobalt composition range of 49 to 90% (Ref 38, 39). A report on the alloys appeared in 1913 (Ref 40). Since that time, cobalt-chromium alloys have been further developed and have been used in applications ranging from aircraft engines to surgical implants. The alloys are noted for high strength, good corrosion resistance, and good wear resistance. The influence of refractory metal additions on strengthening, carbide formation, and intermetallic compound formation is discussed in Ref 41. The cobalt-chromium alloys are used for surgical implants in both the cast and wrought forms, which are typified, respectively, by Haynes Stellite-21, a Co-Cr-Mo-C alloy, and Haynes Stellite-25, a Co-Cr-W-Ni alloy. The cobalt-chromium alloys have various trade names.

Cobalt undergoes a structure transformation at 450 °C (842 °F) and is fcc above this temperature and hexagonal close-packed (hcp) below it (Ref 34). Mixtures of both structures usually exist at room temperature. The cobalt-chromium alloys are strengthened by solution hardening with refractory metals (elements such as molybdenum or tungsten) and by the addition of carbon to form carbide phases that strengthen the material by dispersion hardening and grain-boundary stabilization (Ref 41). The main carbide found in the alloys is $Cr_{23}C_6$, but other carbides, such as Cr_7C_3 and M_6C, are also present. The role of carbide phases in strengthening the material is discussed in Ref 42 and 43. Agglomeration or large amounts of these phases can reduce fatigue life. The nickel addition to the

wrought material stabilizes the fcc phase and increases ductility. Normally, in the cast HS-21 material, both hexagonal (ε) and cubic (α) forms of cobalt can be present, along with some σ phase.

Typical microstructures of the cast, wrought, forged, high-strength, and hot isostatically pressed materials are shown in Fig. 2 to 5. The cast material shown in Fig. 2 has large grains with an interdendritic phase consisting of carbides, cobalt, and σ phase. Voids in cast materials can make the materials weaker. The size and shape of the grain and the location and amount of the carbides depend on the manner of casting and the rate of cooling. Thermomechanical treating of the cast material and annealing at 1065 °C (1950 °F) for 30 min will result in some improvement in mechanical properties (Ref 44).

Figure 3 shows the wrought material of the HS-25 composition. This material is strengthened by deformation, twinning, and small grain size. The forged high-strength alloy shown in Fig. 4 is closely related to the cast material (Fig. 2) in terms of composition. This material has been forged in a manner to produce a small, fine grain size and increased mechanical strength. The hot isostatically pressed material shown in

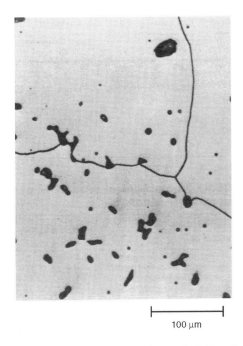

Fig. 2 As-cast microstruc,ture of cast Co-Cr-Mo alloy. Etchant: 20 mL HCl, 10 mL HNO_3, and 3 g $FeCl_3$ for 30 to 60 s

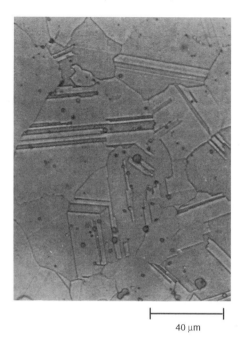

40 μm

Fig. 3 Microstructure of wrought Co-Cr-Ni-W alloy. Electrolytic etch: 100 mL HCl and 0.5 mL H$_2$O$_2$ at 6 V for 10 s

Fig. 5 has a small grain size, a fine dispersion of carbides, and improved mechanical properties.

Porous materials are used as prosthetic devices when there is a need for attachment by ingrowth of soft or hard tissue. In one study, a cobalt-chromium alloy was sintered to produce a material with 30% porosity (Ref 19). This lowered the elastic modulus of the material, but the material was too weak. Another researcher sintered Co-Cr-Mo-C spheres to the surface of a substrate of the same material (Ref 21). This technique is used for the production of prosthetic devices. One problem associated with the production of Co-Cr-Mo-C sintered porous coatings that are sintered in the 1150 to 1300 °C (2100 to 2370 °F) range is the formation of carbide phases during sintering and cooling. An example of the sintered spheres on a solid substrate is shown in Fig. 6.

One extensive study of this problem investigated the relationship of microstructure to mechanical properties of the Co-Cr-Mo-C alloy (Ref 45). These studies of heat treating, cooling, microstructures, and mechanical properties showed that there are two methods of reducing the grain-boundary interdendritic and/or carbide phases responsible for decreasing ductility

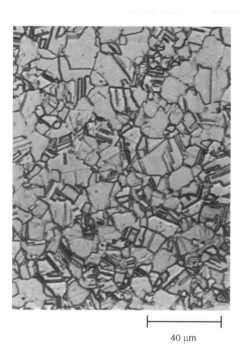

40 μm

Fig. 4 Microstructure of forged high-strength Co-Cr-Mo alloy. Etchant: 20 mL HCl, 10 mL HNO$_3$, and 3 g FeCl$_3$ for 30 to 60 s

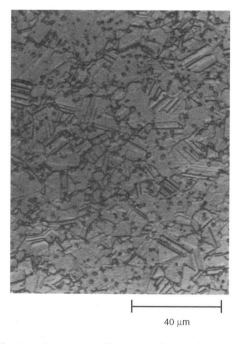

40 μm

Fig. 5 Microstructure of hot isostatically pressed Co-Cr-Mo alloy. Etchant: 20 mL HCl, 10 mL HNO$_3$, and 3 g FeCl$_3$ for 30 to 60 s

and ultimate tensile strength. The first method—cooling the material from a temperature above 1508 K to a temperature below 1508 K, then quenching—is not very practical, and the second method—reducing the carbon content to levels below 0.17%—results in a large decrease in yield strength. In addition, replacing some carbon by nitriding the alloy was found to increase yield strength (Ref 45, 46).

Alloy MP35N (35Co-35Ni-20Cr-10Mo), a cobalt-nickel alloy, has been used for surgical implants for a number of years (Ref 47). Figure 7 shows the microstructure of this alloy in the hardened but aged condition. This material is strengthened by phase transformations induced by deformation, and it has yield strength values ranging from 414 MPa (60 ksi) for annealed material to 2128 MPa (309 ksi) for work-hardened and aged material. Work hardening involves the transformation of a fcc crystal structure to a hcp structure. Aging for 4 h in the 427 to 649 °C (800 to 1200 °F) range results in the precipitation of Co_3Mo and further strengthens the alloy; Co_3Mo has a hexagonal crystal structure and is formed by a peritectic reaction at 1020 °C (1868 °F).

Titanium and titanium alloys are relatively new materials compared to steels and cobalt-chromium alloys. Titanium was discovered in 1790 (Ref 48). The ninth most common element in the earth's crust, titanium occurs as the minerals rutile (TiO_2) and ilmenite ($FeO \cdot TiO_2$), with $FeO \cdot TiO_2$ being found in larger deposits. Titanium is at least as strong as steel and is approximately 50% lighter. This high strength-to-weight ratio has made titanium and its alloys attractive materials for use in aircraft, aerospace, and marine applications.

Titanium is easily fabricated, but contamination with such interstitial elements as hydrogen, nitrogen, and oxygen should be avoided, because these elements have an embrittling effect on titanium. The development of the Kroll process in 1936 for extracting the metal and producing titanium sponge made it possible to produce the metal in commercial amounts (Ref 49); by 1948, it was commercially available in the United States. The Kroll process involves the chlorination of the ore to produce titanium tetrachloride ($TiCl_4$), which is reduced with magnesium metal in a sealed reactor with an inert atmosphere. Magnesium chloride ($MgCl_2$) is drained from the reactor vessel, leaving titanium sponge. The sponge is contaminated with ferric chloride ($FeCl_3$) and $MgCl_2$, which are then leached out. Purer titanium can

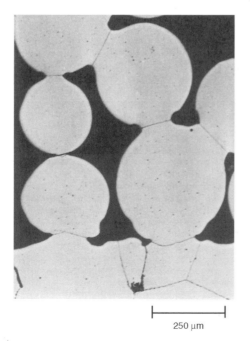

├─────────────┤
250 µm

Fig. 6 Microstructure of sintered porous coated Co-Cr-Mo alloy. Etchant: 20 mL HCl, 10 mL HNO_3, and 3 g $FeCl_3$ for 30 to 60 s

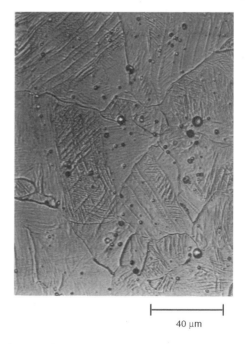

├─────────────┤
40 µm

Fig. 7 Microstructure of MP35N Co-Ni-Cr-Mo alloy. Electrolytic etch: 80 mL $HC_2H_3O_2$ and 20 mL HCl at 6 V for 5 to 60 s

be obtained by decomposing titanium tetraio-dide (TiI$_4$) at high temperatures or by elec-trolytic reduction.

In the 1950s, titanium alloys were developed to answer the need for materials with high strength, low weight, high melting temperature, and high corrosion resistance for jet aircraft engines and airframe components. It was not until the 1960s that titanium alloys were used as surgical implant materials (Ref 10, 50–52). Use of titanium alloys in surgery has been growing steadily since the mid-1970s and continues to increase. An ASTM symposium on the use of titanium for surgical implants was held in 1981 (Ref 53). Figure 8 shows the microstructures of pure titanium, Ti-6Al-4V, and Beta III alloy (Ti-11.5Mo-6Zr-4.5Sn). Mechanical properties of the α-β alloys and the β alloys depend on such factors as heat treatment, quenching, and aging.

Titanium undergoes an allotropic transforma-tion from a hcp structure (α phase) to a bcc structure (β phase) at 882 °C (1620 °F) (Ref 31, 34). As a result of this structural change, tita-nium alloys fall into three classes: α alloys, α-β alloys, and β alloys. Selected alloying additions, such as aluminum, oxygen, tin, and zirconium, are α stabilizers, and other elemental additions, such as vanadium, molybdenum, niobium, chromium, iron, and manganese, are β stabiliz-ers. Aluminum acts as an α stabilizer in amounts up to 8%, but aluminum compositions higher than this can result in an embrittling tita-nium-aluminum phase change. The presence of oxygen as an interstitial element is damaging to toughness.

In one study, porous surface coatings were applied to a solid substrate by using arc plasma spraying (Ref 20). An example is shown in Fig. 9. These coatings and their properties were stud-ied further in another investigation (Ref 54). The pore size of the arc plasma sprayed coating can be varied or can be graduated throughout a given coating. Wire mesh porous coatings are available that are sintered together and then sin-tered to the substrate. Attempts at sintering spherical powders to titanium alloys have not been very successful until recently, because of the need to sinter at high temperatures. Alloy Ti-6Al-4V should not be sintered at tempera-tures above the β transus temperature, because mechanical properties, especially fatigue, are adversely affected.

A titanium-nickel alloy known as Nitinol is used in dentistry and has potential use when a high strain recovery is needed, such as for braces or restraining devices, or when the shape-memory effect of the alloy can be used. According to the shape-memory effect, an alloy wire that is shaped or bent at a given tempera-ture and then reshaped at another temperature will return to the original shape when it is brought back to the shaping temperature. Other alloys, such as gold-cadmium and silver-cad-mium, exhibit this effect (Ref 55).

The shape-memory effect is associated with a martensitic transformation. Shape memory can also occur when the alloy is already in the

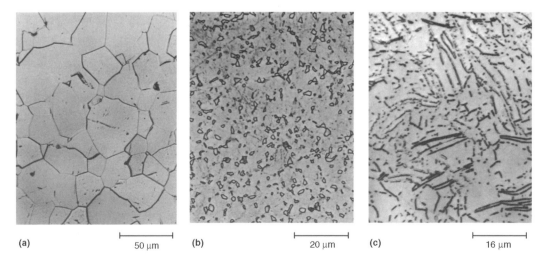

(a)   50 μm   (b)   20 μm   (c)   16 μm

Fig. 8 Microstructures of titanium and titanium alloys. Kroll's etchant: 95 mL H$_2$O, 3.5 mL HNO$_3$, and 1.5 mL HF for 20 s. (a) Unal-loyed titanium. (b) Ti-6Al-4V. (c) Beta III titanium

martensitic condition. In this case, it probably occurs through a rearrangement of the martensitic plates.

There are two temperatures of concern: the transformation temperature and the reverse transformation (A_s) temperature. The transformation temperature, M_s, below which the material transforms to martensite, for stoichiometric titanium-nickel is approximately 650 °C (1200 °F) (Ref 56). The M_s temperature can be lowered by changing the titanium-nickel ratio or by alloying with other elements, such as cobalt. A M_s temperature more compatible with the body can be achieved by alloying titanium-nickel with titanium-cobalt. The reverse transformation temperature, A_s, for titanium-nickel begins at 165.6 °C (330 °F), and that for titanium-cobalt starts at –237.2 °C (–395 °F). The desired shape (for example, a twist in a wire) that the memory will hold is fixed above the M_s temperature, the shape is changed as needed below the temperature transition range (for example, the wire is straightened), the temperature is raised to the A_s temperature, and the original shape returns.

The β-titanium alloys are metastable and are produced by adding alloying elements in sufficient amounts to stabilize the high-temperature bcc structure at room temperature. The mechanical properties of the material depend on the morphology and structure of high-modulus α particles in the low-modulus β matrix. The material can be processed to have a high fracture toughness. There are two types of β stabilizers (Ref 57). The addition of such β stabilizers as molybdenum, vanadium, tantalum, and niobium results in the formation of isomorphous α-titanium from the metastable β. Beta stabilizers such as chromium, manganese, iron, silicon, cobalt, nickel, and copper result in the formation of a eutectoid mixture of α and a compound. The structure and properties of the material can be controlled by alloying and thermomechanical processing. Some β alloys are Beta III, Ti-12 Mo-6 Zr-2Fe, and Ti-13Nb-13Zr. Many other possibilities exist for alloying to produce the β structure.

Pure titanium is used in reconstructive surgery and for purposes not subject to high loads. Pure titanium is also used for coatings.

Significance of Corrosion

Corrosion of metal implants is critical because it can adversely affect biocompatibility and mechanical integrity. The material used must not cause any adverse biological reaction in the body, and it must be stable and retain its functional properties. Corrosion and surface film dissolution are two mechanisms for introducing additional ions to the body. Extensive release of metal ions from a prosthesis can result in adverse biological reactions and can lead to mechanical failure of the device.

Metals used in the human body must have a high corrosion resistance and must not be treated or used in a configuration that would degrade the corrosion behavior. Degradation of metals and alloys used as surgical implant orthopedic devices is usually a combination of electrochemical and mechanical effects. Because surgical implants are being placed in younger people and because the older population is living longer, demands on the materials for good long-term durability and corrosion resistance are increasing.

Biocompatibility is the first consideration for materials of any type that are to be used in the body (Ref 58). Various in vitro and in vivo tests have indicated that selected metals are biocompatible and suitable for use as surgical implants. The long-term effects of metal ions on

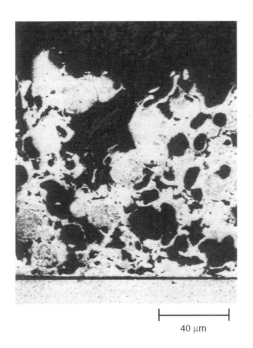

Fig. 9 Microstructure of the arc plasma sprayed coating on porous coated Ti-6Al-4V. Kroll's etchant

40 μm

the body are less well known. Data are being collected, and studies continue in an effort to provide more information. It is desirable to keep metal ion release at a minimum by the use of corrosion-resistant materials. Some effects of incompatible materials include interference with normal tissue growth near the implant, interference with systemic reactions of the body, and transport and deposit of metal ions at selective sites or organs. There is always concern about the carcinogenic effects of foreign materials in the body, both short-term and after periods exceeding 20 years.

The first investigation of tissue tolerance to metals was made by studying wires implanted in dogs (Ref 59). Platinum was concluded to be the least irritating of the platinum, gold, silver, and lead tested. Biocompatibility testing was conducted by implanting metals in rabbits (Ref 60). Minimal tissue reaction was reported to cobalt-chromium alloys, type 316L stainless steel, and titanium. Some tissue reaction was credited to the size and shape of the implant. Some individuals are sensitive to metals, and some develop metal sensitivity at a later time after receiving an implant. Stainless steel implants sometimes cause rashes or pain; this is because of nickel ion release. Metal sensitivity is discussed in Ref 61.

Integrity of the Device. Orthopedic devices must maintain mechanical strength. Load-bearing implants at the lower extremities must support three or four times the body weight. Resistance to cyclic loading is important because the metal would probably be subjected to more than 3×10^6 cycles per year. Corrosion can lead to mechanical failure of the device.

Surface Effects and Ion Release

Metal ion release from surgical implants probably results primarily from corrosion. Another source of metal ions is passive films, which are thick and not stable in body fluids. Titanium is highly corrosion resistant, yet ion release occurs. Titanium ion release is discussed in Ref 62. Titanium that is subjected to various surface treatments comes to the same rest potential in saline solution, indicating that changes have taken place in the surface film (Ref 63). The effects of passivation and sterilization have been studied. Films placed by these methods on stainless steel and cobalt-chromium alloys reduced corrosion currents, but the effects were negligible with Ti-6Al-4V (Ref 64). In all cases, surface films exist that must be stable in the body or must change to a stable form. Metal ion release and retention of ions in the body are discussed in Ref 64 to 67.

Standards

ASTM instituted the F-4 Committee on Medical Devices and Materials. Task forces associated with this committee have developed many approved documents that appear in Ref 17. These documents include specifications for implant metals in terms of composition, mechanical properties, and other factors. Recommended methods for testing corrosion, mechanical properties, and other properties are also available in Ref 17.

Electrochemistry and Basic Corrosion Processes

Corrosion is the result of an electrochemical reaction of a metal with its environment. Chemical dissolution of the surface films does play a role and should not be ignored; however, the principal concern with most forms of corrosion is electrochemical.

Corrosion Reactions. Electrochemical deterioration of the metal occurs as positive metal ions are released from the reaction site (anode) and electrons are made available to flow to a protected site (cathode). The flow of electricity and material loss during this process obey Faraday's laws, resulting in the release of one equivalent weight of metal ions for every 96,500 C of electricity passed through the electrolytic solution.

The electrochemical reaction cell consists of two conducting and electrically connected electrodes in an electrolytic solution. The two electrodes can be dissimilar metals, or they can result from different surface areas of the same metal, defects, impurities, precipitate phases, concentration differences of gas, solution or metal ions, or other variables. A schematic of a corrosion cell is shown in Fig. 10, and a representative oxidation (anodic) reaction and some typical reduction (cathodic) reactions are:

$$\text{Metal (Me)} \rightarrow \text{Me}^{2+} + 2e^-$$

Anodic reaction (loss of electrons)

$$O_2 + 2H_2O + 4e^- \rightarrow 4OH^-$$

$$O_2 + 4H^+ + 4e^- \rightarrow 2H_2O$$

$$2H^+ + 2e^- \rightarrow H_2$$

Cathodic reactions (consumption of electrons)

Thermodynamics of Implant Metal Corrosion. Corrosion occurs because the metal oxide or corrosion product is more stable thermodynamically than the metal. There is always a tendency for metals to corrode, with the driving force being the electrode potential difference between the oxidation and reduction reactions. The thermodynamics and kinetics of corrosion of surgical implant metals are discussed in Ref 68 to 70. Corrosion in general is discussed in Ref 68, 69, and 71 to 74. More information on the thermodynamics and kinetics of aqueous corrosion is available in *Corrosion: Fundamentals, Testing, and Protection*, Volume 13A of *ASM Handbook*.

The change in free energy, ΔG, associated with the electrochemical reaction can be written as:

$$\Delta G = -nFE$$

where n is the number of electrons, F is the Faraday constant (96,500 C), and E is the cell potential. A negative ΔG results in an increased tendency for the electrochemical reaction to occur.

The standard oxidation potentials of metals are measured from a bare metal surface. These potentials can be grouped to indicate active corrosion. This is known as the electromotive force (emf) series (Table 3). The galvanic series (Table 4) is based on reactions of the material with a specific environment. The galvanic series is more practical than the emf series. Table 4 lists the noble or active tendencies of metals in seawater. In one study, measurements were conducted in equine serum; the values are given in Table 5.

The thermodynamic consideration of the relationship of electrode potential to corrosion is shown in Pourbaix diagrams (Ref 76), in which the electrode potential is plotted versus pH for a given temperature and other conditions (Ref 69). Most of these diagrams predict corrosion behavior for pure metals in water at 25 °C (75 °F). The pH of a solution describes the hydrogen ion (H^+) activity and is equal to $-\log[H^+]$. Although these diagrams are for pure metals, the information is useful for determining passivation and the reactions of alloys. These diagrams serve as a guide for determining corrosion, immunity, or passivity; however, they should be used with care, and the information should be correlated with experimental data when possible.

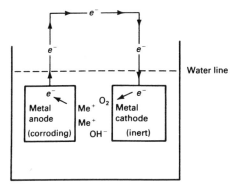

Fig. 10 Schematic of a galvanic-corrosion cell in an aqueous solution

Table 3 Standard electromotive force series of metals

Metal-metal ion equilibrium (unit activity)	Electrode potential versus SHE at 25 °C (75 °F), V
Noble or cathodic	
Au-Au³⁺	1.498
Pt-Pt²⁺	1.2
Pd-Pd²⁺	0.987
Ag-Ag⁺	0.799
Hg-Hg²⁺	0.788
Cu-Cu²⁺	0.337
H₂-H⁺	0.000
Pb-Pb²⁺	−0.126
Sn-Sn²⁺	−0.136
Ni-Ni²⁺	−0.250
Co-Co²⁺	−0.277
Cd-Cd²⁺	−0.403
Fe-Fe²⁺	−0.440
Cr-Cr²⁺	−0.744
Zn-Zn²⁺	−0.763
Ti-Ti³⁺	−1.210
Ti-Ti²⁺	−1.630
Al-Al²⁺	−1.662
Mg-Mg²⁺	−2.363
Na-Na⁺	−2.714
K-K⁺	−2.925
Active or anodic	

SHE, standard hydrogen electrode. Source: Ref 74

Figure 11 shows the Pourbaix diagram for titanium. The known areas of immunity, corrosion, and passivity are indicated. Dashed lines a and b refer to the representative equilibrium reactions $H_2 \rightarrow 2H^+ + 2e^-$ and $2H_2O \rightarrow O_2 + 4H^+ + 4e^-$, respectively. The hydrogen pressure at line a is 1 atm, and the oxygen pressure at line b is 1 atm. Oxygen concentrations in solution will be less below line b, and hydrogen concentration in solution will be less below line a.

Kinetics of Implant Metal Corrosion. The rate at which the corrosion reaction proceeds is related to environmental composition, environmental effects (such as motion or load), and other environmental factors. The rate at which a metal corrodes depends on kinetic factors that are important in determining whether a metal will corrode excessively. For example, there may be a strong driving force or potential difference for a given reaction to proceed, but because of the formation of an impervious surface film or other polarizing action, the reaction rate is slowed or practically stopped. When the polarization occurs mostly at the anode, the system is described as being under anodic control; if the reaction occurs mostly at the cathode, the system is under cathodic control. Figure 12 shows a schematic of an anodic polarization

Table 4   Galvanic series of selected metals and alloys in seawater

Noble or cathodic

Platinum
Gold
Graphite
Titanium
Silver
Chlorimet 3 (Ni-18Cr-18Mo) [Group 1]
Hastelloy C (Ni-17Cr-15Mo) [Group 1]
18–8 stainless steel with molybdenum (passive) [Group 2]
18–8 stainless steel (passive) [Group 2]
Chromium stainless steel 11–30% Cr (passive) [Group 2]
Inconel (passive) [Group 3]
Nickel (passive) [Group 3]
Silver solder
Monel 400 [Group 4]
Cupronickels (Cu-40Ni to Cu-10Ni) [Group 4]
Bronzes (Cu-Sn) [Group 4]
Copper [Group 4]
Brasses (Cu-Zn) [Group 4]
Chlorimet 2 (Ni-32Mo-1Fe) [Group 5]
Hastelloy B (Ni-30Mo-6Fe-1Mn) [Group 5]
Inconel (active) [Group 6]
Nickel (active) [Group 6]
Tin
Lead
Lead-tin solders
18–8 stainless steel with molybdenum (active) [Group 7]
18–8 stainless steel (active) [Group 7]
Ni-Resist (high-nickel cast iron)
Chromium stainless steel, 13% Cr (active)
Cast iron [Group 8]
Steel or iron [Group 8]
Aluminum alloy 2024
Cadmium
Aluminum alloy 1100
Zinc
Magnesium and magnesium alloys

Active or anodic

The alloys in each numbered group are somewhat similar in base composition— for example, copper and copper alloys (group 4). In most practical applications, there is little danger of galvanic corrosion if metals in a given group are coupled or in contact with each other. This is because these materials are close together in the series, and the potential generated by these couples is not great. The farther apart in the series, the greater the potential generated. Source: Ref 67

Table 5   Anodic back series of selected metals and alloys in equine serum

Metal or alloy	Potential versus SCE, V
Titanium	3.5
Niobium	1.85
Tantalum	1.65
Platinum	1.45
Palladium	1.35
Rhodium	1.15
Iridium	1.15
Gold	1.0
Chromium-nickel-molybdenum alloy	0.88
Chromium-nickel-molybdenum alloy	0.875
Chromium	0.75
Chromium-cobalt-molybdenum alloy	0.75
Chromium-cobalt-nickel alloy	0.75
Chromium-cobalt-molybdenum alloy	0.65
Chromium-cobalt-molybdenum alloy	0.65
316L stainless steel	0.48
Nickel-chromium-iron alloy	0.35
Nickel-chromium-iron alloy	0.35
Zirconium	0.32
Nickel-chromium-iron alloy	0.25
Nickel	0.20
Nickel-chromium-aluminum-molybdenum alloy	0.16
Tungsten	0.12
Silver	0.11
Molybdenum	−0.020
Copper-nickel alloy	−0.020
Copper	−0.030
Vanadium	−0.070
Aluminum bronze	−0.080
Tin bronze	−0.090
Nickel silver	−0.10
Admiralty brass	−0.10
Brass	−0.11
Tin	−0.20
Antimony	−0.25
Nickel-molybdenum-iron alloy	−0.30
Nickel-molybdenum-iron alloy	−0.33
Cobalt	−0.35
Indium	−0.40
Aluminum-copper alloy	−0.50
Aluminum	−0.60
Cadmium	−0.65
Aluminum-magnesium alloy	−0.65
Zinc	−0.95
Manganese	−1.08
Magnesium	−1.55

SCE, standard calomel electrode. Source: Ref 75

curve for metals that exhibit an active-passive transition.

The physiological environment contains chloride ions (Cl⁻) and is controlled at a pH level of 7.4 and a temperature of 37 °C (98.6 °F). Following surgery, the pH can increase to 7.8, decrease to 5.5 (Ref 77), then return to 7.4 within a few weeks. Infection or hematoma can cause variations in the pH from 4 to 9. Physiological solutions are oxygenated and contain organic components in addition to the salts. These solutions are electrical conductors.

Surface films on the metals are dominated by certain elements—for example, chromium for the stainless steels and the cobalt-chromium alloys and titanium for the titanium alloys. Changes beyond a specified amount in chromium content of these materials can result in reduced corrosion resistance. Other metallurgical variables can influence corrosion behavior. The corrosion resistance of a material is specific to a number of factors, including composition, changes in metallurgical heat treatment, microstructural phases present, and surface finish.

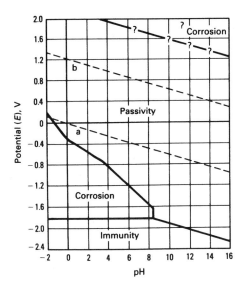

Fig. 11 Pourbaix (potential versus pH) diagram for titanium. Source: Ref 76

Forms of Corrosion in Implant Materials

The metals and alloys used as surgical implants achieve passivity by the presence of a protective surface film that inhibits corrosion and keeps current flow and the release of corrosion products at a very low level (Ref 69). The types of corrosion that are pertinent to the alloys currently used are pitting, crevice corrosion, corrosion fatigue, stress-corrosion cracking (SCC), fretting, galvanic corrosion, and intergranular corrosion. More information on all of these types of corrosion is available in *Corrosion: Fundamentals, Testing, and Protection*, Volume 13A of *ASM Handbook*. Examples of these forms of corrosion can also be found in Chapter 5, "Failure Analysis of Metallic Orthopedic Implants," in this handbook.

Pitting is a severe form of localized corrosion attack that results in extensive damage to the part and in the release of significant amounts of metal ions. Pits may be initiated at breaks in the protective film, defects in the material or protective film, inclusions, voids, and dislocations.

Pit initiation occurs when the protective film is broken by some means and exposes the metal to ions (such as Cl⁻), body fluids, and water. Once the pit has initiated, metal ions form precipitates at the top of the pit and often form a film covering the pit. The film restricts entry of the solution and oxygen into the pit, and this makes repassivation, which would renew the protection, impossible. The small area of the pit and pit tip are anodic to the rest of the material, which is cathodic; this results in a high corrosion current density at the base of the pit. Move-

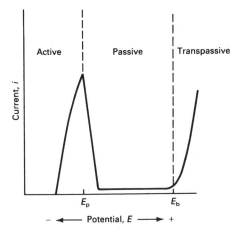

Fig. 12 Schematic of a potentiostatic polarization curve. E_p, protection potential; E_b, breakdown potential

ment of metal ions or H$^+$ ions from the bottom of the pit is restricted by the film covering the top of the pit. As a result, the pH at the bottom of the pit is lowered to the more acid range, and pitting is accelerated. Figure 13 shows an illustration of a pit and gives selected reactions.

Pitting cannot be tolerated in surgical implant metals. The first corrosion test procedure developed by the ASTM F-4/G-1 Joint Committee on Corrosion of Implant Metals was a test to screen passive metals and alloys for resistance to pitting or crevice corrosion (Ref 78). The document specifies an electrode potential stimulation test that is conducted in 0.9% sodium chloride (NaCl) solution at 37 °C (98.6 °F). A Teflon (E.I. Dupont de Nemours & Co., Inc.) washer is placed on the specimen to create a crevice; therefore, pitting and crevice testing are carried out simultaneously. This test shows that type 316L stainless steel, which was used as a reference material, has a pitting potential of 0 ± 50 mV versus a saturated calomel electrode (SCE). Titanium, Co-Cr-Mo-C, and Ti-6Al-4V do not pit or form crevices in this test, indicating that they are not readily subject to pitting or crevice corrosion.

The importance of assessing pitting corrosion resistance by determining pit propagation rate (PPR) curves is discussed in Ref 79 and 80, which also review the usual tests for pitting. These tests involve anodically polarizing the specimen to a breakdown potential, E_b, at which pitting ensues. If the potential is reversed and in the opposite direction, a protection potential, E_p, is reached, below which pits repassivate. If the corrosion potential, E_{corr}, is below E_p, pitting

does not occur: if E_{corr} is above E_p, pitting occurs immediately on immersion. Pitting resistance based on determinations of E_b and E_p have the disadvantage that the value of E_p changes, depending on the amount of pit growth and the length of time of pitting.

The PPR curves are an accurate technique for collecting pitting corrosion data. The PPR data are obtained by applying to the specimen a preselected potential between E_b and E_p and holding at this potential for 10 min. No pitting should have occurred, and the recorded current should be from general corrosion. The applied potential is then increased beyond E_b until a nominal current of 10 mA/cm^2 (64.5 mA/in.^{2}) is reached. The next step is to decrease the applied potential to the same preselected potential and hold there for 10 min. The recorded current is a measure of the rate of general corrosion in the nonpitted areas plus the rate of pit growth. The pits can be repassivated by returning the applied potential to the value of the cathodic potentials, E_c, for 5 min. The process can then be repeated. Some assessment of the pitted area can be made microscopically to determine pit growth area and average pit propagation current densities. This technique can also be used to study crevice corrosion. Application of this method to the study of implant metals is reported in Ref 81.

In one study, hysteresis effects were found on reversing the applied potential in the polarization scanning when testing passivated cast Co-Cr-Mo alloy (Ref 82). This normally indicates pitting. However, because no pits were observed on the surface and because the hysteresis effect was not present on the unpassivated material, pitting was ruled out, and the hysteresis in the polarization curves for passivated specimens was attributed to a breakdown of the existing surface film, followed by repassivation. Other cyclic polarization measurements on Co-Cr-Mo alloy did not show hysteresis (Ref 81).

In another study, potentiodynamic scans were conducted on cobalt-chromium materials; a marked hysteresis was observed with cast Co-Cr-Mo (Ref 83). It was concluded that the material was subject to crevice attack. However, in vivo experiments of cobalt-chromium crevice corrosion test specimens in dogs and monkeys conducted over a period of 2 years found no evidence of crevice corrosion (Ref 84). In addition, accelerated corrosion tests of the relative corrosion resistance of Co-Ni-Cr-Mo-Ti and Co-Cr-

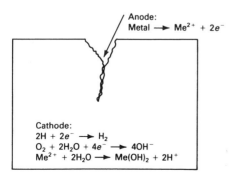

Fig. 13 Schematic of pitting corrosion

Mo alloys showed that the materials have comparable corrosion behavior (Ref 85).

Crevice corrosion is a local attack. It occurs when a metal surface is partially shielded from the environment. Crevice corrosion can occur on metals that would otherwise be resistant to pitting and other corrosion, and it often occurs at a threaded or other type of junction. Damaging ion species accumulate in the crevice, and an environment similar to that of a pit eventually develops. Crevice corrosion problems can often be eliminated by changing the design of a device.

Corrosion fatigue is a fracture or failure of metal that occurs because of the combined interaction of electrochemical reactions and mechanical damage. Corrosion fatigue resistance is an important factor of consideration for load-bearing surgical implant metals or for metals used in cyclic-motion applications. Many corrosion fatigue failures would not occur without the combined, complementary action of these factors. Normally, a failure would not occur, but cracks can initiate from hidden imperfections, surface damage, minute flaws, chemical attack, and other causes. The corrosive environment may result in local corrosive attack that accentuates the effect of the various imperfections. The corrosive attack will be influenced by solution type, solution pH, oxygen content, and temperature.

Stress cycle frequency does not significantly influence the fatigue resistance of materials, and it is convenient and expedient to test at high frequencies. This is not the case for corrosion fatigue. The effects of corrosion depend on the stress cycle frequency, and those effects increase with decreasing frequency. Frequency is an important factor in the evaluation of corrosion fatigue resistance, and materials should be tested at frequencies identical to those encountered in the use of the material (Ref 67). Figure 14 shows an *S/N* curve (stress or applied shear strain amplitude/number of cycles to failure). Corrosion is a dominant process for the material represented by curve B, which does not have a corrosion fatigue limit below which failure would not occur.

Fatigue strength measured in aqueous media is usually less than fatigue strength measured in air, as demonstrated in several investigations. In one study, corrosion fatigue tests were conducted on type 316L stainless steel in synthetic physiological solution held at a temperature of 37 °C (98.6 °F) and with a pH of 7.6 ± 0.2 in axial loading with the stress ratio, $R = 0$, at a frequency of 140 Hz (Ref 86). A 10 to 15% decrease in fatigue strength for a given endurance level resulted when testing in the solution instead of in air at 37 °C (98.6 °F) and 25% relative humidity. Fatigue strength was estimated to be 20 to 30% lower when determined at frequency of 1 Hz. Fatigue bending tests were carried out in Ringer's solution (a lactated 0.9% NaCl solution containing approximately the same concentration of Cl^- ions as body fluids) at a frequency of 1 Hz on type 316L stainless steel and a cobalt-chromium alloy (Ref 87). Results showed a reduction in fatigue strength of both materials when tested in solution:

Alloy	Cycles to failure (40 kg/mm², or 57 ksi load)	
	Air	Ringer's solution
Type 316L stainless steel	5×10^5	9×10^4
Cobalt-chromium	1.5×10^7	3.3×10^5

Other studies involving the determination of crack growth rates in Ringer's solution showed that cast Co-Cr-Mo alloys are susceptible to corrosion fatigue in the human body (Ref 88). Crack growth rates increased, and crack growth threshold levels decreased in solution over the values found for air. Failure was attributed to the synergistic effects of corrosion and cyclic stress, but hydrogen embrittlement was not ruled out. Controlled-potential slow strain rate

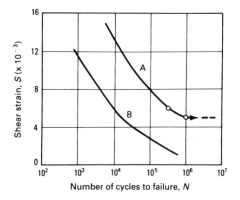

Fig. 14 *S-N* curve. Curve A, the influence of corrosion is small; curve B, corrosion is occurring.

tests conducted in Ringer's solution demonstrated that Co-Cr-Mo alloys are susceptible to hydrogen embrittlement (Ref 89).

Alloy Ti-6Al-4V was studied by using reversible torsion corrosion fatigue testing with a selected applied shear strain amplitude at a frequency of 1 Hz in Hanks's physiological solution at 37 °C (98.6 °F) and pH of 7.4 (Ref 90). The results were compared with those obtained in air (Ref 91) and showed only a slight decrease in fatigue strength in the solution. The tests in air were conducted at a frequency of 0.2 Hz and at a higher shear strain amplitude (±0.020 compared to ±0.18 in aqueous solution). These torsion tests conducted on type 316L, Co-Cr-Mo, and Ti-6Al-4V in Hanks's solution showed Ti-6Al-4V to have superior corrosion fatigue resistance over type 316L and Co-Cr-Mo.

Previous work found this same ranking of the corrosion fatigue resistance in saline solutions (Ref 92). Another study reported that rotating-bending tests at a frequency of 100 Hz in air gave fatigue strengths of 600 to 660 MPa (87 to 96 ksi) for Ti-6Al-4V, 500 to 800 MPa (73 to 116 ksi) for Co-Cr-Mo, and 400 to 780 MPa (58 to 113 ksi) for Co-Ni-Cr-Mo (Ref 93). The wide variation in fatigue strength is due to tests on different materials of the same composition that were heat treated or processed in different ways and shows a range of strength available for these materials. A minimum rotating-bending fatigue strength needed for a hip prosthesis was estimated at 400 MPa (58 ksi) (Ref 93).

Stress-corrosion cracking is a form of localized corrosion that occurs when a metal is simultaneously subjected to a tensile stress and a corroding medium (Ref 94). A single mechanism to explain the process of SCC has not been found, but several mechanisms have been shown to be important in this complex interaction of electrochemical, mechanical, and material factors. One mechanism is the occurrence of preferred anodic dissolution at the crack tip due to high plastic deformation, which causes rupture of the protective film. Another mechanism involves the adsorption of ion species at strained areas in the crack tip, and this results in weak bonds within the metal and the film. In other cases, cracking appears to propagate as a series of brittle fracture events.

Stress corrosion differs from corrosion fatigue in mode of cracking and in the application of the stress. Stress-corrosion cracks are often branched, but fatigue cracks follow a more direct path, with some striations and other microstructural effects. The loading in SCC is static, but the loading in corrosion fatigue is cyclic. Hydrogen embrittlement failure also results from static stress, but in this mechanism of failure, the adsorption of hydrogen and the production of a brittle region at the crack tip are required. Hydrogen can be produced from cathodic reactions. As a result, cathodic protection, which can be used to prevent SCC, cannot be used to stop hydrogen embrittlement.

Stress-corrosion cracking, corrosion fatigue, and hydrogen embrittlement failures can be impeded by a number of methods. The first is to select a material that is not susceptible to this type of failure in the body. Other methods of increasing immunity are to shot peen the surface to produce compressive stresses, to remove surface flaws that could act as crack initiation sites, and to heat treat the material to produce optimal microstructures for resisting mechanical damage.

Fretting occurs when two surfaces are in contact and experience small-amplitude relative oscillatory motion. Fretting corrosion involves wear and corrosion, in which particles removed from the surface form oxides that are abrasive and increase the wear rate. In some cases, the wear debris may be soluble, and increased wear would not occur. Instead, chemical reactions would play a larger role in the deterioration of the material.

Fretting corrosion can have significance for metallic surgical implants because it offers mechanisms of metal ion release in the body and of mechanical failure. Fretting destroys the passive film by which the implant metal achieves its corrosion resistance. Fretting corrosion is extensively discussed and is related to many applications in Ref 95. Fretting corrosion has occurred with plate and screw portions of prosthetic devices, and it could be the cause of fatigue fractures of these appliances (Ref 96). Reference 97 details a test method for measuring fretting corrosion of osteosynthesis plates and screws, and a test method developed for measuring fretting corrosion of modular hip implants is described in Ref 98.

Galvanic corrosion is different from the various forms of corrosion discussed. It concerns the reactions of dissimilar metals. The electrochemical reaction that results when two dissimilar metals are in contact depends on the difference in potential of the two metals; the less noble metal becomes the anode, and the other the cathode. Table 5 (galvanic series) lists the corrosion potentials of implant metals. This information on the corrosion tendency, coupled with measurements of the corrosion rate and other factors, can help predict reactions of these metals in physiological use. The area ratio of the anode to cathode must be taken into account when making this assessment of corrosion behavior. A large anode coupled to a small cathode could produce a low current density, which would indicate a low corrosion rate. The opposite conclusion could be made if the sizes of the anode and cathode were reversed.

The corrosion behavior of coupled metals is discussed in Ref 99, and corrosion tests of coupled metals are reported in Ref 100. These discussions indicate that in some cases, coupled metals can be used for surgical implants. It is possible for the couple to result in enhanced protection; this is the case for titanium with platinum in acid solutions (Ref 67, 69), in which the platinum in the couple causes the potential to be in the passive region of the polarization curve and not active as it was for titanium alone. Expert knowledge of corrosion principles and corrosion testing is required to determine the suitability of coupled metals for surgical implants. If this expertise is not available or if there are any uncertainties, it is best to avoid the use of coupled dissimilar metals.

Intergranular corrosion occurs when the grain boundary becomes anodic or cathodic to the rest of the grain. The change in composition in the grain boundaries may be due to precipitated grain-boundary phases, concentration of impurities, or elemental depletion near the grain-boundary area. The disorder and higher energy of the grain boundaries also provides a means for collecting second phases or contaminating materials that can lead to corrosion.

Synthetic Physiological Solutions (Ref 101)

Two common testing solutions relating to simulated body fluids are Hanks's and Ringer's physiological solutions. These solutions were mentioned earlier in the discussion on corrosion fatigue. The compositions of these solutions are given in Tables 6 and 7, respectively. Proteins, amino acids, serum, or other substances, as appropriate, may be added as needed to these solutions. Ideally, Hanks's and Ringer's solutions have a pH of 7.4, the normal body pH. In cases of wound or infection, the body pH can vary from 5.4 to 7.8.

Corrosion Tests for Evaluating Implant Metals

The experimental apparatus for conducting corrosion measurements can be as simple as that shown in Fig. 15. The components of the apparatus can be altered for making corrosion

Table 6   Composition of Hanks's solution

Solution A	160 g NaCl + 8 g KCl + 4 g MgSO$_4$ 7H$_2$O in 800 mL H$_2$O
Solution B	2.8 g CaCl$_2$ in 100 mL H$_2$O
Solution C	A + B + 100 mL H$_2$O + 2 mL CHCl$_3$ (chloroform)
Solution D	1.2 g Na$_2$HPO$_4$ 7H$_2$O + 2.0 g KH$_2$PO$_4$ H$_2$O + 20.0 g glucose + 2 mL CHCl$_3$ in 800 mL H$_2$O— diluted to 1000 mL
Solution E	1.4% NaHCO$_3$ = 7 g NaHCO$_3$ in 500 mL H$_2$O
Final solution	50 mL C + 50 mL D + 24 mL E + 900 mL H$_2$O + few drops of chloroform

Table 7   Composition of Ringer's and modified Krebs-Ringer solutions

Solution A	8.6 g NaCl + 0.30 g KCl + 0.33 g CaCl$_2$ + water to make 1000 mL
Solution B	To 900 mL of 0.154 mol/L NaCl, add 20 mL 0.154 mol/L KCl and 20 mL 0.11 mol/L CaCl$_2$
Solution C	Krebs-Ringer—100 parts by volume of 0.154 mol/L NaCl + 4 parts 0.154 mol/L KCl + 3 parts 0.11 mol/L CaCl$_2$ + 1 part 0.154 mol/L MgSO$_4$ + 21 parts 0.16 phosphate buffer

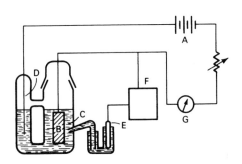

Fig. 15   Schematic of polarization testing apparatus. A, battery or power supply; B, test specimen; C, test environment; D, counterelectrode; E, reference electrode; F, high-impedance volt meter; G, ammeter. Source: Ref 69

fatigue, stress corrosion, or other specific measurements. The measurements can be done manually or automatically.

Corrosion measurements are sensitive to any changes in environment, specimen condition, or electrochemical disturbance. The corrosion process is specific to a given set of conditions. Several factors influence the results of corrosion tests regardless of the type of test being performed:

- Specimens cannot be reused for testing except when the effects of testing can be removed.
- Specimens that have been in solution and then exposed to the air should have the surfaces prepared again before testing.
- Specimens that are accidentally disturbed electrically during the test will not give a reproducible result.
- Surface preparation of the specimen should be kept constant for a given set of experiments; a highly polished surface will be more uniform and will provide a more accurate measure of the surface area.
- The specimen surface should be clean and free of all contaminants, including fingerprints.
- The pH of the testing solution should be monitored at least before and after the test. Solution pH affects the corrosion processes and the stability of the surface films present.
- The oxygen content of the solution should be kept constant by aerating or by deaerating.
- The temperature of the solution should be monitored and kept constant.
- The reference electrode should be handled with care, kept in good condition, and checked for accuracy. Voltages should be given in reference to an electrode, such as the standard hydrogen electrode (SHE) or the SCE.
- All leads should be shielded at the air/solution interface. This is also true for the specimen. It must be totally immersed.
- The amount of time between each step in potential and the voltage increment of each step should be kept constant to obtain reproducible results. The time required to reach a reasonably steady current will vary for different metals. It is possible to step the potential too rapidly, and active regions or other variations in the polarization curve would not be recognized.

- Caution should be exercised and care taken not to touch any electrical leads in all tests and especially in galvanostatic measurements, because the voltage can produce electric shock. The one-hand rule should be observed, and the power always should be turned off before touching the leads and equipment.

Galvanostatic, polarization measurements are performed by applying a current and measuring the resulting potential. This technique is used for Tafel curve and linear polarization measurements, and its applications include corrosion rate measurements. Tafel curves and Tafel slopes are determined by applying currents ranging from 1 μA to 10 mA in small, uniformly spaced increments and recording the steady-state potential after 2 to 5 min. The Tafel slope is evidenced by the straight line portion of this curve. There may be a deviation at the beginning of the curve due to anodic dissolution and a deviation at the latter part of the curve due to concentration polarization and resistance effects between the Luggin probe and the electrode.

The experimental determination and theoretical implications of galvanostatic polarization measurements are discussed in Ref 69. Figure 16 shows a plot of potential versus log current. These curves are obtained by placing the specimen in an aqueous environment, measuring the open-circuit potential after a designated time,

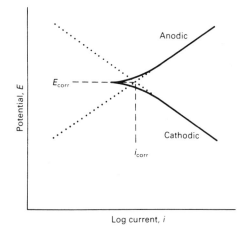

Fig. 16 Schematic of a potential versus log current density curve for anodic and cathodic galvanostatic polarization curves. Source: Ref 69

and then applying a current. This open-circuit potential is also the corrosion potential, E_{corr}. The anodic curve is determined by applying positive currents in small increments and measuring the resulting potential for each increment. The cathodic curve is established in the same manner by applying small negative-current increments and measuring the resulting potential. The linear portions of the curves can be extrapolated and will intersect at E_{corr}.

Further extrapolation of these lines brings them to the potentials for the reversible anodic and cathodic reactions. These reactions determine the signs of the corrosion cell, with the anode being negative and the cathode positive. The extension of the anodic line to the reverse potential brings it to a potential at which the metal is in equilibrium with its ions, and the extension of the cathodic line brings it to the reversible potential for the cathodic reaction. Figure 17 shows plots of these extended lines, known as Evans diagrams.

Polarization resistance measurements are described in Ref 102, which also includes the derivation of an equation to relate polarization resistance and Tafel slopes to corrosion rate. The Stern-Geary equation has been widely used in the determination of corrosion rates. Galvanostatic polarization resistance measurements are described in Ref 103; these measurements do not disturb the system. The use of an alternating current (ac) impedance technique that superimposes a small amplitude overpotential between the test electrode and the reference electrode is discussed in Ref 104 and 105; this superimposition causes a phase shift or perturbation in the current. The ac impedance method is also nondestructive to the specimen and uses the Stern-Geary equation to determine corrosion current density.

Potentiostatic anodic polarization measurements are performed by applying a potential and measuring the resulting current. The applied voltage increment should be small. A recommended rate of applying the potential is 0.006 to 0.012 V/min. This technique is especially suitable for measuring the corrosion behavior of active-passive metals, such as those used for surgical implants. These measurements will show the length of the passive region in terms of applied potential, the breakdown potential, and the magnitude of the current in the passive region. The effects of environment, such as solution pH and organic constituents,

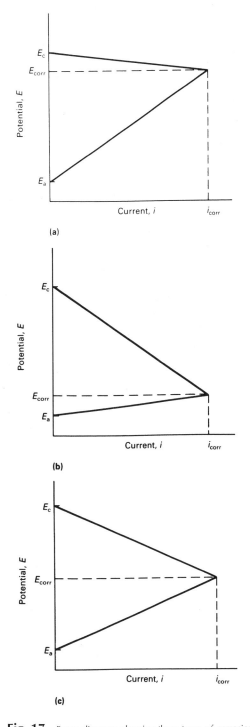

Fig. 17 Evans diagrams showing three types of corrosion rate control. (a) Anodic control (controlled by reactions at the anode). (b) Cathodic control (controlled by reactions at the cathode). (c) Mixed control (controlled by a mixture of both anodic and cathodic reactions). E_{corr}, corrosion potential; E_c, cathodic potential; E_a, anodic potential

can be studied with this method. Figure 12 shows a schematic of an anodic polarization curve.

Another application of the anodic polarization technique involves studies of repassivation kinetics (Ref 106–108). The term *repassivation* was coined to describe events occurring after surface film rupture in SCC. Repassivation involves the formation of a protective film over the abraded or clean metal surface. Repassivation measurements are made in a device that is designed to permit abrasion of the specimen, apply a preselected potential, and take a measurement (after removal of the abrader) of the anodic current transient by using an oscilloscope or a computer. Curve fitting or analysis of the current decay versus time can be carried out to provide information on the kinetics of the film formation and the stability of the film formed.

Other Corrosion Tests and Chemical Analysis. The electrochemical techniques described in the polarization measurements can be used to apply or measure electrode potentials and currents in corrosion fatigue, stress corrosion, pitting, and other tests. Chemical analysis of corroding solutions can be made with atomic absorption, and surface analysis can be made with several techniques, including x-ray photoelectron spectroscopy and Auger analysis. Chemical analysis can provide data on the amount of metal ions released, the oxidation state of the ions, and the nature of the surface film on the metal after testing.

ACKNOWLEDGMENT

The information in this chapter is largely taken from:

• A.C. Fraker, Corrosion of Metallic Implants and Prosthetic Devices, *Corrosion,* Vol 13, *ASM Handbook,* ASM International, 1987, p 1324–1335

REFERENCES

1. C.O. Bechtol, A.B. Ferguson, Jr., and P.G. Laing, *Metals and Engineering in Bone and Joint Surgery,* The Williams and Wilkins Company, 1959
2. C.S. Venable and W.G. Stuck, *The Internal Fixation of Fractures,* Charles G. Thomas, 1947
3. D.C. Ludwigson, Requirements for Metallic Surgical Implants and Prosthetic Devices, *Met. Eng. Q.,* Vol 5 (No. 3), Aug 1965, p 1–6
4. T.P. Hoar and D.C. Mears, Corrosion-Resistant Alloys in Chloride Solutions: Materials for Surgical Implants, *Proc. R. Soc. (London),* SCR.A294 (1439), 1966, p 486–510
5. D.F. Williams and R. Roaf, *Implants in Surgery,* W.B. Saunders, 1973
6. Icart, Letter in Response to the Memorandum of Mr. Pujol, *J. Med. Chir. et Pharm.,* Roux 44, 1775, p 169
7. H. Hansmann, A New Method of Fixation of Fragments in Complicated Fractures. *Verein Deutsches Gesellschaft fur Chirurgie,* Vol 15, 1886, p 134
8. J. Lister, *Br. Med. J.,* Vol 2, 1883, p 855
9. F.H. Jergesen, "Studies of Various Factors Influencing Internal Fixation as a Method of Treatment of Fractures of the Long Bones," National Research Council, Dec 1951
10. G.C. Leventhal, Titanium—A Metal for Surgery, *J. Bone Joint Surg.,* Vol 33, 1951, p 473
11. O.T. Bailey, F.D. Ingraham, P.S. Weadon, and A.F. Susen, Tissue Reaction to Powdered Tantalum in the Central Nervous System, *J. Neurosurg.,* Vol 9, 1952, p 83
12. A.M. Mirowsky, L.A. Hazouri, and D.T. Greener, Epidural Granulomata in Presence of Tantalum Plates, *J. Neurosurg.,* Vol 7, 1950, p 485
13. F. Masmonteil, The Tolerance of Bone for Metallic Foreign Bodies, *Pressé Med.,* Vol 43, 1935, p 1915
14. C.S. Venable, W.P. Stuck, and A. Beach, The Effect on Bone of the Presence of Metals Based on Electrolysis, *Ann. Surg.,* Vol 105, 1937, p 917
15. T.M. Brown, Luigi Galvani, *Encyclopedia Americana,* Vol 12, Grolier, 1984, p 256; B. Dibner, A. Volta, *Encyclopedia Americana,* Vol 28, Grolier, 1984, p 277
16. J. Charnley, *J. Bone Joint Surg.,* Vol 42B, 1960, p 28
17. *Medical Devices,* Vol 13.01, *Annual Book of ASTM Standards,* American Society for Testing and Materials
18. Medical Device Amendments, Public Law 94-295, United States Food and Drug Administration, Bureau of Medical Devices and Radiological Health, 1976

19. J.S. Hirschhorn and J.T. Reynolds, Powder Metallurgy Fabrication of Cobalt Alloy Surgical Implant Materials, *Research in Dental and Medical Materials,* Plenum Press, 1969, p 137–150

20. H. Hahn and W.J. Palich, Preliminary Evaluation of Porous Metal Surfaced Titanium for Orthopedic Implants, *J. Biomed. Mater. Res.,* Vol 4, 1970, p 571

21. R.P. Welsh, R.M. Pilliar, and I. MacNab, Surgical Implants: The Role of Surface Porosity in Fixation to Bone and Acrylic, *J. Bone Joint Surg.,* Vol 53-A (No. 5), 1971, p 963–967

22. J. Galante, W. Rostoker, R. Luek, and R.D. Ray, Sintered Fiber Metal Composites as a Basis for Attachment of Implants to Bone, *J. Bone Joint Surg.,* Vol 53-A (No. 1), 1971, p 101–114

23. A.C. Fraker, A.W. Ruff, A.C. Van Orden, H. Hahn, A.J. Bailey, and C.D. Olson, "Studies of Porous Metal Coated Surgical Implants," NBSIR 85-3166, National Bureau of Standards, June 1985

24. P. Ducheyne, L.L. Hench, A. Kagan, M. Martens, A. Burssens, and J.C. Mulier, Effects of Hydroxyapatite Impregnation on Skeletal Bonding of Porous Coated Implants, *J. Biomed. Mater. Res.,* Vol 14, 1980, p 225–237

25. N.N. Salman, "The Effect of Direct Electrical Current Stimulation on the Bone Growth into Porous Polymeric, Ceramic and Metallic Implants," Ph.D. dissertation, Clemson University, 1980

26. C.T. Brighton, Symposium on Electrically Induced Osteogenesis, *Orth. Clinics N. Am.,* Vol 15 (No. 1), 1984

27. E.P. Lautenschlager, N.K. Sarker, A. Acharya, J.O. Galante, and W. Rostoker, Anodic Polarization of Porous Fiber Metal, *J. Biomed. Mater. Res.,* Vol 8, 1974, p 189

28. H.V. Cameron, R.M. Pilliar, and I. MacNab, Porous Vitallium in Implant Surgery, *J. Biomed. Mater. Res.,* Vol 8, 1974, p 283

29. L.C. Lucas, J.E. Lemons, J. Lee, and P. Dale, In Vitro Corrosion Characteristics of Co-Cr-Mo/Ti-6Al-4V/Ti Alloys, *Quantitative Characterization and Performance of Porous Implants for Hard Tissue Applications,* STP 953, American Society for Testing and Materials, 1987

30. D.F. Williams, *Biocompatibility of Clinical Implant Materials,* Vol 1, CRC Press, 1981

31. M. Hanson and K. Anderko, *Constitution of Binary Alloys,* McGraw-Hill, 1958

32. E.J. Sutow and S.R. Pollack, The Biocompatibility of Certain Stainless Steels, *Biocompatibility of Clinical Implant Materials,* Vol 1, D.F. Williams, Ed., CRC Press, 1981, p 45–98

33. J.W.W. Sullivan, Steel, *Encyclopedia Americana,* Vol 25, Grolier, 1984, p 662–663

34. W.B. Pearson, *A Handbook of Lattice Spacings and Structures of Metals and Alloys,* Pergamon Press, 1958

35. "Standard Recommended Practice for Surface Preparation and Making of Metallic Surgical Implants," F 86, *Annual Book of ASTM Standards,* American Society for Testing and Materials

36. A.T. Kuhn, Corrosion of Co-Cr Alloys in Aqueous Environments—A Review, *Biomaterials,* Vol 2, 1981, p 68–77

37. R. Earnshaw, *Br. Dent. J.,* Vol 8, 1956, p 67

38. E. Haynes, U.S. Patent 873,745, 1907

39. D.F. Williams, The Properties and Clinical Uses of Cobalt-Chromium Alloys, *Biocompatibility of Clinical Implant Materials,* Vol 1, D.F. Williams, Ed., CRC Press, 1981, p 99–127

40. E. Haynes, Alloys of Cobalt with Chromium and Other Metals, *Trans. AIME,* Vol 44, 1913, p 573

41. M.F. Rothman, R.D. Zordan, and D.R. Muzyka, Role of Refractory Elements in Cobalt-Base Alloys, *Refractory Alloying Elements in Superalloys,* J.K. Tien and S. Reichman, Ed., American Society for Metals, 1984, p 101–115

42. J.B. Vander Sande, J.R. Coke, and J. Wulff, A Transmission Electron Microscopy Study of the Mechanisms of Strengthening in the Heat-Treated Co-Cr-Mo-C Alloys, *Metall. Trans. A,* Vol 7, 1976, p 389–397

43. T. Kilner, R.M. Pilliar, G.C. Weatherly, and C. Allibert, Phase Identification and Incipient Melting in a Cast Co-Cr Surgical Implant Alloy, *J. Biomed. Mater. Res.,* Vol 16 (No. 1), 1982, p 63–79

44. T.M. Devine and J. Wulff, Cast vs. Wrought-Cobalt-Chromium Surgical Implant Alloys, *J. Biomed. Mater. Res.,* Vol 9 (No. 2), 1975, p 151–167

45. T. Kilner, "The Relationship of Micro-

structure to the Mechanical Properties of a Cobalt-Chromium-Molybdenum Alloy Used for Prosthetic Devices," Ph.D. thesis, University of Toronto, 1984

46. T. Kilner, *Trans. Soc. for Biomater.,* Vol VIII, 1985

47. C.N. Younkin, Multiphase MP35N Alloy for Medical Implants, *J. Biomed. Mater. Res.,* No. 5, Part 1, 1974, p 219–226

48. J.C. Van Loon, Titanium, *Encyclopedia Americana,* Vol 26, Grolier, 1984, p 785

49. J.C. Van Loon, Titanium (Kroll Process), *Encyclopedia Americana,* Vol 26, Grolier, 1984, p 786

50. D.F. Williams, Titanium and Titanium Alloys, *Biocompatibility of Clinical Implant Materials,* Vol 1, D.F. Williams, Ed., CRC Press, 1981, p 9–44

51. J.A. McMaster, "Titanium for Prosthetic Devices," paper presented at the Dental-Medical Committee Meeting (Cleveland, OH), American Institute of Mining, Metallurgical and Petroleum Engineers, Oct 1970

52. G.H. Hille, Titanium for Surgical Implants, *J. Met.,* Vol 1 (No. 2), 1966, p 373–383

53. H.A. Luckey and F. Kubli, Jr., Ed., *Titanium Alloys in Surgical Implants,* STP 796, American Society for Testing and Materials, 1983

54. H. Hahn, P.J. Lare, R.H. Rowe, Jr., A.C. Fraker, and F. Ordway, Mechanical Properties and Structure of Ti-6Al-4V with Graded-Porosity Coatings Applied by Plasma Spraying for Use in Orthopedic Implants, *Corrosion and Degradation of Implant Materials,* STP 859, A.C. Fraker and C.D. Griffin, Ed., American Society for Testing and Materials, 1985, p 179–191

55. E.W. Collings, *The Physical Metallurgy of Titanium Alloys,* American Society for Metals, 1984

56. L.S. Castleman and S.M. Motzkin, The Biocompatibility of Nitinol, *Biocompatibility of Clinical Implant Materials,* Vol 1, D.F. Williams, Ed., CRC Press, 1981, p 129–154

57. F.H. Froes and H.B. Bomberger, The Beta Titanium Alloys, *J. Met.,* Vol 37 (No. 7), July 1985, p 28–37

58. J.L. Katz, Prosthetic and Restorative Materials for Bone, *Workshop in Bioma-terials,* Battelle Seattle Research Center, Nov 1969

59. Levert, *J. Am. J. M. Sc.,* Vol 4, 1829, p 17

60. P.G. Laing, Compatibility of Biomaterials, *Orth. Clinics N. Am.,* Vol 4 (No. 2), 1973, p 249–275

61. K. Merritt and S.A. Brown, Metal Sensitivity Reactions to Orthopedic Implants, *Int. J. Dermatol.,* Vol 20, March 1981, p 89–94

62. R.J. Solar, Corrosion Resistance of Titanium Surgical Implant Alloys: A Review, *Corrosion and Degradation of Implant Materials,* STP 684, B.C. Syrett and A. Acharya, Ed., American Society for Testing and Materials, 1979, p 259–273

63. A.C. Fraker, A.W. Ruff, P. Sung, A.C. Van Orden, and K.M. Speck, Surface Preparation and Corrosion Behavior of Titanium Alloys for Surgical Implants, *Titanium Alloys in Surgical Implants,* STP 796, H.A. Luckey and F. Kubli, Jr., Ed., American Society for Testing and Materials, 1983, p 206–219

64. R.W. Revie and N.D. Greene, Corrosion Behavior of Surgical Implant Materials: I, Effects of Sterilization; II, Effects of Surface Preparation, *Corros. Sci.,* Vol 9, 1969, p 755–770

65. J. Black, E.C. Maitin, H. Gelman, and D.M. Morris, Serum Concentrations of Cobalt and Nickel After Total Hip Replacement: A Six Month Study, *Biomaterials,* Vol 4, July 1983, p 160–164

66. J.L. Woodman, J.J. Jacobs, J.O. Galante, and R.M. Urban, "Titanium, Aluminum and Vanadium Release from Titanium Based Prosthetic Segmental Replacements of Long Bones in Baboons: A Long Term Study," St. Lakes' Hospital, 1985

67. M.G. Fontana and N.D. Greene, *Corrosion Engineering,* McGraw-Hill, 1967

68. H.H. Uhlig, *Corrosion and Corrosion Control,* 2nd ed., John Wiley & Sons, 1973

69. J. Kruger, Fundamental Aspects of the Corrosion of Metallic Implants, *Corrosion and Degradation of Implant Materials,* STP 684, B.C. Syrett and A. Acharya, Ed., American Society for Testing and Materials, 1979, p 107–127

70. M. Pourbaix, Electrochemical Corrosion of Metallic Biomaterials, *Biomaterials,* Vol 5, 1984, p 122–134

71. U.R. Evans, *An Introduction to Metallic Corrosion,* 3rd ed., Edward Arnold and American Society for Metals, 1981

72. J.C. Scully, *The Fundamentals of Corrosion,* Pergamon Press, 1966

73. J.C. Scully, Ed., *Corrosion: Aqueous Processes and Passive Films,* Vol 23, *Treatise on Materials Science and Technology,* 1983

74. N.D. Thomashov, *The Theory of Corrosion and Protection of Metals,* Macmillan, 1966

75. E.G.C. Clarke and J. Hickman, *J. Bone Joint Surg.,* Vol 35B (No. 3), 1977, p 467

76. M. Pourbaix, *Atlas of Electrochemical Equilibria in Aqueous Solutions,* Pergamon Press, 1966

77. P.G. Laing, Compatibility of Biomaterials, *Orth. Clinics N. Am.,* Vol 4 (No. 2), April 1973, p 249–275

78. "Standard Test Method for Pitting or Crevice Corrosion of Metallic Surgical Implant Materials," F 746, *Annual Book of ASTM Standards,* ASTM

79. B.C. Syrett, Pit Propagation Rate Curves for Assessing Pitting Resistance, *Corrosion,* Vol 33, 1977, p 221

80. B.C. Syrett, The Application of Electrochemical Technique to the Study of Corrosion of Metallic Implant Materials, *Electrochemical Techniques for Corrosion,* R. Baboian, Ed., National Association of Corrosion Engineers, 1977

81. B.C. Syrett and S.S. Wing, Pitting Resistance of New and Conventional Orthopedic Implant Materials—Effects of Metallurgical Condition, *Corrosion,* Vol 34 (No. 4), April 1978, p 138–145

82. L.C. Lucas, R.A. Buchanan, J.E. Lemons, and C.D. Griffin, Susceptibility of Surgical Cobalt-Base Alloy to Pitting Corrosion, *J. Biomed. Mater. Res.,* Vol 16 (No. 6), Nov 1982, p 799–810

83. F.G. Hodge and T.S. Lee III, *Corrosion,* Vol 31, 1975, p 111

84. B.C. Syrett and E.E. Davis, Crevice Corrosion of Implant Alloys—A Comparison of In Vitro and In Vivo Studies, *Corrosion and Degradation of Implant Materials,* STP 684, B.C. Syrett and A. Acharya, Ed., American Society for Testing and Materials, 1979, p 229–244

85. P. Sury and M. Semlitsch, Corrosion Behavior of Cast and Forged Cobalt-Based Alloys for Double Alloy Joint Prostheses, *J. Biomed. Mater. Res.,* Vol 12, 1978, p 723–741

86. J.R. Cahoon and R.N. Holte, Corrosion Fatigue of Surgical Stainless Steel in Synthetic Physiological Solution, *J. Biomed. Mater. Res.,* Vol 15, 1981, p 137–145

87. O.E.M. Pohler and F. Straumann, Fatigue and Corrosion Fatigue Studies on Stainless-Steel Implant Material, *Evaluation of Biomaterials,* G.D. Winter, J.L. Leray, and K. de Groot, Ed., John Wiley & Sons, 1980, p 89–113

88. J.D. Bolton, J. Hayden, and M. Humphreys, A Study of Corrosion Fatigue in Cast Cobalt-Chrome-Molybdenum Alloys, *Eng. Med.,* Vol 11 (No. 2), 1982, p 59–68

89. B.J. Edwards, M.R. Louthan, Jr., and R.D. Sisson, Jr., Hydrogen Embrittlement of Zimaloy: A Cobalt-Chromium-Molybdenum Orthopedic Implant Alloy, *Corrosion and Degradation of Implant Materials,* Second Symposium, STP 859, A.C. Fraker and C.D. Griffin, Ed., American Society for Testing and Materials, 1985, p 11–29

90. M.A. Imam, A.C. Fraker, and C.M. Gilmore, Corrosion Fatigue of 316L Stainless Steel, Co-Cr-Mo Alloy, and ELI Ti-6Al-4V, *Corrosion and Degradation of Implant Materials,* STP 684, B.C. Syrett and A. Acharya, Ed., American Society for Testing and Materials, 1979, p 128–143

91. M.A. Imam, "Effect of Microstructure on Fatigue Properties in Ti-6Al-4V," Ph.D. thesis, The George Washington University, 1978

92. D.F. Bowers, "Corrosion Fatigue: Type 304 Stainless Steel in Acid Chloride and Implant Metals in Biological Fluids," Ph.D. thesis, Ohio State University, 1975

93. M.F. Semlitsch, B. Panic, H. Weber, and R. Schoen, Comparison of the Fatigue Strength of Femoral Prosthesis Stems Made of Forged Ti-6Al-4V and Cobalt Based Alloys, *Titanium Alloys in Surgical Implants,* STP 796, H.A. Luckey and F. Kubli, Jr., Ed., American Society for Testing and Materials, 1983, p 120–147

94. E.N. Pugh, Stress Corrosion Cracking,

Encyclopedia of Materials Science and Engineering, Pergamon Press, 1982

95. R.B. Waterhouse, *Fretting Corrosion,* Pergamon Press, 1972

96. L.E. Slotter and H.R. Piehler, Corrosion Fatigue Performance of Stainless Steel Hip Nails—Jewett Type, *Corrosion and Degradation of Implant Materials,* STP 684, B.C. Syrett and A. Adarya, Ed., American Society for Testing and Materials, 1979, p 173–195

97. "Standard Test Method for Measuring Fretting Corrosion of Osteosynthesis Plates and Screws," F 897, *Annual Book of ASTM Standards,* American Society for Testing and Materials

98. "Standard Practice for Fretting Corrosion Testing of Modular Implant Interfaces: Hip Femoral Head-Bore and Cone Taper Interface," F 1875, *Annual Book of ASTM Standards,* Vol 13.01, ASTM

99. D.C. Mears, The Use of Dissimilar Metals in Surgery, *J. Biomed. Mater. Res.,* Vol 9 (No. 4), 1975, p 133–148

100. C.D. Griffin, "An In Vitro Electrochemical Corrosion Study of Surgical Implant Materials," M.S.E. thesis, University of Alabama at Birmingham, 1979

101. A.C. Fraker, Medical and Dental, *Corrosion Tests and Standards: Application and Interpretation,* R. Baboian, Ed., ASTM, 1995, p 705–715

102. M. Stern and A.L. Geary, Electrochemical Polarization: A Theoretical Analysis of the Shape of Polarization Curves, *J. Electrochem. Soc.,* Vol 104, 1957, p 56–63

103. D.A. Jones, The Advantages of Galvanostatic Polarization Resistance Measurements, *Corrosion,* Vol 39 (No. 11), 1983, p 444–448

104. K.J. Bundy and R. Luedemann, Characterization of the Corrosion Behavior of Porous Biomaterials by AC Impedance Techniques, *Quantitative Characterization and Performance of Porous Implants for Heart Tissue Applications,* STP 953, American Society for Testing and Materials, 1987

105. L. Lemaitre, M. Moors, and A.P. Van Peteghem, AC Impedance Measurements on High Copper Dental Amalgams, *Biomaterials,* Vol 6, Nov 1985, p 425–426

106. J.R. Ambrose, Repassivation Kinetics, *Corrosion: Aqueous Processes and Passive Film,* Vol 23, *Treatise on Materials Science and Technology,* J.C. Scully, Ed., Academic Press, 1983, p 175–204

107. J.R. Ambrose and J. Kruger, Tribo-Ellipsometry: A New Technique to Study the Relationship of Repassivation Kinetics to Stress Corrosion, *Corrosion,* Vol 28 (No. 1), 1972, p 30–35

108. P. Sung and A.C. Fraker, Repassivation Kinetics of Ti (6Al)-4V, 316L Stainless Steel, Co-Cr (Cast) and Co-Ni-Cr (MP35N), *Transactions of the Seventh Annual Meeting of the Society for Biomaterials,* Vol IV, 1981, p 28

CHAPTER 5

Failure Analysis of Metallic Orthopedic Implants

EXPOSURE OF ORTHOPEDIC IM-PLANTS to the biomechanical and biochemical forces and interactions between the implants and the biological environment may lead to failure due to mechanical or biomechanical reasons. Fatigue or corrosion fatigue damage is one of the major causes for failure of implant devices. Local loading conditions produce the fatigue stresses. Dynamic loading in the presence of body liquid can also cause surface attack by fretting, fretting corrosion, or wear at implant junctions, such as screw heads and plate holes. A combined attack of fatigue with stress corrosion can also cause implant breakdown.

The normal pH of the body fluids is almost neutral, with a mean value of approximately 7.4. At injured sites, the pH shifts to acidic values as low as 4.0, especially in hematoma. Of all the ionic components of blood plasma and interstitial fluids, the chlorine ions are typically the most aggressive to metal implants. Several types of chloride-induced corrosion attacks have been reported to affect implants; pitting, intergranular corrosion, and crevice corrosion have all been observed.

Various types of forces act on the implants and the bone. In the intact musculoskeletal system, the acting forces are balanced. When a bone is fractured, the balance of forces is destroyed, and the muscle forces pull the bone fragments in various directions. During operative reconstruction of a fractured bone, attaching the fragments to orthopedic implants stabilizes the fracture. If the bone is perfectly reduced, the entire implant is supported by bone, the acting forces are again in equilibrium, and only relatively small and uncritical loads are exerted on the implant. However, if the bone is not perfectly reconstructed, if fracture gaps are present, or if fragments of bone

are missing, the weight-bearing forces are not completely balanced, and the loads may be unevenly distributed.

As a result, bending and torsional stresses can concentrate in areas of the implant where bone support is missing. The implant undergoes cyclic loading in these zones, and the risk of fatigue damage may increase. It is not necessary for the implant to be loaded in the plastic deformation range for fatigue cracks to develop. Local stress concentrations may be sufficient to initiate fatigue cracks in the surface of the implant. The development of fatigue damage depends on the number of load cycles and the intensity of loading. An estimate of the number of cycles that an implant may undergo in a given time period varies from 54,000 cycles per month (assuming 1 h motion per day) to 324,000 cycles per month (with 6 h motion per day). Fatigue is a frequent cause of hip-fracture-fixation device failure.

Types of Orthopedic Devices

Depending on the duration of their function, the two major categories of such devices are prostheses and internal fixation implants. Prosthetic devices (Fig. 1) are implants designed to remain in the body for a lifetime. They serve as joint replacements (replacing the total joint or only one component) or as bone replacements (replacing larger sections of bone, for example, after tumor resection). Internal fixation devices (Fig. 2) are implants designed to provide temporary stabilization. They are used for maintaining the shape of the reconstructed bone for treatment of fractures or for corrective orthopedic operative procedures. After healing, internal fixation devices, having served their purpose, are commonly removed.

Prosthetic Devices

Artificial joints are mainly used to replace painful joints that are degenerate and inflicted with diseases. Severe joint injuries are occasionally treated with prosthetic components.

When prostheses replace the entire joint, two artificial joint surfaces are anchored at the bone ends that remain after resection, and the prosthesis simulates the joint motion. Occasionally, only one joint surface, such as the femoral head, is replaced by an artificial component, which works against a natural articulation surface. Most joint replacements are performed on the hip. Because the normal femoral head is almost spherical, its

motion is relatively easy to simulate. More complicated is the articulation of the knee and the various types of knee prostheses that compromise the original motion range. Prostheses are also available for the humeral head (shoulder), elbow and finger joints, the ankle, and the jaw (Fig. 1).

Most total joint systems have articulation components made from dissimilar materials so that, for example, metal or ceramics work against a plastic material, such as polyethylene (Ref 1). Finger joints, as well as some other prostheses, are made completely from plastics or metal-reinforced plastics (Ref 2).

Many prostheses are anchored by using a bone cement in a bed that has been mechanically prepared in the remaining bone. Recently, various designs have been developed for the

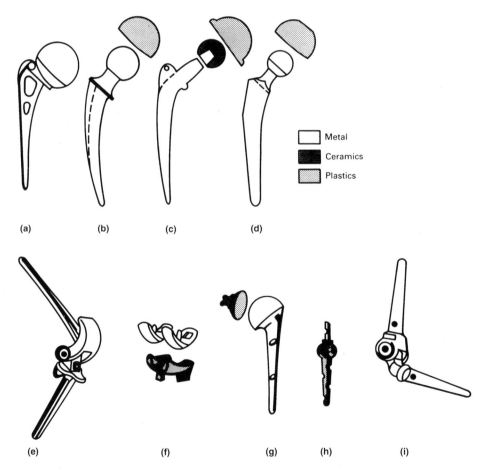

Fig. 1   Typical examples for joint prostheses (schematic). (a) Classic Moore hip endoprosthesis. (b) Müller total hip prosthesis (metal against polyethylene acetabular cap). (c) Weber total hip prosthesis with movable head and metal, ceramic, and polyethylene components. (d) Müller total hip prosthesis with straight stem. (e) Hingelike knee joint prosthesis; metal against metal (G.E.U.P.A.R.). (f) Sliding knee joint prosthesis; metal against plastic (Geomedic). (g) Total shoulder joint prosthesis; metal against plastic (St. Georg). (h) Total finger joint prosthesis with metal and plastic components (St. Georg). (i) Total elbow joint prosthesis; metal-to-metal (McKee)

cementless anchoring of prostheses by a tight fit. Certain prosthesis systems have porous surface coatings on their shafts to increase the surface area and to allow microanchorage of the bone. Developments in the field of joint prostheses are progressing rapidly. In this chapter, only metallic components are considered.

In tumor resections, large defects are created by extensive bone and joint removals, which are often bridged with custom-made

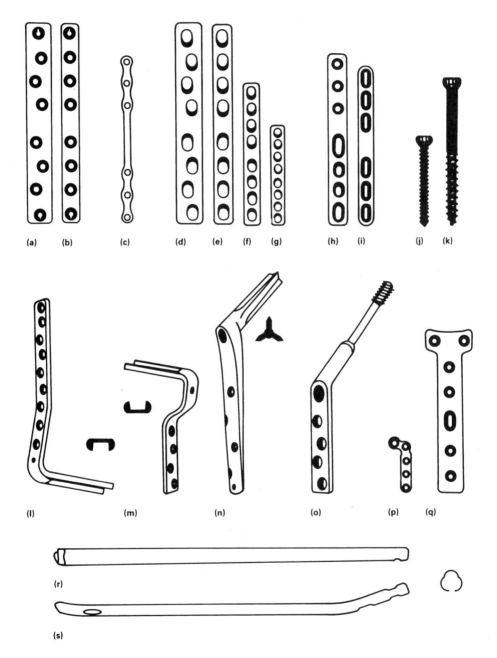

Fig. 2 Typical examples for orthopedic internal fixation devices (schematic). (a) and (b) Round hole bone plates (can be used with compression devices). (c) Classical Sherman bone plate. (d) to (g) Dynamic compression plates of various sizes. (h) Compression bone plate with glide holes. (i) Classical Bagby compression bone plate. (j) Cortical bone screw. (k) Cancellous bone screw (with shaft to produce compression). (l) Condylar angle blade plate. (m) Hip plate for osteotomies. (n) Jewett nail plate with three-flanged nail. (o) Two-component dynamic hip screw plate. (p) Miniature L-plate—for example, for hand surgery. (q) T-plate for the humeral and tibial head. (r) Straight Küntscher intramedullary femoral nail. (s) Intramedullary tibia nail. Note cloverleaf profile on both (r) and (s).

prostheses, modified standard joint prostheses, or fracture-treatment implants. Bone cement and/or other filling materials are sometimes added to the reconstruction for more stability. In the treatment of tumor resections, the surgeon is often forced to be inventive and to choose unorthodox techniques of reconstruction. Frequently, the remaining bone has been irradiated and lacks its normal regenerative vitality.

Implants for Internal Fixation

Implants for internal fixation are characterized by their versatility (Fig. 2). They are used to maintain the shape of the reconstructed bone in fracture treatment of the injured patient or, in corrective orthopedic surgery, to stabilize osteotomies (sectioning and realignment of bone) or to perform arthrodeses (stiffening of joints by fusion of bones). Various types and sizes of bone plates, bone screws, intramedullary rods (nails), pins, and orthopedic wire are available (intramedullary refers to use of the marrow space of the bone for support). Some implants have very specific uses; others have a wide range of applications with different functions.

Under the impact of a trauma, bones can fracture in any configuration and combination. In each patient, the fractures are unique and require individual treatment. This explains the necessity of versatile implants. Nevertheless, certain fracture classifications and methods for the treatment of typical fracture configurations have been established (Ref 3). In the selection of the appropriate implants and operation technique, not only the type of fracture and its location but also the condition of the soft tissue, the structure and consistency of the bone, the age and condition of the patient, and any present complication must be considered. Even when the best possible reconstruction has been achieved, the weight-bearing stability of an internal fixation device can vary widely, and the weight-bearing schedule of the patient must be correspondingly adjusted.

Depending on the situation, the patient may be allowed one of the following postoperative modes of motion: exercise only, partial weight bearing, or full weight bearing. The rate of bone healing depends on different factors and determines the further course of postoperative weight bearing. Because of the previously mentioned complexity, the possibility of an implant-related complication is comparably higher in fracture treatment than in corrective surgery or joint replacement, which are both usually carried out under standard conditions. Unless a pathological situation is present, the surgeon can achieve primarily stable biomechanical conditions when performing a corrective osteotomy or a joint replacement. When these conditions remain, the probability of an implant failure is minimal. The stabilization difficulties can be listed in ascending order, as follows:

- Joint replacements (endoprostheses)
- Corrective orthopedic surgery
- Fracture treatment
- Tumor resection (most difficult)

Complications Related to Implants

Internal fixation or joint replacement procedures can fail for such reasons as:

- Failure of the bone to heal
- Bone resorption
- Breakage of bone
- Loosening of implants
- Bending of implants
- Breakage or disintegration of implants

These events can be interrelated and usually require an intervention with reoperation to effect clinically successful results.

The term *implant failure* can be misleading. Therefore, in this chapter, the term *implant failure* is used to indicate that an implant has broken or disintegrated in a manner such that it cannot fulfill its intended function. Implant failure is not identical with a faulty implant, because there can be purely biological and biomechanical reasons for implant breakage or malfunction. In most cases, only a thorough analysis of the clinical conditions under which an implant failed can explain the reason for failure.

As stated in the introductory paragraph to this chapter, implants can undergo surface attack by fretting, fretting corrosion, or wear. These types of attack can be relatively mild; they often occur only on the microscopic level, do not interfere with the functioning of the implant or the healing of the bone, and do not require reoperation. On prosthetic devices, however, wear of the articulation surfaces has occasionally been found to be so intense that the components have had to be replaced. Corrosion of implants involving dissolution that requires intervention is found only with materials that are excluded by the official standards for materials for orthopedic implants. In this chapter, the term *degradation* is associated with the surface attack of implants.

Metallic Implant Materials

A number of metals and alloys have proven to be satisfactory as implant materials during years of surgical application. They are specified as implant materials by standards of ASTM International and the International Organization for Standardization (ISO), as listed subsequently, and by other national standards. These materials are corrosion resistant and well accepted by body tissues (biocompatible) and therefore satisfy two of the basic requirements for implants. These two properties are generally related because the less substance the metal surface releases, the better the material is accepted by the tissue. Experimentation has proven that the different pure metals of the periodic table exhibit cell toxicity at different concentrations in tissue and organ-culture tests (Ref 4–6). Some of the metals play important roles in the body metabolism, although they can become toxic beyond certain concentrations (Ref 7). For other metals that behave indifferently in the body, such as titanium, no metabolic function is yet known.

Fatigue resistance is another general requirement for implants, but the critical loading is different for the various types of implants and applications. The required mechanical strength of orthopedic implants also varies and depends on the shape of the implant and the application. Good ductility (discussed subsequently) is often desired.

The following is a list of some of the major ASTM standards for implant materials:

- Austenitic stainless steels: F 138/139 (type 316L), F 1314 and F 1585 (nitrogen-strengthened stainless steels)
- Unalloyed titanium: F 67 (ASTM grades 1, 2, 3, and 4)
- Titanium alloys: F 136 (Ti-6Al-4V extra-low interstitial, or ELI), F 1295 (Ti-6Al-7Nb), F 1713 (Ti-13Nb-13Zr), F 1813 (Ti-12Mo-6Zr-2Fe)

- Cast cobalt alloy: F 75 (Co-28Cr-6Mo)
- Wrought cobalt alloys: F 90 (Co-20Cr-15W-10Ni), F 562 (Co-35Ni-20Cr-10Mo), F 799 (Co-28Cr-6Mo), F 1058 (Co-20Cr-15.5Ni-7Mo-Fe)

Certain applications, for example, in the skull, involve the use of tantalum or niobium, both of which have high corrosion resistance and are biologically well accepted. Additional ASTM standards specify cast and forged conditions for stainless steels and other materials; they are among other implant-related standards in Ref 8.

The Body Environment and Its Interactions with Implants

The Biochemical Environment. Orthopedic implants are exposed to the biomechanical and biochemical forces of the body, and certain interactions take place between the implants and the biological environment. Figure 3 indicates the ionic composition of blood plasma and interstitial and intracellular fluids. Of the components shown, the chlorine ions are the most critical for metal implants. As stated previously, the normal pH of the body liquids is approximately neutral—in the range of 7.2 to 7.4 pH (Ref 10). At injured sites, the pH shifts to acidic values of approximately 5.2; in hematoma, it can drop to 4.0. In cases of infection, the pH shifts to alkaline values (Ref 11). At sites of local fretting corrosion, the environment can also become acidic through corrosion products and thus enhance further corrosion.

Chromium steels, low-grade austenitic stainless steels, and sensitized stainless steels are not sufficiently corrosion resistant in the body environment. This has been observed on retrieved implants that were manufactured 20 to 40 years ago. High-grade austenitic stainless steels as specified in the standards (ASTM F 138/139) exhibit overall corrosion resistance and are presently the materials most frequently used for internal fixation devices.

The Dynamic Environment. Various types of forces act on the implants and the bone. In the intact musculoskeletal system, the acting forces are balanced. The macroscopic shape and the microscopic structure of the bone are adjusted to the forces of normal motion and loading. Muscles and tendons counteract bending forces that would overload the bone. When loaded physiologically under weight bearing, the bone undergoes small elastic deformations, which act as a fine stimulus that keeps the bone in a healthy condition. For example, a trained athlete develops heavier and stronger bones than an untrained person, or if a patient is bedridden for a long period of time, his bone structure becomes porous because it is not exposed to the normal loading forces.

When a bone is fractured, the balance of forces is destroyed. This can be well studied on the dislocations of injured bones; in these cases, the muscle forces pull the bone fragments in various directions. After operative reconstruction of a fractured bone, the fragments are stabilized with implants. If the bone is perfectly reduced, the entire implant is supported by bone, and the acting forces are again in equilibrium. Relatively small and uncritical loads are then exerted on the implant, and the risk of implant-related complications is minimal.

However, if the bone is not completely reconstructed—that is, fracture gaps are present or fragments of bone are missing—the weight-bearing forces are not completely balanced and evenly distributed. As a result, bending and torsional stresses can concentrate in areas of the implant where bone support is missing. Under weight bearing, the implant undergoes cyclic

loading in these zones, and a potential risk of fatigue damage may arise. For fatigue cracks to develop, it is not necessary for the implants to be loaded in the plastic deformation range. Local stresses that occur under loading in the elastic deformation range of the material are sufficient to initiate fatigue cracks in the surface of the implant.

The development of fatigue damage depends on the number of load cycles and the intensity of loading. In clinical terms, this means that implant fatigue depends on the width of the bone gaps, on the length of the lever arms, and on the intensity and duration of the weight bearing, if a critical fatigue condition develops.

Table 1 gives an estimation of the number of cycles an implant may undergo during a given time period, during which a certain amount of motion per day is anticipated. To estimate the loading, static and dynamic forces must be considered. In one study, a maximum force of 2600 N (585 lbf) was determined on the femoral head in the loading phase during a test of a 60 kg (135 lb) patient (Ref 12). This is more than four times the body weight.

As long as bone healing progresses normally, an implant will not undergo fatigue fracture, because the loading decreases successively as the bone becomes more supportive. Normal

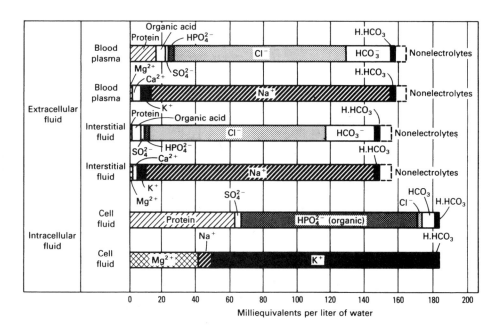

Fig. 3 Ionic compositions of blood plasma, interstitial fluid, and intracellular fluid. Source: Ref 9

bone has a remarkable inherent regeneration potential. However, certain conditions must be fulfilled so that the bone heals and regenerates. The course of bone healing is not fully predictable and depends on various factors.

Bone Healing. Normal bone regenerates continuously at a relatively slow rate. Approximately 3% of the Haversian systems of the bone structure are usually in a stage of remodeling (Ref 13, 14). In the injured bone, the remodeling and regenerative processes are highly activated. Figure 4 shows a microradiograph of the cortical bone structure in the remodeling stage. One important precondition for bone healing is immobilization. Bone tissue tolerates only minimal amounts of elastic motion, particularly during repair. This explains the high success of operative fracture treatment by internal fixation. Even in severe joint injuries, functional healing is achieved.

Depending on the local conditions, different bone repair mechanisms can occur (Ref 13, 14). Generally, one can distinguish secondary and primary bone healing. Secondary bone healing takes place if relatively wide fracture gaps exist and a certain amount of mobility is present. The bone heals through callus formation; that is, fibrous tissue and cartilage form first, followed by bone. Under too much motion, complications can arise because bone does not form, and nonunion, or pseudarthrosis, develops (pseudarthrosis is the formation of a false joint between bone fragments). If this happens and an implant is present, enough load cycles can accumulate at the fracture zone to cause the implant to fail through fatigue. In most such cases, a reoperation is inevitable to treat the nonunion—for example, by application of compression—regardless of whether a broken implant is present or not.

Example 10 in this chapter discusses a case in which the implant was removed to treat a nonunion. Microscopic analysis revealed that a fatigue crack had already developed at the hole of the plate, which was situated near the unstable fracture site. Another plate was inserted under compression, and the bone healed without further complications.

Primary bone healing develops without callus formation, if the bone fragments are in contact with each other and are rigidly stabilized with implants. The bone fragments unite by means of transmigrating blood vessels and subsequent remodeling of the bone structure. These healing processes can be disturbed if the patient has a pathological bone condition, if an infection is present, or if necrotic (dead) bone fragments are resorbed.

Necrosis (the pathological death of living tissue) occurs when the blood supply of the bone fragments is damaged by the injury. Such fragments lose their nourishment and vitality. Complications can arise when necrotic fragments are resorbed: the fracture gap widens, relative motion increases, and bone healing is prevented or significantly delayed. Again, an implant can be subjected to a long period of increasing cyclic loading with a chance of fatigue failure. To treat such a situation and to enhance bone healing, implantation of cancellous (spongy) bone grafts and compression of the fracture site may be indicated. Although a second operation involves discomfort for the patient, it is sometimes necessary in order to ensure bone healing and satisfactory functional results.

Bone Resorption Through Motion. Clinical and experimental observations indicate that persistent motion beyond a certain degree causes bone resorption when mechanical instability is present (Ref 15, 16). Thus, fracture gaps can

Table 1 Estimation of load cycles for one leg during walking

For these calculations, it is assumed that one load cycle per leg takes 2 s, which means that every second one step is made with alternating legs (other authors estimate 1 to 2.5×10^6 load cycles per year per leg).

Motion per day, h	Cycles per day	Cycles per 1 month	Cycles per 4 months	Cycles per year
1	1,800	54,000	216,000	657,000
3	5,400	162,000	648,000	1,971,000
6	10,800	324,000	1,296,000	3,942,000

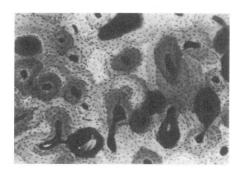

Fig. 4 Microradiograph from thin section of cortical bone. The varying x-ray density of the Haversian systems and the enlargement of some blood vessel cavities indicate that the bone is in a stage of remodeling. 77×

widen, and implants, or portions of implants, can become loose. The widening of fracture gaps means increased cyclic loading of the implant unless weight bearing is reduced. Implant loosening can cause either local stress concentration, with increased risk of fatigue, or relaxation of the stresses in the implant. Under the latter conditions, the chance of implant failure is reduced. Local bone resorption followed by mechanical degradation of bone cement and partial loosening of prosthesis stems is a typical sequence of events that is responsible for fatigue failures of prostheses.

Mechanical Properties of Bone. As a construction material, bone has properties that differ from those of metals. Bone is viscoelastic, can resorb or regenerate, and thus may change its mechanical properties and volume with time. Comparative mechanical measurements show that the ultimate tensile strength, the fatigue strength, and the elastic modulus of cortical bone are approximately ten times less than that of cold-worked stainless steel. Cancellous bone is spongy and much softer than cortical bone and exhibits mechanical behavior that is different from that of cortical bone but has a higher healing rate (Ref 17). Bones derive their overall strength from their geometric configuration. The typical compressive strength of bone is the result of the composite structure of organic collagen and apatite crystals.

Combined Dynamic and Biochemical Attack. Dynamic loading in the presence of body liquids can cause wear and fretting corrosion at implant junctions, such as screw heads and plate holes, or at artificial articulation surfaces. Extensive research has been devoted to the study of wear on artificial joints and its degradation products. Corrosion fatigue is always a subject of argument and is discussed in the section "Fatigue Properties of Implant Materials" in this chapter.

It is generally agreed that stress-corrosion cracking is not a concern in high-quality implant materials. It can be observed only in combination with other failure modes, such as fatigue.

Design of Internal Fixation Devices

Leading internal fixation systems contain different types of devices that are available in various configurations and sizes. Some major implant types are specified by standard-bearing organizations, such as ASTM and ISO, but many established implants are not standardized. Figure 2 shows a selection of characteristic internal fixation devices.

Straight bone plates (a to i, Fig. 2) often must be contoured to fit the curvature of the bone. This requires ductility and moderate rigidity of the plates. In many fracture situations, it is necessary to compress the fracture site with the aid of the bone plate to achieve stability and to promote bone healing. Therefore, certain plates have specially formed screw holes (compare d to g, Fig. 2) that allow compression of the fracture gap while the screws are inserted. Certain types of plates can be applied with compression devices to achieve the same effect. One-piece angled plates, two-component angled plate systems, and plates with specially formed heads (1 to q, Fig. 2) are designed for the fixation of short fragments at the bone ends, specifically the femur.

Bone screws have two characteristic types of threads (j and k, Fig. 2), depending on intended use in cortical or cancellous bone. Intramedullary nails (r and s, Fig. 2) are inserted in the bone cavity. They are increasingly used in an interlocking fashion for comminuted fractures, in which the bone is splintered or crushed into numerous pieces. Pins and wires of various dimensions belong to the standard equipment of the orthopedic surgeon. A variety of implants exist, and some are for specific fracture types and corrective operations.

When implants are designed, the following factors must be considered:

- General anatomy and its individual deviation
- Operative approach
- Operative technique
- Available space at the fracture site
- Variability of the fracture situation
- Local bone consistency
- Healing tendency of the particular bone regions
- Probable complications
- Physiology and biomechanics
- Dynamic loading and weight-bearing conditions
- Response of the bone to the implant
- Properties of the implant material

Due to all the physiological restrictions, the ideal implant design, from an engineering point of view, is sometimes not feasible. In such cases, only the best possible compromise can be reached.

In addition to biological compatibility, the endurance of the implant is one of the basic requirements. Because of the previously listed factors, implants cannot be designed with high mechanical safety factors for all possible loading conditions, because the volume and rigidity would exceed the biological limits. For example, a bone plate displaces soft tissue; in areas where the soft tissue coverage is thin, a plate with too large a cross section could cause soft tissue damage and complications. An implant designed only for high mechanical and fatigue resistance could become very rigid and would shield the bone from the physiological loading stresses. Consequently, rarefaction of the bone structure could occur. If the elasticity of the plate and the screws are not in the right proportion to each other or to the bone, screws could be pulled out of the bone or could break. On the other hand, if a plate is too flexible, nonunion could occur. If too large an area of the bone surface is covered with a plate, the blood supply may be impaired.

Usually, implants are so designed that they maintain their shape unless a dramatic event takes place, such as a second trauma. As discussed previously, the fatigue strength of implants is not unlimited. Stresses in the elastic loading range are sufficient to initiate fatigue. As long as the well-reduced bone fragments are in contact, the implants are supported. Critical cyclic loading occurs only when the internal fixation is unstable in the presence of fracture gaps and bone defects. Specific surgical techniques were developed to achieve stable fixation (Ref 3). Figure 5 shows the different degrees of stability in internal fixations.

There are clinical situations in which comminution (reduction to particles) or loss of fragments does not allow stable fixation. Implantation of bone grafts is then indicated to promote bone healing and to develop stability.

Analysis of Failed Internal Fixation Devices

The metallurgical investigation of failed implants can reveal the failure mechanism. Because of the complexity of the biological conditions discussed earlier in this chapter, the cause of implant failure can, in most cases, be assessed only when the clinical history and the corresponding radiographs are analyzed by a clinical expert. This is particularly true in cases of fatigue failure. One should be cautious not to mistake small deviations from material standard specifications or small flaws as the reason for an implant failure when the real cause is heavy cyclic overloading. As experiments demonstrate, fatigue cracks can initiate on the implant surface without the presence of flaws. Judging the implant design as a possible cause of failure necessitates biological, biomechanical, and surgical knowledge.

Implants should be disinfected before examination. Although implants are usually rinsed in the hospital, biological residues can adhere to the surface and obscure the details of the fracture surface. Ultrasonic cleaning with 10% oxalic acid, a clinical disinfectant, or an enzymatic digestion is suitable for the highly corrosion-resistant implants. Probable corrosion products must be detected before such a procedure. However iron-rich blood residues should not be mistaken for rust if local microanalysis of the chemical composition is performed.

Under the microscope, electropolished implant surfaces usually exhibit small craters where inclusions were dissolved. Occasionally, these structures are erroneously interpreted as corrosion pits.

During the internal fixation and later at the retrieval, implants are handled with metallic tools, and this handling results in scratches and mechanical marks on the implant. It is often not possible to determine whether the marks were produced during retrieval or fixation.

ASTM standards on testing and evaluation of implant devices may be taken as a guideline for the analysis of failed implants. Not all portions of the suggested investigation protocol are equally applicable for the different implants.

Failure Analysis Examples

The failure analysis examples, or case histories, included in this chapter are broken down into six categories:

- Failures related to implant deficiencies (Examples 1 to 7)
- Failures related to mechanical or biomechanical conditions (Examples 8 to 12)
- Failures related to implant degradation (Examples 13 to 16)
- Failures related to inadequate design (Example 17)
- Fractures of total hip joint prosthesis (Example 18)

- Fractures of total knee prosthesis (Example 19)

Table 2 provides a summary of the types of devices, materials, and failure mechanisms described in these examples.

The three primary sources for these examples were:

- *Failure Analysis and Prevention,* Vol 11, *Metals Handbook,* 9th ed.
- *Handbook of Case Histories in Failure Analysis*
- The journal *Practical Failure Analysis*

All are published by ASM International. More detailed information on these sources can be found in the Acknowledgments at the conclusion of this chapter.

Failures Related to Implant Deficiencies

Most of the failed implants submitted for analysis are manufactured from high-quality implant materials and are free of metallurgical defects. Implant breakage of current materials is usually due to mechanical or biomechanical reasons. However, there are occasionally implants received that are manufactured from inadequately processed materials or that were produced many years ago when metallurgical

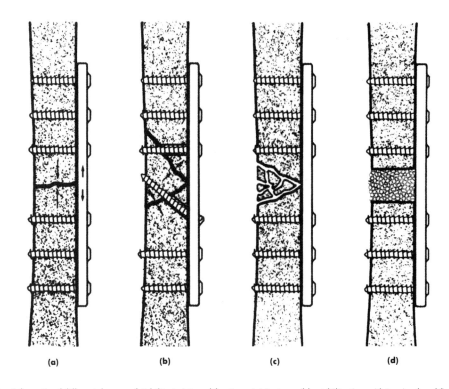

Fig. 5   Schematic of different degrees of stability in internal fixations. (a) Best possible stabilization with tension band fixation. The plate is on the tension side of the bone. The fracture site is compressed by means of the plate, which was applied under tension. If the bone surface is straight, the plate is prebent at the center to exert compression and on the opposite cortex when the plate is put under tension. (b) Good stability. The two screws that stabilize the small third fragment are inserted in lag screw fashion and compress the fracture gaps. If no bone defects are present, the reduced bone and the plate support each other. See Ref 3 for techniques. (c) Unstable situation where plate has only adapting and bridging functions, because the fragments are too small to be stabilized individually. Primary bone grafting may be indicated. This situation does not differ significantly from that shown in (d). (d) Plate has bridging function in leg-lengthening procedure. The gap between bone ends has been created intentionally for lengthening. Except for very young patients in whom a bone regenerate appears spontaneously, the gap is filled with bone grafts. Implant breakage has been rarely reported for this technique.

techniques were less advanced. Examples 1 through 7 in this section document such cases.

Example 1: Severe General Corrosion on Historic Lane Plate Made from Chromium Steel

Background and Discussion. The four-hole Lane plate shown in Fig. 6(a) was inserted 46 years ago and remained in the body for 26 years. A large portion of the plate disintegrated and consisted mainly of corrosion products. Figure 6(b) shows the extensive corrosion holes on a metallographic section of the plate. The plate, manufactured from a chromium steel, exhibited transformation structures and carbides. The screws, which are formed similar to wood screws, were made from a soft austenitic 304 stainless steel and exhibited minimal surface corrosion. The corrosion products of the plate impregnate the surrounding tissues, as seen on the microprobe analysis shown in Fig. 6(c).

Conclusion. This is a case of general corrosion due to improper materials selection. The corrosion may have been enhanced because of the austenitic stainless steel screws. In contrast, a recently retrieved intramedullary tibia nail of the type shown in Fig. 2(s), which had been in the body for 24 years, showed no signs of corrosion. This nail was produced from a low-carbon remelted type 316L stainless steel.

Example 2: Failure of a Stainless Steel Hip Fracture Fixation Device

Background. A Jewett nail hip implant failed after 2 months of service. Fracture occurred through the first of five screw holes in the plate section.

Table 2 Summary of failure analysis examples (case histories)

Example number	Type of device	Material	Failure mechanism
Failures related to implant deficiencies			
1.	Lane plate	Chromium steel	General corrosion due to improper materials selection
2.	Jewett nail	Type 316L stainless steel	Low-cycle fatigue failure due to repair welding
3.	Bone screw	Cast Co-Cr-Mo alloy (ASTM F 75)	Fracture due to casting defects
4.	Femoral head	Cast type 316L stainless steel	Fatigue failure due to coarse grain size
5.	Moore pins	Co-Cr alloy	Brittle fracture due to grain-boundary separation
6.	Bone plate	Type 316L stainless steel	Corrosion-fatigue fracture due to a nonmetallic inclusion
7.	Cerclage wire	Type 304 stainless steel	Intergranular corrosion due to sensitization
Failures related to mechanical or biomechanical conditions			
8.	Cortical bone screw	Type 316LR stainless steel	Shearing fracture
9.	Fixation device screws	Type 316LR stainless steel	Fatigue failure due to unstable fixation
10.	Bone plate	Type 316LR stainless steel	Fatigue-crack initiation and fretting corrosion due to implant instability
11.	Bone plate and screw	Type 316 stainless steel	Fatigue cracking due to placement of bone plate
12.	Angled blade plate	Type 316L stainless steel	Fatigue fracture possibly due to inadequate plate size
Failures related to implant degradation			
13.	Bone screw	Type 304 stainless steel	Pitting corrosion due to improper materials selection
14.	Bone plate	Type 316LR stainless steel	Fretting and fretting corrosion
15.	Screw head	Titanium	Fretting and fretting corrosion
16.	Bone screws	Type 316L stainless steel	Fracture due to combined pitting corrosion and fatigue
Failures related to inadequate design			
17.	Bone plate	300-series stainless steels	Fatigue failure due to improper design
Fractures of total hip joint prosthesis			
18.	Femoral head	Cast Co-Cr-Mo alloy (ASTM F 75)	Fatigue fracture at a gas pore and fretting corrosion
Fractures of total knee prosthesis			
19.	Tibial tray	Ti-6Al-4V (extra-low interstitial, or ELI)	Fatigue fracture due to improper process control during sintering of coating and subsequent heat treatments

The Jewett nail implant is widely used to assist in immobilizing the femoral head in cases where femoral neck fracture has occurred. The nail portion of the appliance is inserted through the neck, across the fracture, and into the head. The plate portion rests on the shank of the femur and is affixed to it with screws.

The applicable specification at the time of manufacture was ASTM F 55-66T, which pertains to stainless steel bars and wires for surgical implants.

Specimen Selection. Three samples were cut from the plate portion of the implant, two in the vicinity of the fracture and one away from the fracture. These samples were mounted in a cold-setting resin and used for metallographic examination and microhardness testing. A small section was cut from the plate section for chemical analysis.

Visual Examination and Macrostructural Analysis. Figure 7 shows the as-received device. Failure resulted from fracture of the plate section across the first screw hole. This is the area of maximum cyclic bending stress during service.

Figure 8 shows the mating fracture surfaces. It is evident that failure initiated at the outside (convex) surface of the plate and progressed through its thickness. The fracture morphology is characteristic of fatigue, in that it is flat and brittle in texture.

The inside surface of the plate section on the nail side is shown in Fig. 9. Note the beveled, burnished area in the final fracture zone caused by rubbing of the screw after fracture occurred. This burnishing indicates that the implant had been fractured for some time prior to its failure, which occurred within a relatively short time after implantation. The cyclic stresses in the fracture area were very high relative to the strength of the material, and failure required relatively few stress cycles.

Metallography and Microstructural Analysis. Metallographic examination of samples cut from the plate section of the implant revealed a series of repair welds on the inside surface of the plate in the vicinity of the fracture. These welds had been ground and polished and were not apparent until the implant was sectioned. Figure 10 shows two metallurgical

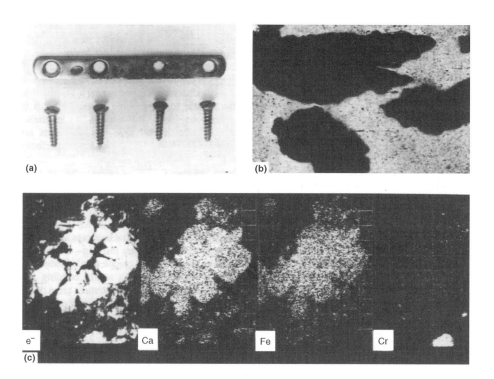

Fig. 6 Failed historic Lane plate. (a) Heavily corroded Lane plate from chromium steel. Implant was retrieved after 26 years. (b) Longitudinal section parallel to plate with large corrosion holes. 190×. (c) Microprobe analysis of tissue surrounding the plate. Chromium and iron corrosion products have impregnated the tissue. At the location shown, the question is whether the corrosion products penetrated bone structures or the impregnated tissue mineralized.

mounts of samples taken near the fracture. The repair welds are clearly delineated. The fracture surface is on the right in Fig. 10(a) and on the left in Fig. 10(b) and is approximately 2.5 mm ($^1/_{10}$ in.) from the welds. The microstructure in one of these semilenticular areas is shown in Fig. 11.

Figures 12 and 13 depict the microstructures observed away from the weld (and fracture) and near the weld (and fracture), respectively. Figure 12 shows the structure observed approximately 13 mm ($^1/_2$ in.) from the fracture shown in Fig. 10(b). This structure was unaffected by the heat of welding and was generally present in the plate material (strain-hardened austenite). The hardness of this material was determined to be 30 to 34 HRC, which is consistent with the observed microstructure.

The structure shown in Fig. 13 is recrystallized austenite. This structure was adjacent to the welds and at the fracture surface and was the direct result of repair welding, which created an annealed, softened zone. The hardness of this material was 80 to 86 HRB.

Chemical Analysis/Identification. The chemical composition of the implant material was analyzed as type 316L stainless steel, which was within specification for ASTM F 55-66T.

Discussion. The process of repair welding changed the condition of the material adjacent to the welds and substantially reduced yield strength, tensile strength, and attendant fatigue strength. The welds were placed at the point on the plate that experienced the most severe bending stresses in service. Thus, the plate was made weakest in the area where it should have been strongest.

Conclusion and Recommendations. The hip implant contained a series of hidden repair welds located on the inside of the plate section between the first and second screw holes. The plate material was recrystallized by the heat of welding, causing a severe loss in strength that led to low-cycle fatigue failure.

Manufacturers should never attempt to salvage this type of critical device by welding or any other procedure that might compromise its integrity.

Example 3: Retrieved Bone Screw Made from Co-Cr-Mo Alloy with Casting Defects

Discussion. Portions of the threads of the screw shown in Fig. 14(a) had broken off, and other threads had cracked. The screw was made from a cast Co-Cr-Mo alloy. A longitudinal section through the screw revealed gas porosity,

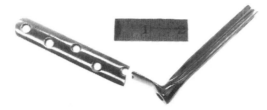

Fig. 7   As-received Jewett nail implant

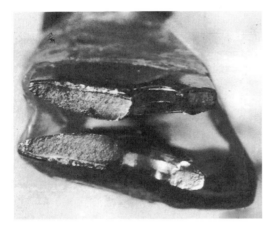

Fig. 8   Mating fracture surfaces. 14.24× Failure initiated on the outside (convex) surface and progressed across the plate thickness by low-cycle fatigue. ~15×

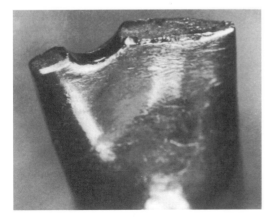

Fig. 9   Inside surface of the plate section on the nail side. The beveled zone was caused by rubbing of the screw head after fracture occurred.

segregation of primary inclusions, and oxides (Fig. 14b, c). The screw threads broke because of mechanical weakness from gas holes, brittleness, and dissolution of oxides.

Conclusion. With today's advanced casting techniques and testing methods, such implant defects can be avoided and eliminated.

Example 4: Fracture of a Cast Stainless Steel Femoral Prosthesis

Background. A cast 316L stainless steel femoral head replacement prosthesis failed midway down the stem within 13 months of implantation. This type of prosthesis is used to replace the femoral head and neck in cases of arthritic or other degenerative diseases of the hip.

The manufacturer specified a minimum yield strength of 240 MPa (35 ksi) and a minimum tensile strength of 480 MPa (70 ksi).

The substitution of cast stainless steel for the traditional wrought stainless steel or cast cobalt-chromium alloy in this application caused a dramatic reduction in strength and an attendant increase in the likelihood of mechanical failure. Cast stainless steel possesses roughly half the yield and tensile strengths of the other two materials.

Specimen Selection. Two samples were cut from the lower section of the stem, one at the fracture surface and the other from the bottom end. The samples were mounted to show longitudinal cross sections. Drillings from the lower section of the stem were used for chemical analysis.

Another prosthesis with identical grain sizes was obtained from the same manufacturer. Two substandard-sized tensile bars were machined, one from the bottom of the stem and the other from the body of the stem where the subject prosthesis fractured.

Visual Examination. Failure of the implant occurred approximately midway down the stem (Fig. 15). Severe "orange peel" was present around the fracture on the concave (compression) side of the stem. This effect (Fig. 16, see arrows) is indicative of an underlying coarse grain size. The surface markings on the portion of the stem on the right in Fig. 16 were made by the tool used to remove the stem from the femur after fracture.

Figure 17 shows the mating fracture surfaces. The fracture texture was coarse and faceted, again reflecting the underlying internal structure. Note that the orange peel was confined to the concave side of the stem. There was a complete absence of this effect on the convex (tensile) side of the fracture (indicated by arrows). Fracture in this area initiated and propagated via fatigue, culminating in overload failure of the remainder of the cross section accompanied by gross plastic deformation (orange peel).

Metallography and Microstructural Analysis. Metallographic examination of the two samples cut from the stem verified that the implant was a casting and that the grain size was extremely large. Figure 18 shows the mounted sections in the etched condition. There were only four grains through the entire section at the fracture.

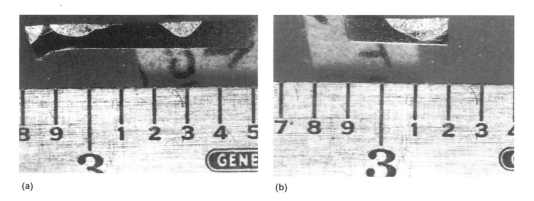

(a) (b)

Fig. 10 Metallurgical mounts of samples cut from the plate section at the fracture. The fracture surface is on the right in (a) and on the left in (b). The divisions on the scale are 2.5 mm ($^1/_{10}$ in.).

Figure 19 shows a secondary crack propagating from the convex side of the stem 13 mm ($\frac{1}{2}$ in.) from the main fracture. There was no plastic deformation in the material adjacent to this crack, characteristic of fatigue. The general microstructure consisted of a matrix of austenite with particles of ferrite, a structure commonly found in cast stainless steel.

Chemical analysis of the prosthesis showed that the material conformed to the requirements

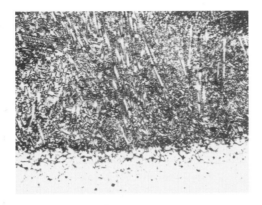

Fig. 11 Microstructure of one of the semilenticular areas in Fig. 10(a), clearly showing it to be a weldment. 61×

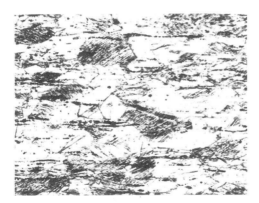

Fig. 12 Microstructure of material away from the repair welds. 122×

Fig. 13 Microstructure of material adjacent to the weld and at the fracture surface shown in Fig. 10(b). 122×

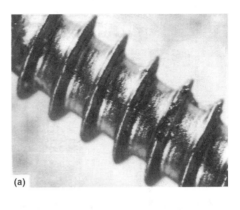

(a)

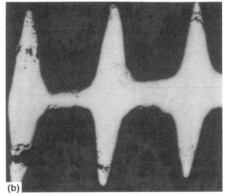

(b)

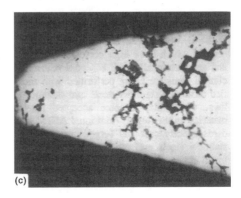

(c)

Fig. 14 Retrieved screw of cast Co-Cr-Mo alloy (type ASTM F 75). (a) Defective screw threads from casting deficiencies. (b) Longitudinal section through threads showing porosity. 15×. (c) Enlarged thread of section shown in (b) with gas holes, segregation of primary phases, and dissolved oxides. 155×

for type 316L stainless steel. It did not conform to any of the cast stainless steel alloys.

Mechanical Properties. Standard Rockwell tests conducted on the stem of the fractured prosthesis showed the hardness to be 70 to 71 HRB both at the end of the stem and near the fracture.

Tensile tests conducted on samples machined from the sample prosthesis supplied by the manufacturer yielded the following results:

Property	Sample taken from stem end (finer grain)	Sample taken from midstem (coarser grain)
0.2% offset yield strength, MPa (ksi)	211 (30.6)	173 (25.1)
Ultimate tensile strength, MPa (ksi)	460 (66)	418 (60.6)
Hardness, HRB	70–71	70–71

The prosthesis did not meet the manufacturer's stated strength criteria in the portion of the stem that fractured. It is interesting to note that the hardness did not reflect the difference in strength between the coarser- and finer-grained materials.

Discussion. It was evident that the prosthesis was incapable of sustaining the high cyclic stress imposed during service and failed via fatigue. Loads on the hip joint increase up to five times body weight during the heel-strike phase of walking. In addition, abnormal activity of the patient and/or deterioration of the fixation cement can result in increased stresses. Therefore, it is imperative that biocompatible materials of the highest possible strength be used for

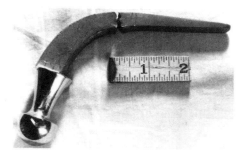

Fig. 15 Failed femoral head prosthesis

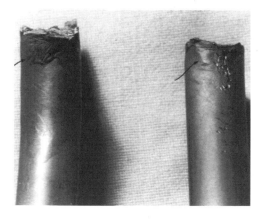

Fig. 16 Concave side of stem, showing gross orange-peel surface (arrows)

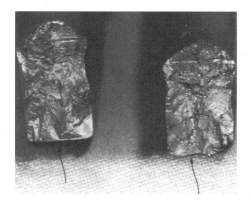

Fig. 17 Mating fracture surfaces. Fatigue fracture initiated on the convex (tensile) side of the stem (arrows).

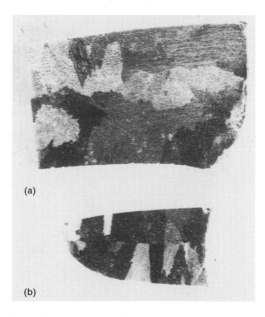

Fig. 18 Macrographs of the metallographic samples taken at (a) the fracture and (b) the stem end. The fracture surface is on the right in (a). 3×

prostheses so that the highest possible stresses can be tolerated. In this instance, a class of materials was chosen that was probably margin-

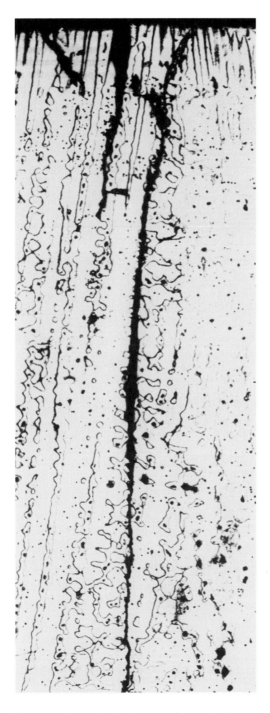

Fig. 19 Micrograph showing a secondary crack adjacent to the main fracture at the tensile surface of the stem. The crack is typical of fatigue. The general microstructure consists of a matrix of austenite with particles of ferrite. 81×

ally biocompatible but that possessed less than half the strength of the wrought stainless or cast cobalt-chromium alloys traditionally used.

The casting procedure produced an inordinately large grain size in the area that experienced the highest stress, further exacerbating the danger of failure. The well-known relationship between grain size and strength was effectively illustrated by the tensile tests performed on the sample prosthesis. Moreover, the tests showed that neither the fine- nor the coarse-grained material conformed to the manufacturer's own strength requirements.

Conclusion and Recommendations. The conditions of service are unknown, and the question as to whether or not the prosthesis would have failed even if a higher-strength material had been used cannot be answered. Therefore, the most probable cause of failure was the low strength of the prosthesis material, which resulted in fatigue failure in a relatively short period of service. The large grain size in the stem also must be considered a major factor in the reduced strength.

Whether failure would have occurred if the grain size had been less coarse is arguable. However, the class of material used for this application was mechanically weaker than those traditionally used.

Example 5: Broken Adjustable Moore Pins Made from Cobalt-Chromium Alloy

Background and Discussion. Two of four adjustable Moore pins, which had been used to stabilize a proximal femur fracture, were broken and deformed at their threads. The pins were made from a cobalt-chromium alloy and were not in the same condition. One pin contained brittle precipitates in the grains and grain boundaries. Correspondingly, the fracture occurred partially along the grain boundaries (Fig. 20a). Scanning electron microscopy (SEM) showed grain-boundary separation (Fig. 20b).

The nut used with the pin was made from a cast Co-Cr-Mo alloy and had segregations in the microstructure and gas holes and precipitates in the grain boundaries (Fig. 20c). The nut was not specifically loaded and did not fail.

The other broken pin was made from a cold-worked cobalt-chromium alloy. The grain boundaries contained few precipitates, but lines of primary inclusions were randomly distributed (Fig. 20d). The fracture surface exhibited a mixed fracture mode with intermingled dimples and fatigue striations (Fig. 20e). The pins did not exhibit any corrosion.

Conclusion. This example demonstrates how the different conditions of cobalt-chromium alloys affected failure behavior. In one of the Moore pins, brittle fracture was aided by grain-boundary separation.

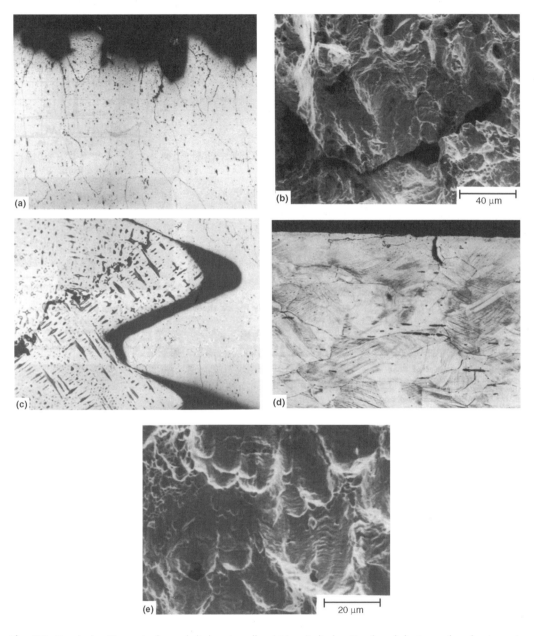

Fig. 20 Two broken Moore pins from cobalt-chromium alloy. (a) Longitudinal section through fracture surface showing grain-boundary precipitates and a partially intercrystalline fracture. 63×. (b) SEM fractograph indicating grain-boundary separation. Compare with (e). (c) Longitudinal section through screw and nut. The nut shows as-cast structures of Co-Cr-Mo alloy (type ASTM F 75). 160×. (d) Longitudinal section of the other broken pin in the cold-worked condition with fewer grain-boundary precipitates, lines of primary inclusions, and a small surface crack (there were more cracks along the surface). 100×. (e) Corresponding fracture surface with dimples and fatigue striations. Compare with (b).

Example 6: Microstructural Analysis of Failure of a Stainless Steel Bone Plate Implant

Background. In April 1999, a young patient received a stainless steel plate implant for a femoral fracture in the third medial left femur. Sixteen days later, the patient was urgently readmitted to the hospital because of "pain and functional impotence of the left femur." Radiography of the femur showed that the stainless steel bone plate had fractured and that no bone callus had formed.

The bone plate was a nine-hole dynamic compression device, typical of the orthopedic internal fixation devices used to stabilize fractured femurs. The plate was made of type 316L stainless steel and was correctly positioned on the tension side of the bone (Fig. 21).

The plate had fractured at the fourth hole from the top (Fig. 21) and had separated into two pieces: the top portion of the plate (as sketched in Fig. 21) is identified as part "A," and the bottom portion (the longest portion) is identified as part "B."

Materials Characterization. In order to investigate and to identify the causes of the implant failure, a certain number of samples were taken from the two portions: samples "a," "b," "c1," "c2," and "d," as indicated in Fig. 22. A series of analyses were performed to classify the material used to produce the plate and to valuate the correspondence to standard requirements. The referring standard was ASTM F 138 for implant materials, "Standard Specification for Wrought 18 Chromium-14 Nickel-2.5 Molybdenum Stainless Steel Bar and Wire for Surgical Implant (UNS S31673)." In accordance with the requirements reported in the standard specification, the stainless steel used to fabricate the plate was analyzed to determine the alloy composition and the morphology of secondary phases and nonmetallic inclusions.

The alloy composition was determined by microprobe electron analysis energy-dispersive x-ray spectroscopy coupled with a SEM. The secondary phases and nonmetallic inclusions were evaluated on metallographic cross sections (sections "c1" and "c2") of the plate after etching with Murakami solution. The concentration of inclusions was estimated referring to standard ASTM E 45, method A, reference II. The mechanical properties of the stainless steel were measured by Vickers micro-hardness tests. Sample "d" was tested for susceptibility to intergranular corrosion by following the practices recommended in ASTM A 262 section E. Sample "d" was also used for grain size determinations by following the practices recommended in ASTM E 112. The results of elemen-

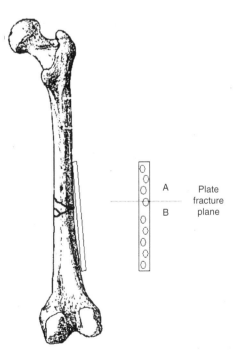

Fig. 21 Schematic of bone fracture and bone plate positioning

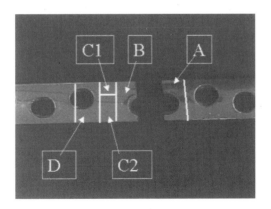

Fig. 22 Identification of bone plate samples used for failure analysis

tal analysis are reported in Table 3. The ASTM F 138 limit compositions are reported in the same table as reference. The plate composition is compatible with the ASTM specifications for type 316L, except for a slightly elevated manganese content. The silica content was below the maximum allowed by the specification.

The metallographic investigation for secondary phases did not reveal the presence of delta ferrite, and the nonmetallic inclusions were generally aluminum oxides, magnesium-aluminum spinel, and calcium aluminates. The more diffuse oxide inclusions found had globular form (named "type D" in ASTM E 45), and an average index of 0.8 was calculated. This inclusion index is lower than the allowable maximum of 1.0. It is important to note that some inclusions of not negligible dimensions were found next to the surface of the analyzed samples.

The average microhardness (Brinell scale) was 295 HB, which is slightly higher than the maximum accepted for hot-rolled bar (250 HB). This higher hardness suggests that the plate fabrication process caused minimal cold work to the implant. Sample "d" passed the intergranular corrosion test, proving absence of sensitization and a grain size number (5.17) that is higher than the minimum (5.0) allowed by ASTM E 112.

Discussion. The SEM images of the fractured surfaces of parts b and a are shown in Fig. 23 and 24. The fracture morphology is consistent with a brittlelike failure as consequence of a fatigue and/or corrosion fatigue. Fatigue striations are evident throughout most of the fracture surface (Fig. 23, part 1). Fatigue bands and secondary fractures orthogonal to the primary fracture surface are apparent in some locations (Fig. 23, part 2), as is a fracture terminated by ductile rupture or microvoid coalescence (Fig. 23, part 3). Additionally, several areas of surfaces a and b show clear evidence of plastic deformation caused by rubbing of the mating surfaces subsequent to the plate rupture.

Table 3 Elemental composition of bone plate (energy-dispersive x-ray spectroscopy microanalysis)

Element	Composition, wt%	ASTM F 138
Si	0.63 ± 0.03	0.75 max
S	<0.1	0.01 max
Cr	18.92 ± 0.09	17.00–19.00
Mn	2.31 ± 0.06	2.00 max
Ni	13.81 ± 0.11	13.00–15.00
Mo	2.84 ± 0.27	2.25–3.00
Fe	bal	bal

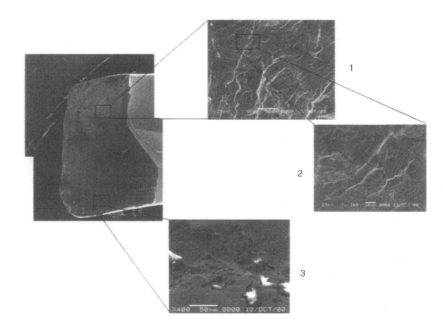

Fig. 23 SEM micrographs of surface fracture b. See text for details.

On the major section of the fractured surface of part a, it was possible to distinguish the initiation or origin of the crack that led to the collapse of the plate. The initiation site was a superficial surface inclusion that happened to have an internal inclusion in close proximity (Fig. 24).

Using the fractographic indications, it was possible to develop the progression of events that led to the fracture of the bone plate (Fig. 25). The fracture initiated at the point marked "1" (Fig. 25) and, because of bending stresses, propagated through the bone plate, as shown by the lines and arrows (marked "2"). The stresses on the nonfractured portion of the plate section increased as the crack grew, and when one side of the plate had fractured, the stress on the opposite side of the plate became significant. The increased stress on the nonfractured side of the plate was sufficient to cause the initiation of several fatigue cracks. The propagation of one of these cracks (marked "3") caused the formation of a new fracture surface (marked "4") and led to the complete fracture of the bone plate. The final fracture was in the region marked "5" in Fig. 25.

This crack-propagation sequence is corroborated by the observations on the external (thigh side) and internal (bone side) surface of the two portions of the fractured plate. The SEM of the external side of the plate showed a system of secondary cracks that developed orthogonally to the fracture surface (Fig. 26, part 1) and several other fatigue cracks on the top edge of the screw hole (Fig. 26, parts 2 to 4). These cracks were only on the side of the plate opposite the initiation site (marked with an arrow on Fig. 26). Final fracture of the plate occurred by the propagation of one of these flaws, as described previously.

In Fig. 27, micrographs of the plate surface on the bone side of the implant are shown. It is evident that the fracture features were practically obliterated because of rubbing after the final fracture. The observed zones correspond to the external edges of the final section of rupture (Fig. 25, marked "5").

Failure of plate fixation implant is not an unusual event. The failure frequency is approximately 13% for titanium implants and 1% for stainless steel implants.

In the absence of metallurgical defects or anomalous stress conditions, a properly installed 316L bone plate can last over 20 years in the human body. The most common damage mechanism is fatigue and/or corrosion fatigue. The fatigue is a phenomenon that, through cyclic loads, generates a small surface flaw that

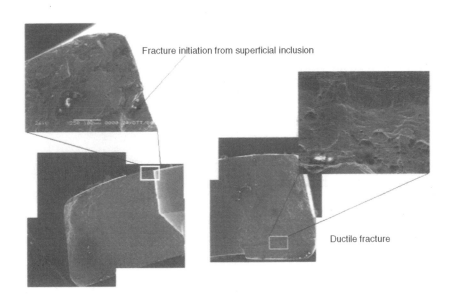

Fig. 24   SEM micrographs of surface fracture a with identification of fracture-initiation site. See text for details.

subsequently propagates to failure. The rate of propagation depends on the loading (stress) conditions but generally increases with time. The crack-propagation velocity can be very high and cause the rupture of a component in a few days or a few hours (depending on the load and cycle frequency). At low stresses, flaw initiation is generally very difficult in a part with a

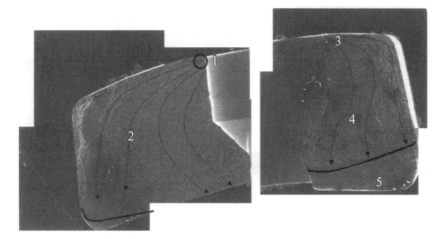

Fig. 25 Evolution of crack front on fracture surface a. See text for details.

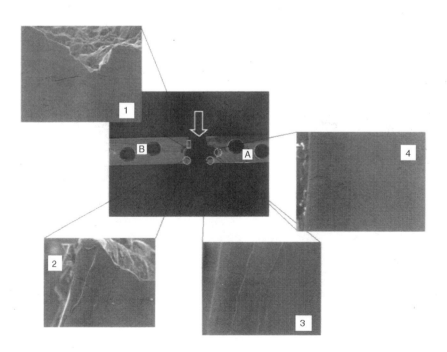

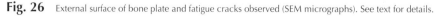

Fig. 26 External surface of bone plate and fatigue cracks observed (SEM micrographs). See text for details.

well-polished, inclusion-free surface. Under these conditions, the crack-initiation process may control the fatigue life of the component. However, in this case, the initiation event was bypassed because an existing inclusion served as the initiation site. The short time to failure is attributed to the ease of initiation and increased fatigue crack-propagation rates due to the presence of the low-pH, chloride-containing body fluids surrounding a fresh wound.

Conclusion. The femoral plate analyzed in this example failed because a nonmetallic (silica-alumina) inclusion on the plate surface and near a screw hole served as a crack-initiation site and significantly shortened, or eliminated, the crack-initiation time. This allowed the crack-propagation process to begin as soon as any cyclic loads were placed on the implant. Under these circumstances, the very aggressive environment (chlorides and pH 4 solution) typical of a fresh wound caused the propagation of a corrosion-fatigue flaw. Thus, the failure occurred under conditions that would not have been so onerous if the inclusion had not been present.

Additionally, the bone fracture reduction may not have been perfect, and relative movement between the two bone sections may have occurred. Such motion could cause the plate to be subjected to high bending stresses. The screw hole provided a stress concentration that, when added to the effect of the inclusion, was sufficient to make the activity associated with assisted perambulation drive the fatigue pro-

cess. The situation became progressively worse as the crack propagated, and a complete fracture of the implant required a very short period of time. This example illustrates the importance of steel cleanliness to the behavior of orthopedic implants.

Example 7: Intergranular Corrosion on Cerclage Wire of Sensitized 304 Type Stainless Steel

Background. The wire was used with two screws and washers for a tension band fixation (Ref 3) in a corrective internal fixation (Fig. 28). The cerclage wire was found broken at several points and corroded when it was removed after 9 months (Fig. 29a).

Metallographic analysis revealed that the wire was made of type 304 stainless steel without molybdenum, as seen in the energy-dispersive x-ray analysis (Fig. 29b); this material does not comply with the standards. The screws and washers were intact and were made of remelted implant-quality type 316L stainless steel, corresponding to the standards. The microstructure of the wire, which was in the soft condition, as

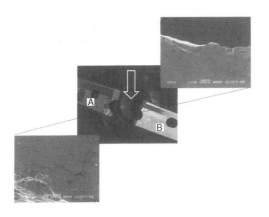

Fig. 27 Internal surface of bone plate (bone side) and fatigue cracks observed (SEM micrographs)

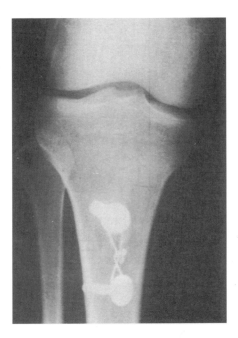

Fig. 28 Radiograph showing a tension band fixation containing a cerclage wire, two screws, and washers beneath the screw heads. See also Fig. 29.

required, showed signs of sensitization, with chromium carbide precipitates at the grain boundaries (Fig. 29c). Typical intergranular corrosion with pitted grains was evident through SEM fractography (Fig. 29d).

Conclusion. For this internal fixation, orthopedic wire of an insufficient stainless steel type was used. Improper heat treatment of the steel led to intergranular corrosion and implant separation. The wire came from a source different from that of the screws and washers and did not meet current standards for orthopedic wire.

Failures Related to Mechanical or Biomechanical Conditions

Bone screws fracture in two modes—by mechanical forces during insertion or removal or by fatigue failure. Examples for both are given as follows.

Mechanically forced shearing fractures are a typical failure in screws (see Example 8 in this chapter). Although stainless steel bone screws are normally manufactured from cold-worked material, their shearing ductility is usually considerable. Ductile shearing fractures are characterized by a spiral texture of the fracture surface, flow lines at the fracture edges, overload dimple structure on the fracture surface, and heavily deformed microstructure at the fracture edge in longitudinal sections. Occasionally, screw heads can be sheared off by repeated tightening, particularly when the cortex (dense outer bone wall) is thick, because the thicker the cortex, the higher the retention of the screw. Excessive oblique positioning of the screw in a plate hole can also cause fracture if the screw head is bent by the plate hole during insertion.

Fatigue Failures of Screws. As discussed in Example 9 in this chapter, fatigue failure at varying thread levels is also a problem sometimes encountered. One of the causes of such failures is unstable fixation.

Fatigue Damage of Bone Plates. Most broken plates have been loaded under unilateral

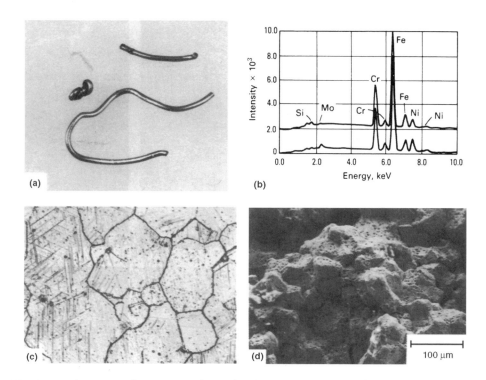

Fig. 29 Intergranular corrosion of a type 304 stainless steel cerclage wire. (a) Broken cerclage wire. (b) Energy-dispersive x-ray analysis under the SEM. Lower spectrum: reference material type 316L screw material. Upper spectrum: type 304 steel with less nickel content and no molybdenum from investigated implant wire. (c) Cross section of sensitized wire, with grain boundaries and deformation lines heavily attacked by etching because of chromium carbide precipitates. 180×. (d) Fracture surface under SEM indicating intergranular corrosion with pits on grain surfaces

bending, because bone defects in the opposite cortex are a typical cause of instability and breakage. Thus, tensile and shearing stresses are created in the top surface of the plate. Correspondingly, this is the surface where crack initiation is usually found. Depending on the fracture situation and the location, torsional stresses can also be created. This is especially true in forearm fractures because of the rotational motion that takes place. Examples 10 to 12 in this chapter show three stages of fatigue damage on bone plates.

Example 8: Shearing Fracture of a Type 316LR Stainless Steel Screw

Background and Discussion. The cortical bone screw shown in Fig. 30 broke during the internal fixation procedure. The fracture surface (Fig. 30a) exhibited extensive spiral deformation. Figure 30(b) shows the dimple structure characteristic of a ductile failure mode. The dimples are oriented uniformly in the deformation direction. Figure 30(c) shows a magnifica-

tion of the flow lines at the fracture edge. The longitudinal metallographic section perpendicular through the fracture surface (Fig. 30d) exhibited a zone of heavily deformed grains at the fracture edge. The microstructure and the hardness of the screw corresponded to the standards.

For comparison, the shearing fractures of a commercially pure titanium screw and a cast Co-Cr-Mo alloy (ASTM F 75) screw are shown in Fig. 31 and 32. The spiral-textured fracture surface of the titanium screw was smooth (Fig. 31a) and had uniform, shallow shearing tongues and dimples indicative of a ductile fracture mode (Fig. 31b).

In contrast, the fracture surface of the cast Co-Cr-Mo alloy screw had an erratic structure (Fig. 32a), which can be explained by the large grain size and the tendency of the grains to fracture along crystallographic planes. Figure 32(b) shows such fracture planes of differently oriented grains. These planes exhibited crystallographically oriented mixed shearing structures and dimples (Fig. 32c), as well as traces of slip (Fig. 32d). Gas holes with dendritic freezing

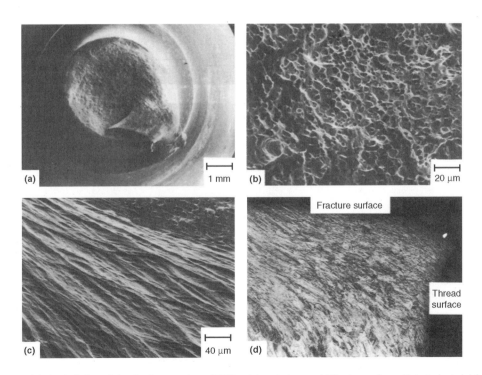

Fig. 30 Mechanically forced shearing fracture of type 316LR stainless steel screw. (a) Fracture surface with typical spiral deformation texture. SEM. (b) Closeup of fracture surface with shear dimples oriented in twisting direction. (c) Fracture edge with flow lines. (d) Longitudinal metallographic section through fracture surface. Deformation zone from shearing is adjacent to the fracture edge. Original deformation structure of the screw is visible at the bottom of the micrograph. 62×

surfaces are shown in Fig. 32(e). In the longitudinal section of a similar screw (Fig. 32f), large grains can be observed, along with deformation between the threads, which leads to shear rupture. Figure 32(g) shows a starting shear crack propagating along slip planes.

Conclusion. The shear fracture most likely occurred because the screw was inserted very obliquely in the screw hole and therefore sheared off.

Example 9: Characteristic Observations on Type 316LR Stainless Steel Screws That Failed by Fatigue

Discussion. Fatigue fracture can occur on different thread levels, depending on the loading situation (Fig. 33a). No deformation zone was created at the fracture site shown in the longitudinal metallographic section in Fig. 33(b). Occasionally, the initiation of secondary fatigue cracks is found parallel to the fracture plane or in a nearby thread groove. Figure 33(c) shows one of the fracture surfaces with fatigue striations.

Corresponding to the energy-dispersive x-ray analyses, the screws (Fig. 33a) were manufactured from cold-worked remelted (R) type 316L stainless steel and showed no structural or manufacturing defects. The material meets ASTM F 138 Special Quality specifications. The screws were used with a relatively rigid plate to treat a fracture complication in the upper end of the femur.

Conclusion. Radiographs indicated various signs of unstable fixation, which explains the fatigue failures. The two screws were situated at the distal end of a compression screw plate, where the proximal lever arm was the longest, compared to the other screws.

Example 10: Fatigue Initiation on Type 316LR Straight Bone Plate

Background. The plate shown in Fig. 34(a) and (b) was used to treat a pseudarthrosis in the proximal femur. Because healing did not progress, the plate was removed and submitted for investigation. The bone was replated with an angled blade plate, and compression was exerted on the pseudarthrosis to promote bone healing.

Investigation. The plate seemed to be macroscopically intact. At higher magnification, fatigue cracks were apparent on the top surface of the small section of the plate (Fig. 35) at the fifth screw hole indicated on Fig. 34(a). In the background of the surface, slip systems are visible, partially in conjunction with initial cracks.

From crack-initiation studies, it is known that persistent slip systems appear first on the surface that is loaded under critical cyclic stresses. Precracks and initial cracks develop from these slip systems. Some of the initiation cracks propagate further and become major cracks that penetrate the cross section. The extent of this

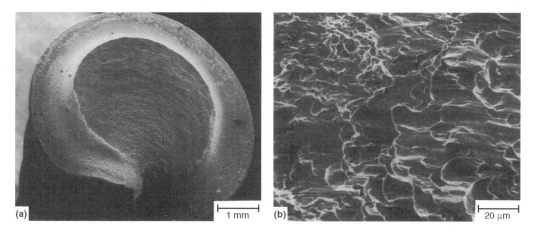

(a) 1 mm   (b) 20 µm

Fig. 31 Shear fracture of a commercially pure titanium screw. (a) SEM fractograph showing spiral-textured fracture surface of sheared-off screw. Typical deformation lines are fanning out on the thread. (b) Uniformly distributed shearing tongues and dimples

fatigue surface damage is representative for the stress intensity.

Figure 35 shows structures as were described previously for the fatigue-initiation process. The intensity of these structures, compared to results of systematic crack-initiation experiments, sug-gested that the plate was rather heavily loaded. Morphological comparison and fatigue-initiation curves indicated that a local stress concentration of 500 to 600 MPa (72 to 87 ksi) was present. This load would still be below the elastic limit of the cold-worked stainless steel. No

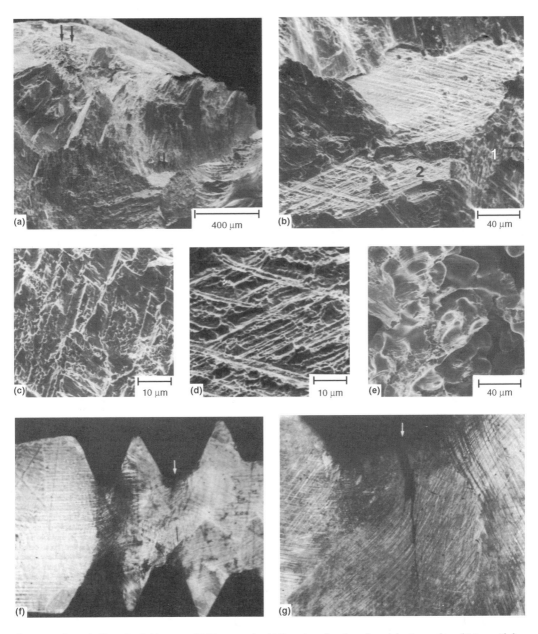

Fig. 32 Sheared-off cast Co-Cr-Mo screw. SEM fractography. (a) Overview of portion of rough fracture surface. (b) Area with fracture planes of three differently oriented grains (single arrow, Fig. 32a). (c) Shearing structures and dimples in grain identified by the numeral 1 in Fig. 32(b). (d) Slip traces in grain identified by the numeral 2 in Fig. 32(b). (e) Gas holes with dendritic freezing surfaces (double arrows, Fig. 32a). (f) Longitudinal section through identical screw with starting shearing damage. 10×. (g) Shearing crack (arrow, Fig. 32f). 130×

fatigue cracks were visible on the broad section of the asymmetrically placed hole. Thus, fatigue damage occurred earlier in the portion with the smaller cross section. In addition, rotational forces are to be expected in this area.

Fatigue-bending tests on such broad plates showed that the fatigue life of plates with asymmetrically arranged holes is at least as long as for plates with holes situated in the center. At a centered screw hole, fatigue initiates at approximately the same time on both sides of the hole. At the asymmetrically placed holes, fatigue begins at the large section only after a fatigue crack begins to propagate into the small plate section.

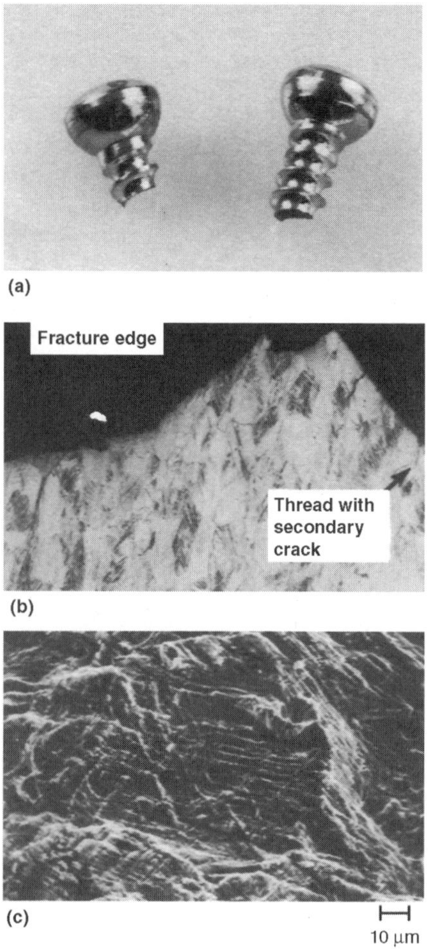

(a)

Fracture edge

Thread with secondary crack

(b)

(c)   ⊢―⊣
                                        10 μm

Fig. 33 Type 316LR stainless steel screws that failed by fatigue. (a) Fatigue fractures at different thread levels. (b) Longitudinal section perpendicular to fracture surface without deformation zone at fracture site. A small secondary crack is shown at thread site (arrow). 55×. (c) Fatigue striations on fracture surface

Discussion. Although fatigue cracks are observed more frequently at the edges of the plate holes, crack initiation often takes place on the total surface area adjacent to the middle section of the plate hole. This is demonstrated on another broken plate (Fig. 36), in which a large secondary crack had developed parallel to the main crack in the center of the surface. Another small crack was visible on the edge of the plate hole. A large portion of the plate surface at the fracture edge showed deformation from fatigue damage. Crack initiation does not take place in the plate holes and is not related to the fretting that may occur between the screw head and plate. An exception may be some special plate hole designs for which corrosion fatigue was reported (Ref 18).

In Fig. 35, no crack initiation is visible at the pits caused by electropolishing. In addition, mechanical marks from the plate bending did not act as stress raisers. The stainless steel has no particular notch sensitivity, and the fatigue behavior is forgiving with respect to mechanical damage.

In the radiographs shown in Fig. 34(a) and (b), extensive bone deficiency is present in the area where two plate holes were not filled with screws. In Fig. 34(b), a wide gap is visible. The empty screw hole (No. 6 from the top) situated directly over the defect does not show fatigue damage, but hole No. 5, which sits at the edge of the proximal bone fragment, has the described fatigue cracks. Because screw hole No. 5 was situated at the transition between the supporting bone and the defect, stress concentration was higher here than at the empty hole No. 6, where the elastic deformation could occur more uniformly. In the defect zone of the original fracture, between screws No. 4 and 7, the plate is not supported by the bone, and the load is transmitted only through the plate, which caused cyclic loading of the implant and fatigue-crack initiation.

It is also characteristic that fretting corrosion occurred at the screw/plate interface at screw hole No. 7. This screw was closest to the bone defect and was secured only in one cortex. Compared to all the other screws, this one was the most likely to undergo relative motion. As outlined in the legend in Fig. 34(a), at all other contact areas between screw head and plate hole either minimal or no fretting, or fretting corrosion and mechanical damage, was found.

Conclusion. For this analysis, only the two radiographs shown in Fig. 34 were available. They are not adequate to estimate the clinical postoperative history, but they are sufficient to explain the fatigue-crack initiation due to insta-bility.

Example 11: Fatigue Crack on a Type 316 Stainless Steel Bone Plate and Corresponding Broken Screw

Background. A narrow bone plate was used to stabilize an open midshaft femur fracture in an 18 year old patient.

Investigation. As seen in Fig. 37(a), a radiograph taken 13 weeks after the operation, the plate had a crack at a plate hole next to the fracture site. The plate was slightly bent in the horizontal plane, and the fracture gap was con-siderably open. In the lateral view, a broken screw is visible at the second plate hole above the fracture gap (Fig. 37b).

The screws and plate shown in Fig. 37(c) were supplied by three different manufacturers.

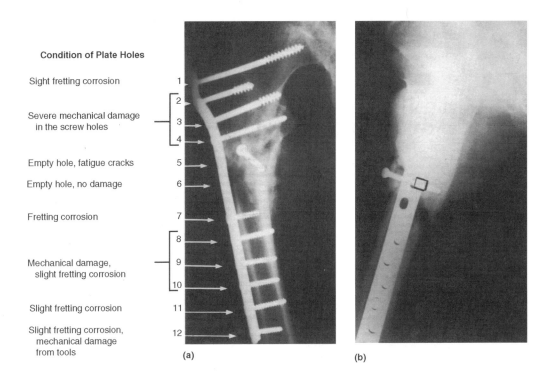

Condition of Plate Holes

Sight fretting corrosion — 1

2

Severe mechanical damage — 3
in the screw holes

4

Empty hole, fatigue cracks — 5

Empty hole, no damage — 6

Fretting corrosion — 7

8

Mechanical damage, — 9
slight fretting corrosion

10

Slight fretting corrosion — 11

Slight fretting corrosion, — 12
mechanical damage
from tools

(a)   (b)

Fig. 34   Crack initiation on type 316LR stainless steel dynamic compression plate. (a) Anterior-posterior radiograph. The plate was used to treat the nonunion of a fracture between the fourth and seventh screws. The plate was bent intraoperatively to fit the contour of the bone. (b) Radiograph with lateral view showing wide bone gap, indicating instability. The boxed area indicates the location of initiating fatigue cracks.

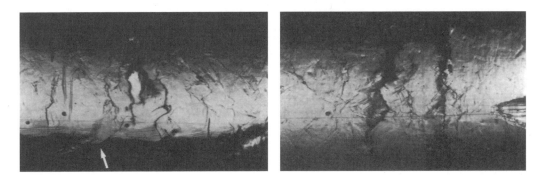

Fig. 35   Two views of the plate surface with fatigue cracks at the fifth hole shown in Fig. 34(a). White arrow (left) indicates tool mark from bending that does not interfere with fatigue damage structure. See text for further description. Both 110×

The compression holes of the plate are a modification of those of other implant systems. Energy-dispersive x-ray analyses indicated that all implants were made of type 316 stainless steel. However, the microcleanliness of the materials was different. The minimal primary inclusion content found in the plate and in one of the screws was typical of high-quality re-

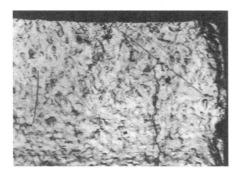

Fig. 36 Top surface of broken plate of type 316LR stainless steel. Fatigue cracks parallel to the fracture edge and a wide area exhibiting primary fatigue deformation are visible. 65×

melted steel that meets the requirements in ASTM F 138. The remaining screws from a different source, including the broken screw, had a high primary inclusion content and did not comply with this standard.

Figure 38(a) shows a longitudinal section perpendicular to the fracture surface of the broken screw. The local crack formation appeared to have been influenced by the presence of larger inclusions. From the striations found on the fracture surface under the SEM, it was concluded that the screw failed through a fatigue mechanism. In addition to the fatigue striations, many dimples were present (Fig. 38b), which were created primarily through inclusions. In areas with final overload structures, the dimple formation was also influenced by inclusions (Fig. 38c).

The crack in the plate originated at the upper, outer corner of the plate, as seen from the beach marks in Fig. 38(d). This indicates the action of asymmetric bending and rotational forces. The beach marks were oxidized, and the fracture surface was covered with fatigue striations (Fig. 38e).

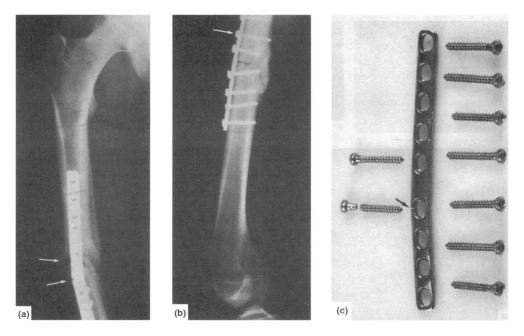

Fig. 37 Stainless steel bone plate with fatigue crack and broken screw. (a) Radiograph taken 13 weeks after operation. Anterior-posterior view. Arrows indicate crack in plate and open fracture gap. (b) Corresponding lateral view. Arrow indicates broken screw. (c) Bend in plate in the horizontal plane at the unfractured side of a screw hole (arrow). Deformation was due to dorso-lateral acting forces. Screws are not placed at original position. See also Fig. 38.

Discussion. Not all clinical details of this case are known, but from a biomechanical viewpoint based on the radiographs (Fig. 37a, b), the fatigue failures of the plate and screw can be attributed to the unusual placement of the narrow bone plate. Because of the open fracture situation with severe soft tissue damage, the narrow plate was placed on the frontal aspect of the femur, which is not a typical configuration. A broad plate is usually applied at the lateral side of the femur if plate fixation is indicated. Physiologically, the lateral side of the femur is under tension, and if the plate is mounted laterally, exerting compression on the fracture site creates a tension band effect, which provides excellent stability (see Fig. 5a and Ref 3).

In this case, the plate was not on the tension side, and obviously, no compression (or not enough compression) had been applied. Because of the anatomic conditions and the fracture configuration, the plate was loaded under asymmetric bending and torsional forces, which created maximum stresses at the lateral edge of the plate hole near the fracture site. This is confirmed by the location of the fatigue-crack origin shown on the fracture surface in Fig. 38(d).

The instability of the internal fixation was indicated by the callus formation, by the rounded edges of the fracture ends, and by some screw loosening. The first screw over the fracture gap was definitely loose, as deduced from the resorption hole in the cortex beneath the plate. This caused additional loading on the next screw, which failed by fatigue. Because of the different sources of the implants, the head design of some of the screws was not compatible with the screw hole geometry of the plate. This did not cause the instability but may have hastened its progress. Similarly, the inclusion content of the screw did not cause the fatigue failure but may have reduced the fatigue strength to some extent.

Conclusion. This example shows that a smaller plate and an unusual positioning had to be chosen because of the critical soft tissue con-

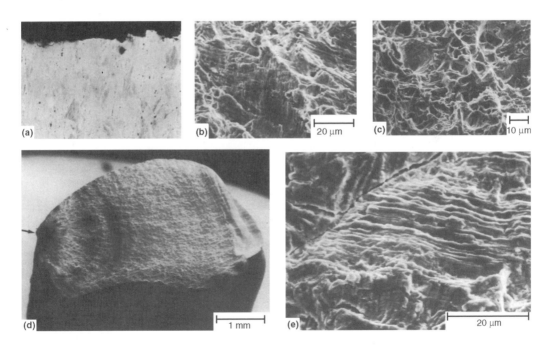

Fig. 38 Fracture surfaces of the failed screw and bone plate shown in Fig. 37. (a) Longitudinal section through fractured screw showing edge of fracture surface and high inclusion content. A large slag inclusion was present at the void under the fracture edge. 55×. (b) Fracture surface of screw showing fatigue striations (containing secondary cracks) and dimples. (c) Fracture surface of screw and zone showing overload fracture containing large dimples partly caused by inclusions. (d) Plate fracture surface. Arrow points to crack origin, which is indicated by beach marks. (e) Fatigue striations from center of plate fracture surface (running originally transverse to loading direction)

dition, which leads to decreasing stability and eventual fatigue failure. It is important to realize that at the time of injury, the soft tissues have priority because of the risk of serious complications. After plate removal, the fracture was stabilized with an intramedullary nail, and bone healing proceeded.

Example 12: Fatigue Fracture of a Type 316L Stainless Steel Angled Plate

Discussion. Figure 39(a) shows a broken angled plate that was applied to the proximal femur. The fatigue fracture occurred at a plate hole. The fatigue damage at the fracture edge at the top surface of the plate indicated that symmetric cyclic bending forces had acted. Figure 39(b) shows slip bands produced on the surface during cyclic loading. Figure 39(c) reveals fatigue striations.

The microstructure of the plate had a high degree of cleanliness (Fig. 39d). The deforma-

tion structure showed that the material was in the cold-worked condition, which was confirmed by Vickers hardness tests. Energy-dispersive x-ray analysis indicated a chemical composition corresponding to a type 316 stainless steel (the carbon content was not determined).

Conclusion. The plate material corresponded to the current standards for surgical implants and was not the cause of the implant failure. Because no radiographs or other clinical details were available, it could not be evaluated if the plate size was adequate for the clinical conditions.

Fatigue Properties of Implant Materials

Remelted Type 316LR Stainless Steels. Because metal fatigue accounts for most implant fractures, some fatigue properties of type 316LR stainless steel, based on experimental studies (Ref 19, 20), are addressed.

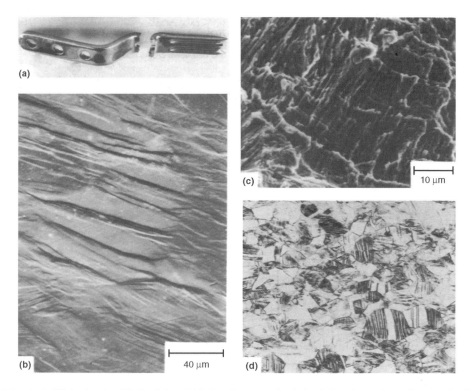

Fig. 39 Angled blade plate that failed by fatigue. (a) Fatigue fracture at plate hole. (b) Top plate surface at fracture edge showing intense fatigue surface damage (slip bonds), indicating that the plate was heavily loaded. (c) SEM of fracture surface. Fatigue striations can be seen in the grain at the lower right-hand corner. Other fracture features are crystallographically oriented. (d) Microstructure of cross section reveals that plate was made from cold-worked stainless steel of high microcleanliness. 80×

The *S-N* (stress-number of cycles) fatigue curves for the steel in recrystallized and cold-worked conditions are shown in Fig. 40. As shown in Fig. 40(a), the fully reversed bending tests were performed on flat specimens in air and in Ringer's solution (a lactated 0.9% sodium chloride solution that contains approximately the same concentration of Cl^- ions as body fluids). The improved fatigue strength in the cold-worked condition is of particular interest for implants. Plates, screws, pins, and certain nails are produced mainly from cold-worked material. The fatigue limits determined in rotating-bending beam tests on the same materials are comparably higher than those found in the bending tests (Ref 19).

In the recrystallized condition, the fatigue strength of the steel is not significantly affected by Ringer's solution. In the cold-worked condition, fatigue life in the high-cycle range is reduced in Ringer's solution. Corrosion fatigue in the usual sense, however, does not occur, because, morphologically, no signs of corrosion are detectable by optical microscopy and SEM. Ringer's solution appears to accelerate the individual fatigue stages. This complies with observations of fracture surfaces of broken plates that do not show a corrosive component combined with their fatigue structures and which do not differ from structures produced experimentally in air.

Additions of 0.25% clottable fibrinogene to the Ringer's solution have been shown to neutralize its fatigue-life reducing effect. The corresponding *S-N* fatigue curves were similar to those generated in air (Ref 21).

On retrieved implants, however, it has been found that fatigue-fracture surfaces can secondarily corrode when crevice or fretting conditions develop in the fracture gap. Such corrosion structures can be locally observed. In the transition areas, fatigue striations with superimposed corrosion pits can be seen (Fig. 41a, b).

Implants rarely fail under conditions where fatigue loading exceeds the yield stress and plastic deformation takes place. Table 4 lists the relationships between the ultimate tensile stress, yield stress, and fatigue limits for the recrystallized and cold worked stainless steel used to generate the fatigue curves shown in Fig. 40(a).

The fatigue endurance limit of the cold-worked stainless steel corresponds to approximately 30% of the yield stress, whereas that of the recrystallized steel condition corresponds to approximately 67% of the yield stress. If, at stresses below the yield stress, deformation structures develop on the specimen surface before fatigue cracks form, one must conclude that these deformation structures are created by local repeated elastic deformations. Examination of test specimen surfaces during the fatigue tests described previously shows how fatigue cracks develop from cumulative surface damage (Ref 20). This is illustrated on replicas of a recrystallized stainless steel specimen that was fatigued in Ringer's solution (Fig. 42a to d). The following stages of fatigue surface damage were observed: formation of persistent slip steps, slip bands, increasing quantities of multiple slip systems, precracks, short secondary

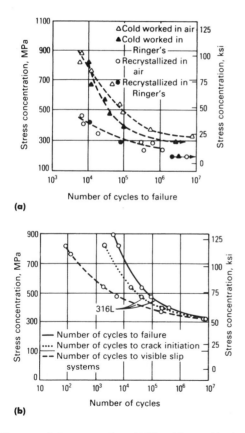

(a)

(b)

Fig. 40 Fatigue curves of type 316LR stainless steel implant material tested in bending mode. (a) *S-N* curves for stainless steel in cold-worked and soft condition that was tested in air and aerated lactated Ringer's solution. (b) Fatigue curve for number of cycles to failure as shown in Fig. 40(a) for cold-worked stainless steel that was fatigued in air. The two additional curves show the number of cycles to initiation of visible slip systems and the number of cycles to crack initiation. Source: Ref 20

cracks, and one or several major cracks. A main crack will then propagate through the cross section of the specimen. The same processes are morphologically observed on specimens fatigued in air; however, they proceed more slowly in air. This mechanism explains how fatigue cracks initiate without flaws or particular stress raisers.

The slip bands created by fatigue often have the character of extrusions that are accompanied by intrusions. These intrusions can act as micronotches and initiate cracks. On retrieved broken stainless steel implants, the fatigue damage structure described previously is preserved on the surface in the vicinity of the fracture edge.

From the systematic evaluation of test specimens during the fatigue process, S-N curves of early fatigue damage were generated (Ref 20). As shown in Fig. 40(b) for the cold-worked

stainless steel, curves for the number of cycles to visible slip system formation and crack initiation are similar to the S-N curve for the number of cycles to failure. The curves indicate that the lower the load, the longer the time spent in the initiation stage.

Micrographs of failed fatigue specimens of the cold-worked stainless steel show that the intensity of fatigue surface damage adjacent to the fracture edge depends on the load (Fig. 43a to c). At low stress levels, few glide systems develop. This surface morphology can be used to estimate if an implant was loaded in the high- or low-cyclic fatigue range.

On stainless steel implants, fatigue striations are abundant on the fracture surfaces, unless the surface has been subjected to secondary mechanical damage. In addition to fatigue striations, crystallographic fracture structures are found. The latter appears before a stable crack

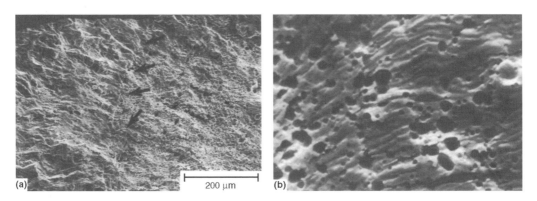

Fig. 41 Secondary corrosion attack on fatigue-fracture surface. (a) Fracture surface of 5 mm (0.2 in.) long crack in an intramedullary tibia nail made of cold-worked type 316LR stainless steel. The crack developed during the early postoperative stage when the fixation was unstable and bending and rotational forces acted on the nail. The crack did not impair fracture healing or nail removal. The fracture surface was covered with fatigue structures except for a small zone where shallow corrosion pits superimposed the fatigue structures. Locally, critical crevice conditions must have developed in the crack. Under weight bearing, small relative motion can take place in the gap, damaging the passive film. In addition, stagnation and acidification of the body liquid is possible. Arrows indicate the transition between fatigue and corrosion structures. The microstructure of the nail showed no irregularities and was not connected with the corrosion. (b) Shallow secondary corrosion pits superimposed on fatigue striations.

Table 4 Relationship between the ultimate tensile stress, yield stress, and fatigue limit for cold-worked and recrystallized type 316LR stainless steel

Material condition	UTS(a)		Yield stress(b)		Fatigue limit		Ratio of fatigue limit to UTS	Ratio of fatigue limit to yield stress
	MPa	ksi	MPa	ksi	MPa	ksi		
Cold worked	1050	152	994	144	300	43.5	0.28	0.30
Recrystallized	590	85.5	266	38.5	180	26	0.30	0.67

(a) UTS, ultimate tensile stress. (b) Yield stress = $\sigma_{0.2\%}$ yield stress

front forms. Secondary cracks, which run parallel to fatigue striations, do not indicate stress corrosion or corrosion fatigue (Ref 19).

Wrought Type ASTM F 563 Cobalt Alloy. The fatigue-crack-initiation mechanism in wrought cobalt alloys was assessed with the same type of tests described for stainless steel. Morphologically, the process is the same as that for stainless steel, but all initiation steps are shifted to higher stress values because of the higher strength and fatigue resistance of alloy ASTM F 563.

Compared to stainless steels, the morphology of the fatigue-fracture surfaces is characterized by very dense patterns of fatigue striations. These patterns superimpose the normally dominating crystallographic structures. It is sometimes difficult to distinguish fatigue striations from glide or tearing structures. This is particularly true when the glide systems have an orientation that accommodates the formation of striations (Fig. 44a to c). The toughness of these types of wrought cobalt alloys is assumed to account for this behavior.

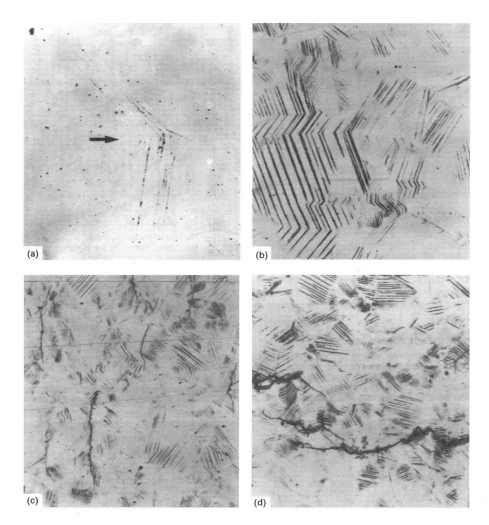

Fig. 42 Free surface replica showing the development of fatigue surface damage on recrystallized type 316LR stainless steel in aerated Ringer's solution at 38 °C (100 °F), at applied stress of 250 MPa (35.5 ksi). (a) The first visible slip systems developed at a triple point (decorated persistent slip steps) after 500 load cycles. 225×. (b) Increased density of multiple slip systems after 29,500 cycles. 275×. (c) Short cracks that developed in a zigzag pattern between glide systems after 40,700 cycles. Loading axis is horizontal to the micrograph. 110×. (d) Major cracks that were partially developed through coalescence of short cracks after 60,000 cycles. Loading axis is vertical to the micrograph. 90×. The specimen failed after 69,113 cycles.

Commercially Pure Titanium. The morphology of fatigue initiation and propagation of titanium is more complex than that of stainless steel. The limited number of glide systems of the hexagonal close-packed crystal structure of titanium is assisted by twinning processes to

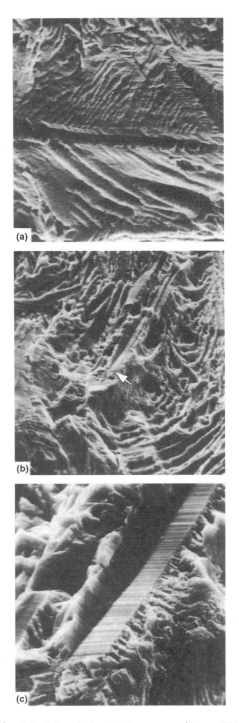

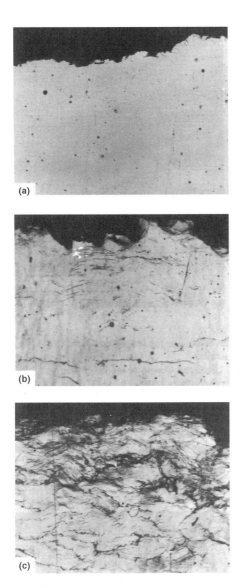

Fig. 43 Cold-worked type 316LR stainless steel that was fatigued in air at different stress levels. Surfaces of broken specimens at fracture edge are shown. (a) Failure at an applied stress of 330 MPa (47.8 ksi) after 7,682,434 load cycles. Only a few glide systems adjacent to the fracture edge are visible. 70×. (b) Failure at an applied stress of 600 MPa (87 ksi) after 105,308 cycles. Multiple glide systems and additional cracks near the fracture edge are shown. 55×. (c) Failure at an applied stress of 800 MPa (116 ksi) after 5308 cycles. Heavy deformation structure and multiple additional cracks appear. 55×

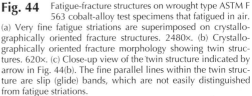

Fig. 44 Fatigue-fracture structures on wrought type ASTM F 563 cobalt-alloy test specimens that fatigued in air. (a) Very fine fatigue striations are superimposed on crystallographically oriented fracture structures. 2480×. (b) Crystallographically oriented fracture morphology showing twin structures. 620×. (c) Close-up view of the twin structure indicated by arrow in Fig. 44(b). The fine parallel lines within the twin structure are slip (glide) bands, which are not easily distinguished from fatigue striations.

allow plastic deformation (Ref 22). Correspondingly, the range of ductile behavior of titanium is more limited than that of stainless steel.

The corrosion resistance of titanium in the body and its tissue compatibility are excellent. There have been no reported cases of allergies to titanium. Unfortunately, the wear properties of titanium and its alloys are poor; therefore, they are not usually chosen as material for the articulation surfaces of prostheses.

The same fatigue experiments described for type 316LR stainless steels were performed on commercially pure titanium specimens. For comparison, Fig. 45 shows the fatigue surface damage on a broken titanium test specimen. The polarized light reveals that twinning, wavy glide, and grain-boundary distortion contribute to the fatigue damage on the specimen surface.

The fatigue-fracture surfaces of titanium can show very different features, depending on overall and local stress conditions, crystallographic orientation, and material conditions. Figures 46(a) to (c) show fractographs of the surface of a cold-worked titanium specimen fatigued at a stress level of 600 MPa (87 ksi). Depending on local stress distribution and grain

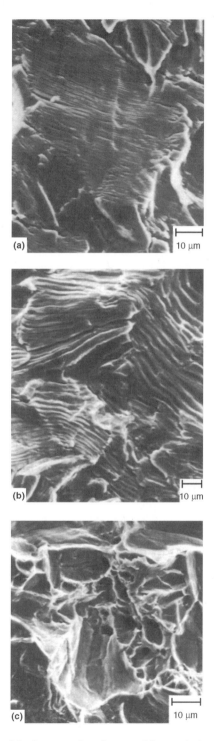

(a)   10 μm

(b)   10 μm

(c)   10 μm

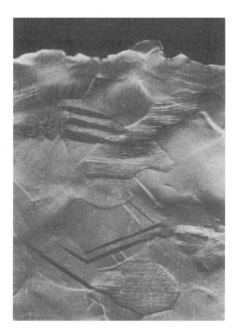

Fig. 45   Specimen surface of recrystallized titanium at fracture edge. Specimen was fatigued at a stress of 600 MPa (87 ksi) in air. Twinning, wavy glide deformation, and grain-boundary distortion are visible on this relatively heavily loaded specimen. Polarized light. 330×

Fig. 46   Fracture surface of commercially pure titanium test specimens that failed at an applied stress level of 600 MPa (87 ksi) in air. (a) Very fine fatigue striations. (b) Coarse fatigue striations probably in transition to glide bands. (c) Overload tearing structures

orientation at the crack front, extremely finely spaced fatigue striations (Fig. 46a) can form in the vicinity of very coarse striations (Fig. 46b), which appear to be in transition to glide formation. Figure 46(c) shows an area of overload fracture with prismatic and dimple tearing structures. These fatigue structures indicate ductile behavior.

Figures 47(a) and (b) illustrate an area of the fracture surface of a titanium bone plate that suffered fatigue failure in an unstable internal fixation situation. The bone plate showed mixed fracture structures, such as fatigue striations, tearing structures, and terraces. Figure 47(a) shows an overview, and Fig. 47(b) shows ledges and tearing structures of the terrace.

Failures Related to Implant Degradation

Metallic substance can be released from implants by such mechanisms as:

- General corrosion
- Galvanic corrosion
- Intergranular corrosion
- Maintenance of passive film of highly corrosion-resistant implant materials
- Stress corrosion combined with fatigue
- Pitting corrosion combined with fatigue (Example 16 in this chapter)

- Corrosion fatigue
- Crevice corrosion
- Fretting corrosion
- Fretting
- Wear

Reports on in vivo and in vitro studies and discussions of the degradation and corrosion of implants are found in Ref 23 to 25.

Implant degradation can lead to mechanical failure of the implant when severe disintegration takes place, as illustrated in Example 7 in this chapter. However, with the use of improved implant materials and metallurgical processing, visible general corrosion, intercrystalline corrosion, and galvanic corrosion are seldom observed today.

Combined attack of fatigue with stress corrosion, fretting, or fretting corrosion can also cause implant breakdown, but these failure modes are rare. Slight branching of cracks found on broken implants may not indicate stress corrosion but can be explained by fatigue-propagation processes. In experiments with magnesium chloride solution, stress-corrosion cracks in type 316L stainless steel are characterized by extensive branching. The fracture surfaces of these cracks exhibit facets and multiple fine cracks that, in most cases, are crystallographically oriented (Ref 19, 23). The combination of fatigue with stress corrosion has been

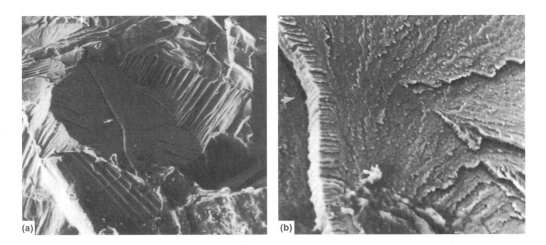

Fig. 47 Fatigue-fracture surface of broken commercially pure titanium bone plate with mixed fracture morphology. (a) Fracture surface shows fatigue striations, terraces, and tearing ridges, depending on the local crystallographic orientation. 250×. (b) Higher-magnification view of the area indicated by arrow in (a) showing large and small ledges with partial tearing configurations. 1250×

observed in few cases on type 316L stainless steel. Very little metal is released into the tissue by this form of attack.

The generation of wear, fretting, or corrosion products can evoke local physiological reactions that may necessitate reoperation. This is, however, seldom experienced. Local reactions in relation to fracture-treatment implants are occasionally reported but usually cease after resting of the limb and after routine removal of the implant on healing of the fracture. The systemic effects of metals that are released from implants are the subject of much research and speculation. Unambiguously diagnosed general allergies to implant metals are rarely reported. However, mere contact with the metal is sufficient to create such reactions in patients susceptible to allergies. If implants remain in the passive condition, the release of metal ions is very low, corresponding to the current density related to the corrosion potential of the passive stage. These metal traces are usually below the concentrations that are detectable with modern analytical techniques.

Crevice corrosion, fretting corrosion, fretting, and wear typically occur at the contact areas of multiple-component implants. Wear is found on the articulation surfaces of prostheses. In a long-term study on total hip prostheses that were in the body for approximately 8.3 years, up to 2.8 mm (0.11 in.) of material loss was found, amounting to a wear rate of 0.34 mm/year (0.013 in./year). These wear rates were measured on radiographs and involve the abrasion of the metal head and the polymer acetabular cup, and the polymer creep.

The wear behavior of a prosthesis depends on the surface finish, the contact area, the loading, the loading directions, and the wear properties of the material. Many improvements have been made to minimize the wear on artificial joints, and researchers and producers have designed various wear simulators (Ref 26, 27). If prosthesis stems become loose, wear and fretting or, sometimes, shallow fretting corrosion can take place at various areas of the stem (compare Fig. 59c and d in Example 18 in this chapter).

The contact areas between screw heads and plate holes are usually susceptible to fretting and fretting corrosion when relative motion occurs between the screw and the plate. Compared to artificial joint surfaces, the contact areas between screws and plates are smaller and therefore are subject to higher surface pressures.

Thus, it is difficult to prevent fretting at screwhead/plate-hole junctions by using special surface treatments. Mechanical attack is found on all implant materials at such junctions, but the degree of additional corrosion varies with the local condition and the type of material.

On commercially pure titanium, mechanical abrasion is found with oxidation of the wear particles (Example 15 in this chapter). On Ti-6Al-4V alloys, wear and wear fatigue are found; in these cases, wear fatigue is indicated by cracking of the worn material surface layers. Because fretting easily destroys the passive film, stainless steel can develop pitting corrosion in connection with fretting. In addition, the geometry between the plate hole and the screw head provides crevices. The intensity of pitting corrosion in connection with fretting depends on the quality of the steel. For example, type 304 stainless steel or steel with a high inclusion content is prone to more severe pitting than a type 316LR steel (compare Examples 13 and 14 in this chapter). On high-quality stainless steels, mechanical attack and shallow pitting corrosion are observed. On screw-plate combinations in wrought cobalt alloys, pitting is observable only with SEM. Also, on cast Co-Cr-Mo alloys, fretting and slight corrosive attack have been observed.

On two-component hip-screw plates, fretting and fretting corrosion can also be observed. Reference 23 provides the results of analyses of fretting and fretting corrosion conditions on retrieved implants made from various materials. Examples 14 and 15 in this chapter illustrate fretting and fretting corrosion conditions on screwplate junctions for stainless steel and titanium.

Example 13: Heavy Pitting Corrosion on a Type 304 Stainless Steel Screw

Discussion. Figure 48 shows a screw head that exhibits heavy pitting corrosion attack. Deep tunnels penetrated the screw head (Fig. 48a) and followed the inclusion lines (Fig. 48b). This screw was inserted in a plate made of type 316LR stainless steel that showed some mechanical fretting and very few corrosion pits.

Conclusion. This is another example where type 304 stainless steel is not satisfactory as an implant material and where inclusion lines contribute to corrosion, which is also observed on steels of higher quality but with larger amounts of primary inclusions.

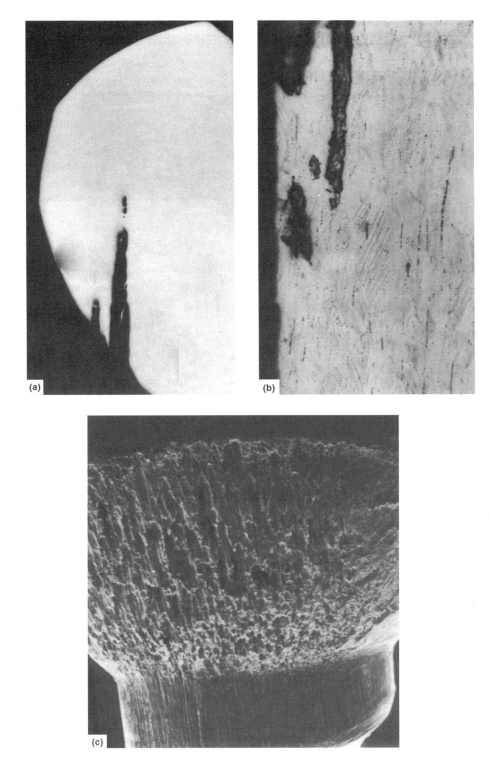

Fig. 48 Heavy pitting corrosion on type 304 stainless steel bone screw. (a) Longitudinal section through head of bone screw showing corrosion tunnels. (b) Etched longitudinal section showing the many primary inclusion lines and corrosion tunnels that follow the inclusions. (c) SEM overview of corrosion attack on screw head

Example 14: Screw Hole with Fretting and Fretting Corrosion of a Type 316LR Stainless Steel Plate

Discussion. Figure 49 shows a plate hole with the area that was in contact with the screw head. In contrast to Example 13, the attack on this high-quality type 316LR stainless steel was only shallow. Figure 49(a) shows an overview indicating that a large portion of the contact area exhibited only mechanical grinding and polish-

ing structures. The fine corrosion pits in the periphery are shown at a higher magnification in Fig. 49(b). The intense mechanical material transfer that can take place during fretting is visible in Fig. 49(c) and (d). In front of this structure is a corrosion pit that is surrounded by a burnished surface texture. The burnished surface may have broken open at this point. Observation of other implant specimens confirms that material layers are smeared over each other during wear and can be attacked by pitting corro-

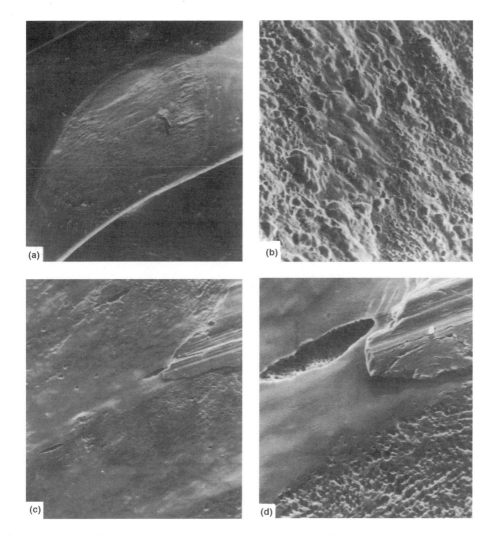

Fig. 49 Fretting and fretting corrosion at the contact area between the screw hole of a type 316LR stainless steel bone plate and the corresponding screw head. (a) Overview of wear on plate hole showing mechanical and pitting corrosion attack. 15×. (b) Higher-magnification view of shallow pitting corrosion attack from periphery of contact area. 355×. (c) Contact area showing the effects of mechanical material transport (material tongue in right upper corner), fretting and wear (burnished areas), and corrosion (shallow pitting). 355×. (d) Higher-magnification view of Fig. 49(c). 650×

sion. These pits are then covered by a new burnished material film that can break open again. Thus, the material is worn and degraded.

Figure 50 illustrates how the corrosion and wear products are transported in the tissue. These products are found extracellularly and phagocytized in the fibrocytes of the connective tissue in this example.

Conclusion. Examples 13 and 14 show the importance of proper implant materials selection. Pitting and fretting corrosion are much less severe when a high-quality stainless steel (type 316LR) is selected over a conventional stainless steel, such as type 304.

Example 15: Titanium Screw Head with Fretting Structure at Contact Area with Plate Hole

Discussion. Figure 51(a) shows a portion of a titanium screw head with a lip of material that was transported by fretting at a plate-hole edge. A flat fretting zone is visible on the screw surface over the material lip, which is magnified in Fig. 51(b). A cellular wear structure containing wear debris is present. Figure 51(c) shows material destruction and the formation of the thin flakes of wear debris. Mechanical deformation is superimposed on wear structures in Fig. 51(d).

Conclusion. No morphological signs of corrosion have been observed in connection with fretting structures. This has been typically found on all contact areas of plate holes and screw heads of titanium that were investigated.

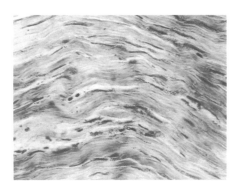

Fig. 50 Connective tissue near stainless steel bone plate with impregnation of corrosion products. These products are found extracellularly and in the connective tissue cells. 230×

Example 16: Failure of Type 316L Stainless Steel Bone Screws Because of Combined Pitting Corrosion and Fatigue

Background. Two type 316L stainless steel orthopedic screws broke approximately 6 weeks after surgical implant. In this instance, the screws had been employed to fasten a seven-hole narrow dynamic compression plate to a patient's spine.

The screws (Fig. 52) had a cancellous configuration and were manufactured in accordance with ASTM F 138. The screws were 38 mm (1.5 in.) in length, with a 6.4 mm (0.25 in.) diameter between thread peaks and a 3.2 mm (0.125 in.) diameter between thread roots. They were made of type 316L stainless steel in the work-hardened condition, having a specified hardness range of 30 to 35 HRC, which is within the one-half to three-fourths hard range.

Specimen Selection. The broken screws, along with screws of the same vintage and source, were subjected to examination. The broken screws were cleaned in acetone using ultrasonic agitation.

Visual Examination. Visual and low-power microscopic examination revealed that the broken screws were relatively clean, with what appeared to be only superficial corrosion products, while the unused screws were meticulously clean. The plane of the fracture surface of the broken screws was normal to the screw axis, and no noticeable plastic deformation was evident.

Macrofractography. Examination of the fracture surfaces at low magnification using an optical microscope showed that, for the most part, the fracture surfaces had been rubbed out by the attrition of the broken surfaces. This surface condition indicated that the fracture mode was fatigue.

Scanning Electron Microscopy/Fractography. Transverse cross sections of the broken screws were metallurgically polished. Figure 53 shows the plan view of the surface of a broken screw. Figure 54 is a magnified side view of the fracture surface, revealing the corrosion pits that served to initiate fatigue fractures.

Discussion. Fractography established that fracture was by fatigue and that the fatigue cracking originated at corrosion pits. Therefore, corrosion resistance of the screws was a major factor.

From a fatigue standpoint, the screws should not have been specified in the cold-worked condition. It has been established that cold-worked austenitic stainless steels lose their fatigue strength when notched. It has also been established that austenitic stainless steels in the annealed condition are not sensitive to notches. Cold-worked material is very notch sensitive, with notches decreasing the fatigue strength from approximately 760 to 170 MPa (110 to 25 ksi). In contrast, the notch-insensitive annealed material has an approximate fatigue strength of 230 MPa (33 ksi) at room temperature, which is approximately 33% greater than that of the notched cold-worked material. Thus, in an aggressive environment such as body fluids, which generate corrosion pits while the body simultaneously provides fatigue loading, the annealed austenitic stainless steels have a greater resistance to fatigue failure than the specified cold-worked material.

Conclusion. The primary cause of the fracture was pitting corrosion, which provided initiation sites for fatigue cracks. Because of the notch sensitivity of the cold-worked material to fatigue fracture, it provided no advantage over annealed material. In addition, a higher-alloy-content stainless steel, such as type 317L, should

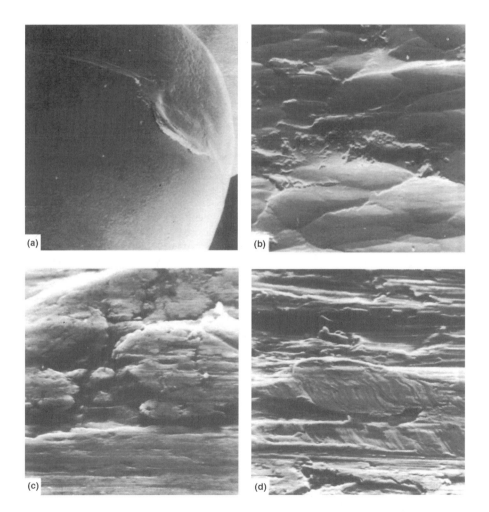

Fig. 51 Wear on head of titanium screw. (a) Material transport and fretting zone. (b) Close-up view of wear structures showing fine wear products. 120×. (c) Wear structures showing generation of small wear particles. 1200×. (d) Wear structures with additional fretting structures. 305×

be considered. Type 317L has a decided advantage over type 316L from both a pitting-resistance and notch-sensitivity standpoint. Type 317L has slightly higher chromium, nickel, and molybdenum contents than does 316L.

Failures Related to Inadequate Design

The use of surgically implantable biomedical fixation devices to stabilize fractured bones into proper alignment for subsequent healing is a widely accepted medical practice. Thousands of these devices have been inserted into human beings within the last half-century. In the form of tubes, rods, or plates, these orthopedic devices are surgically implanted and affixed to bones, usually with screws of the same alloy composition. Fixation implants usually remain in the human body until the broken bone has healed sufficiently to sustain normal loading without the additional support provided by the implant. After several weeks or months, the fixation implant is usually surgically removed, because the presence of the higher-elastic-modulus metal support may hinder the repaired bone development if it is retained in place.

From the mechanical/metallurgical perspective, in addition to the basic requirement of excellent biocompatibility, these implants must possess high strengths and exhibit exceptional resistance to fatigue. It has been estimated that fixation implants may be subjected to repeated stressing in excess of 10^6 cycles per year. Chemically, the resistance to all forms of localized and general corrosion processes is also absolutely essential for stability and patient comfort. Unfortunately, some fixation devices are applied in locations where the structural design of the implant (its overall size, shape, and the location of holes for the attachment to bone with screws) does not always lend itself to satisfactory mechanical/metallurgical design practice. Circumstances that inhibit optimal design may be dictated by the patient's anatomy and physiological conditions. These may create

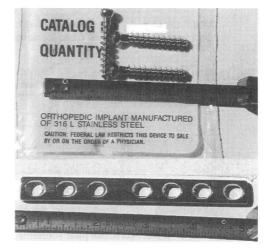

Fig. 52 Cancellous bone screws and the seven-hole narrow dynamic compression plate

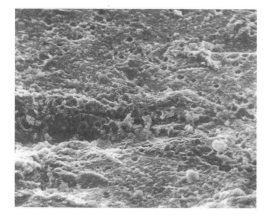

Fig. 53 Scanning electron micrograph showing plan view of corrosion pits on surface at the origin of the fatigue fracture in the thread root of a screw. 640×

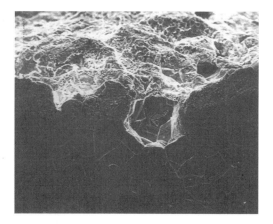

Fig. 54 Scanning electron micrograph showing a corrosion pit cross section at the origin of the fatigue fracture. 256×

an undesirable situation for even the short-term survival of the fixation device after implantation. The following example describes how inadequate design can lead to failures of implant fixation devices.

Example 17: Fatigue Failures of Austenitic Stainless Steel Orthopedic Fixation Devices

Background. Four 300-series stainless steel implant fixation devices that experienced premature failures while in place and attached to healing broken bones were examined. All four failures were remarkably similar in nature, indicative of a design inadequacy. These failed implant devices required surgical removal to alleviate pain of the patient. Typically, the failed implant was replaced with a more robust substitute of a similar design and the same alloy composition.

It is evident that the success of an orthopedic fixation surgical implant is highly dependent on the mechanical/metallurgical performance of that device. These factors are intrinsic to the device itself. Obviously, the skill of the surgeon during the implantation operation is also critically important. The alignment of the fixation device with the broken bone as well as the bone itself and the uniform setting of the attachment screws to the bone are all critical features. For example, it may be important to set all of the screws equally to distribute or balance the loading. However, this analysis is not concerned with those surgery-related issues. This analysis only addresses the intrinsic metallurgical/mechanical factors as they affect the failure process. The design of the implant and the location of screw holes for attachment to the bone are of concern.

Because of the critical nature of the properties of the implant, the material that the implant is made of was also considered.

As stated in Example 6 in this chapter, a properly installed austenitic stainless steel implant can perform satisfactorily for more than 20 years in the human body. That length of time is rarely, if ever, required for any fixation implant. However, it does serve as a benchmark to emphasize the gross inadequacy of those implants that fail prematurely after only a brief duration. These short-term, premature failures, often after only a few days or weeks of service, suggest that something is amiss with the implant material or its design. It is not surprising that the patients, the victims of these failed implants, often turn to the courts for redress.

Analysis. Although different alloys and materials are used for the thousands of orthopedic fixation devices, this analysis reports on four different failures that occurred for 300-series austenitic stainless steel implants. The use of austenitic stainless steels is separately addressed following the analysis and discussion of the failure modes of the four implanted fixation devices. Figures 55(a) and (b) are scanning electron micrographs of the fracture surfaces of two of the four different failed implants. The fracture surfaces contained regions that were practically obliterated by the flow, wear, and repeated rubbing after the device failure within the patient. However, there were also some fracture surface regions that appeared nearly pristine.

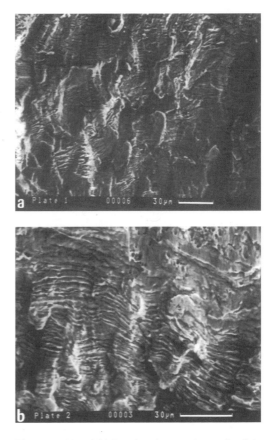

Fig. 55 (a) and (b) Scanning electron micrographs of the fracture surfaces of two of the failed stainless steel fixation implant devices. Note the numerous parallel striations heralding the crack advance during repeated stressings, indicative of fatigue failure.

Those pristine regions on all four of the implant failures have one surface feature in common: the existence of numerous fatigue striations on the fracture surfaces. The numerous striations are evident in these scanning electron micrographs and clearly herald the fact that the implants failed by fatigue.

The four implant fixation devices were applied at four different locations in four different human beings. Because the locations of these bone fracture fixation devices were different, the conditions of loading are expected to have been different for each device. These factors, along with the varying anatomical features of the patients, suggest that the actual stress conditions to which the implant fixation device was subjected are likely to have been different. The actual states of stress for the individual implants were undoubtedly quite complicated while these devices were in place. In spite of these differences, each of these devices experienced an obvious fatigue failure. The numerous fracture surface fatigue striations in Fig. 55 are indisputable evidence.

It must be noted that fatigue is not the only possible failure mechanism for orthopedic implants. Simple overload failures may occur if the fixation device does not possess sufficient strength. Corrosion is also of concern, especially in the presence of a galvanic couple when different alloys are mistakenly used for the device and its attachment screws. However, fatigue was undeniably the cause of failure in each of these four austenitic stainless steel fixation devices.

Fatigue is not restricted to implanted orthopedic devices. Mechanical/metallurgical design practices to reduce or eliminate fatigue are well understood. This is true from both the theoretical and practical perspectives. Unfortunately, the examination of these four orthopedic fixation implant devices did not reveal a strict adherence to fundamentally accepted design practices to limit or reduce the possibility of fatigue failure. Adherence to these well-established design practices, including fatigue life assessment, could have significantly minimized the possibility of the fatigue failure of these four fixation devices.

The process of fatigue failure occurs in two stages: the initiation of a fatigue crack, and crack propagation to failure with repeated cyclic loading. The electron micrographs of the fracture surface striations in Fig. 55(a) and (b) are indisputable evidence of the crack-propagation or -extension process. The striations are a record of the incremental fatigue-crack-extension process under repeated loading conditions. The presence of extensive regions of wear—the plastic flow and smoothing, although they are not depicted in the previously mentioned figure—are further evidence of repeated loading of the failed implant device after the crack had initiated and during the crack-growth process. These processes all occurred while the fixation device remained implanted within the patient.

The primary issue of concern is the cause of the failure of the implant fixation device itself. The extensive wear regions on the fracture surfaces relate to the period of time after fatigue-crack initiation, or perhaps even after total fracture, that the device remained in the patient prior to its replacement. The wear also reflects the particular conditions to which the specific implant was subjected.

Figures 56(a) and (b) reveal that the implant device fracture or failure occurs at the reduced cross section of one of the screw attachment holes that are used to insert screws to affix the implanted device to the bone. All four of these implant fixation devices failed at that precise location: the reduced cross section at the screw attachment holes. This is not surprising, because it is well known that initiation sites for fatigue cracks are regions of stress concentration, such as sharp radii, reduced cross sections, and metallurgical inclusions. The presence of inclusions and their deleterious effects in orthopedic implants is well known and documented (see Example 6 in this chapter). It is the reason for ultraclean metallurgical processing, often involving multiple vacuum remelting of the metals and alloys before they are used to manu-

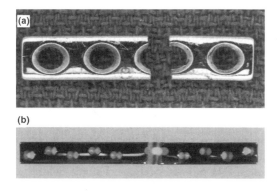

Fig. 56 (a) and (b) Macroscopic views of two of the failed fixation device implants. Note the failures at the reduced cross sections of the screw attachment holes.

facture these devices. However, metallurgical processing defects of the nature mentioned previously are not the only causes for premature fatigue-crack initiation. Scratches and/or gouges of the device surface during surgical procedures may also serve as the source or origin of fatigue-crack initiation. However, there was no evidence of surgically induced damage to the four implant devices or any evidence suggestive of inclusion effects. Figures 56(a) and (b) illustrate failures that occurred at the reduced cross sections of the devices associated with the location of the screw holes.

The presence of the substantially reduced cross sections, associated with the screw holes for the attachment of the fixation device to the broken bone, is an obvious design weakness. These holes are a source of stress concentration and create an initiation point for the fatigue cracks in the reduced cross sections. The fatigue failures initiated from the attachment screw holes in each of the four different fixation devices. The size and positioning of the screw holes can be considered to be a serious design fault. Numerous examples of orthopedic internal fixation devices with different arrangements of the screw attachment holes have been illustrated earlier in this chapter. It is readily apparent even to the casual observer that, for many of these, the screw attachment holes constitute a significant fraction of the implant device cross section. As such, they are expected to be locations of stress concentration and fatigue-crack initiation.

Unfortunately, the large screw holes are more than just a point for fatigue-crack initiation. To the implant fixation device, the severely reduced cross sections are a source of double jeopardy: crack initiation and growth. The presence of the screw hole during loading creates a stress concentration that is highly conducive to fatigue-crack initiation. Cracks invariably initiate at the edges of these holes, in spite of the manufacturer's attempts to reduce the occurrence of that event by chamfering and polishing the screw hole inside edges. The presence of this preventive treatment is a clear indication of the manufacturer's concerns for the role that these screw holes may have in the fatigue failure of these types of fixation implant devices. Equally or perhaps even more detrimental is the stress gradient that the screw hole produces during normal loading of the implant during the patient's daily activities. The presence of stress gradients is highly conducive to fatigue-crack

growth. Stress gradients in the vicinity of holes are expected to accelerate crack growth once the fatigue crack has initiated. Thus, the attachment screw holes actually contribute a twofold reduction to the life of the implant. Not only do the holes serve as the sites where fatigue cracks initiate, but they also create a significant stress gradient to accelerate the fatigue-crack growth process and hasten the ultimate fatigue failure of the device at the reduced cross section. Clearly, it comes as no surprise that all four of these surgical implant fixation devices failed from fatigue cracks originating at the reduced cross sections at the attachment screw holes.

It must be concluded that the mechanical/metallurgical design of these fixation implant devices leaves much to be desired from an engineering perspective. The presence of large screw attachment holes that constitute a considerable fraction of the load-bearing cross section creates severe stress concentrations. These screw attachment holes are an obvious weakness and a location for fatigue-crack origination. This design weakness often leads to the initiation of cracks from the screw attachment holes. The cracks subsequently propagate by fatigue to failure. This process was the mechanism of the device failure in all four of the implants investigated.

Materials Selection. One cannot separate the design and the material used for the design. Their interdependence for implant fixation devices is discussed in the following section. The 300-series austenitic stainless steels are frequently used materials for fixation implants of this type. Austenitic stainless steels have considerable merit from the corrosion point of view. When properly processed, in a metallurgical sense, the 300-series austenitic stainless steels are practically corrosion-free in the human body environment. However, these alloys do leave much to be desired from the viewpoint of fatigue resistance. Austenitic stainless steels are well known to exhibit a low proportional limit, a characteristic that leads to the initiation and propagation of fatigue cracks. Other materials are superior to austenitic stainless steels from the viewpoint of fatigue resistance, including titanium and titanium alloys, cobalt alloys, the 400-series stainless steels, and custom-processed high-carbon steels.

The conditions for a premature fatigue failure are present when a material that is highly susceptible to fatigue is combined with a weak mechanical design that promotes fatigue.

Fatigue failures are practically inevitable under this combination of conditions. All four of the fixation implant devices observed in this study failed in a similar fashion from just such fatigue. From the metallurgical/mechanical design perspective, these fixation implant devices are simply not a compatible material/design combination. This type of fatigue-sensitive design with an austenitic stainless steel should never have been instituted for a mechanical device and should not be tolerated in a medical application where the comfort and well-being of an injured human is at issue.

Would simply a material change prevent fatigue failures of the type observed in these fixation devices? Of course, it can never be predicted with absolute certainty that a failure will not occur. However, there are obvious materials selection processes that can be instituted to improve the implant performance and reduce the likelihood of fatigue failure. The metallurgical literature suggests material choices that are superior to the austenitic stainless steels not only for fatigue resistance but for corrosion resistance in the body environment as well. The material cost of the implantation device is a rel-atively insignificant portion of the total cost of the surgical procedure to insert it. Therefore, the choice and use of a superior material for use as an internal fixation implant device in humans is easy. Titanium or one of the titanium alloys are obvious choices superior to austenitic stainless steels.

Finite-Element Analyses. To quantitatively compare the fixation device attachment screw hole design and the materials selection for the type of fixation implants that were observed to have failed by fatigue, a finite-element analysis of the implant design was undertaken. The commercial code ABAQUS was applied to calculate the linear elastic response of two distinctive types of fixation plates: one of austenitic stainless steel and the other of a titanium alloy. Two designs/geometries were chosen to address the screw hole attachment configurations and to contrast the asymmetric and symmetric screw hole alignments.

Two common plate geometries are illustrated in Fig. 57(a) and (b). Fixation plate "a" has an asymmetric attachment screw hole pattern, with several of the screw holes offset toward one edge of the fixation plate. Type "b" plate is slightly

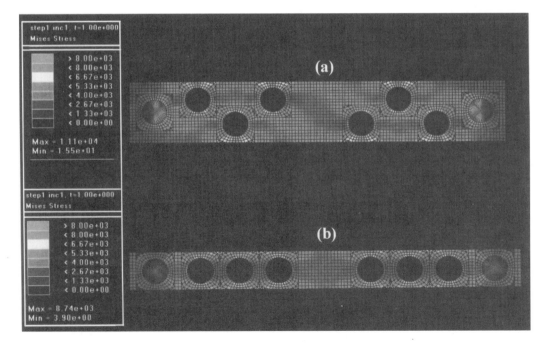

Fig. 57 Finite-element analysis meshes for two bone plate fixation device designs with a unit displacement imposed in the axial direction of the plates. (a) Asymmetric design. (b) Symmetric design. The original figure, which was reproduced in color, clearly showed that the asymmetric screw attachment hole design developed much higher stress concentrations than did the symmetric design. See text for details.

narrower and has the holes aligned along the length of the implant device on the plate centerline.

An austenitic stainless steel and a titanium-alloy device were both examined to compare responses for the two implant device designs. In this analysis, typical austenitic stainless steel properties and titanium-alloy properties were used. The austenitic stainless steel was assigned a yield stress of 250 MPa (36 ksi), a tensile strength of 600 MPa (87 ksi), and an elastic modulus of 210 GPa (30,460 ksi). The titanium alloy was assigned a yield stress of 800 MPa (116 ksi), a tensile strength of 900 MPa (131 ksi), and an elastic modulus of 116 GPa (16,820 ksi). The higher yield strength and lower elastic modulus of the titanium alloy have significant beneficial effects on the resulting stresses and stress concentrations experienced by the fixation device. However, in these linear finite-element analyses, the strengths of the alloys were not used; only the elastic moduli enter into the calculations.

The finite-element meshes for each plate are shown in Fig. 57(a) and (b). The majority of the elements in each of the meshes are second-order quadrilateral (eight-node) plate elements. Some second-order triangular (six-node) elements were used for transitioning. Second-order elements are well suited for use near stress concentrations, because their ability to accurately model stress gradients is superior to that of first-order elements. Applying the finite-element code, two cases were examined for the two designs and materials considered for the fixation implant device. The first was that of a unit stress on the gross cross section of the fixation plate (not shown in Fig. 57). The second was a unit displacement in the axial direction of the plate. This latter result is presented in Fig. 57(a) and (b). To load or constrain the plates, the end screw attachment holes on the plate centerline were fixed. The remaining six screw attachment holes in each case were not restrained.

These two cases were not chosen to precisely simulate the actual loading of a fixation device that may be expected in service in the human body. For the most part, that loading is a complex situation relating not only to the fixation device but also to the particular bone and the details of the coupling, the attachment of the implanted device to the bone, and the anatomy of the specific patient. Rather, the two distinct conditions mentioned previously were chosen to investigate the screw attachment hole design

and the material of which the fixation device was constructed. The purpose is to directly compare those features for the two common design features: hole asymmetry and hole symmetry.

Quantitative estimates of the stress-concentration factors associated with the screw attachment holes and the reduced cross sections were obtained. These quantitative estimates show that the asymmetric design of the offset attachment screw holes is slightly less desirable from the stress-concentration perspective. However, there is actually a double negative effect, because the volume of more highly stressed material is also larger for the asymmetric screw hole design. This factor further increases the susceptibility of the asymmetric hole design to fatigue failure. It is evident that the asymmetric hole design, which leaves a significantly reduced cross section near to the device edge, is much less desirable from a fatigue design perspective than the design that places the holes aligned symmetrically along the implant device centerline. However, as previously shown in Fig. 55(a) and (b), fatigue failures occurred in implants of both designs. This is not surprising, considering the stress concentrations from the screw hole sizes and their placements.

The von Mises equivalent stress contours for the linear elastic unit displacement analyses of the two plate designs are shown in Fig. 57(a) and (b). Because the model was linear elastic, the stresses can simply be scaled according to the displacement. In this situation, the displacements of the structure and the stiffness of the materials determine the stresses that develop in the structure. It is evident from the stress contours in Fig. 57 that higher stresses are developed and that a larger volume of highly stressed material develops in the fixation plate with the asymmetric hole design. That stress concentration occurs dominantly, although not completely, directly adjacent to the hole surface displaced toward the edge of the fixation plate. Because the von Mises stress contours can be interpreted as contour lines, the onset of material yielding may be predicted from this analysis. Yielding occurs when the von Mises equivalent stress reaches the yield strength of the material.

For displacement-controlled situations, it is the displacement of the structure and the stiffness of the materials that determine the stresses and the stress concentrations that develop. If all other conditions are equal and titanium were substituted for austenitic stainless steel, then the stresses in the structures would be reduced by an amount related to the ratio of the elastic moduli of the two materials. If titanium were substituted for stainless steel, the stresses would be reduced by a factor of 116 to 220, their elastic moduli ratio. When this is combined with the much higher yield stress of the titanium alloy, 800 MPa (116 ksi) compared with just 250 MPa (36 ksi) for the stainless steel, it is quite obvious that from a mechanical-property perspective, titanium is far superior to austenitic stainless steel for these fixation implant devices. Not only are the stresses in the fixation device reduced for equivalent displacement loading, but the yield stress of the titanium is considerably higher, thus inhibiting yielding and serving as a deterrent to fatigue failures. Completely aside from the fatigue-failure prevention, the lower elastic modulus of the titanium also presents a much closer, although still somewhat removed, elastic modulus match with that of the bone and thus potentially better performance in terms of its biocompatibility.

Conclusion. Four failed austenitic stainless steel orthopedic fixation implant devices were examined. Scanning electron microscopy revealed that all four failed by fatigue, as evidenced by the presence of numerous fatigue striations on their fracture surfaces. In each of the four implants, the fatigue cracks initiated from the screw attachment holes at a location toward the outside surface of the device. This eventually caused fracturing across the narrow region of the reduced cross section that is created by the screw attachment hole design.

The screw attachment hole design was examined by finite-element analysis. The asymmetric location hole design, where the screw holes are offset toward the device edge, was contrasted with the symmetric design, where the screw holes are aligned on the centerline of the implant device. The finite-element analysis was also used to compare the use of austenitic stainless steel with a titanium alloy, because the material elastic modulus is incorporated within that analysis. Titanium was judged to be a superior choice to the austenitic stainless steel.

It is concluded that the failure of these implant fixation devices was a result of the design of the large attachment screw holes creating a stress concentration and significant weakness in the device. This design weakness is highly susceptible to fatigue. The symmetric screw attachment hole design is slightly superior to the asymmetric one in this respect. These

implant fixation devices could be significantly improved by the substitution of titanium or a titanium alloy for the austenitic stainless steel. The higher strength and the lower elastic modulus of titanium suggest that it would be much more resistant to the fatigue-failure process observed in these failed implant fixation devices and may be more biocompatible as well.

Fractures of Total Hip Joint Prostheses

The hip joint prosthesis is the most common joint replacement. The function of the normal hip joint, the design of the hip joint prosthesis, and the related complications have been extensively studied, compared to other joints.

A retrospective multicenter study on the performance of 39,000 total hip replacements over a period of 10 years was published in 1982 (Ref 28). A biomechanical concept of the total hip prosthesis based on clinical experience that gives a background for the understanding of complications can be found in Ref 29.

One of the complications encountered in total hip replacements is the fracture of prosthesis stems. Lateral bending and torsional forces act on the prosthesis stem when it is not supported. All fractures of the hip prosthesis stems are reportedly caused by a fatigue-failure mechanism (Ref 27). The fracture of prosthesis stems is a secondary event that follows loosening of the stem.

Different factors, which can also act in combination, promote stem loosening. These factors include bone resorption, degradation of bone cement, and unfavorable positioning of the prosthesis (see Example 18 in this chapter). Blood clot inclusions, holes in the cement, and overheating of the bone can also contribute to stem loosening.

Information on the performance and testing of hip stem material can be found in Ref 27 and 30 to 32. Standard techniques for the cyclic bending test of hip prosthesis stems have also been developed (Ref 30).

Example 18: Broken Stem of Femoral Head Component of Total Hip Prosthesis Made from Cast Cobalt-Base Alloy

Background. In a 65 year old male patient, radiotranslucency was visible around the collar of the femoral head prosthesis on radiographs taken 5 months after implantation. One month later, the bone cement was broken at the distal end of the prosthesis stem, and a small indentation on the lateral contour of the stem was visible where the stem had broken 2 weeks later.

Investigation. Figure 58(a) shows a radiograph illustrating the broken prosthesis. The dislocation of the fragment of the prosthesis indicated the degree of loosening and implant loading.

Under weight bearing, the proximal prosthesis fragment was pushed toward lateral, and the loosening in the medio-lateral plane can be seen as a gap between the lateral stem contour and the bone or cement. The upper arrow in Fig. 58(a) indicates the loosening at the collar. The bottom arrow marks the crack in the bone cement plug at the end of the stem. Figure 58(b) shows an overview of the broken prosthesis component. Because of the loosening, the end of the stem was heavily worn in contact with the bone cement (Fig. 58 c, d).

In analyses of broken prosthesis stems, such wear or fretting traces are good indicators of the presence of motion and loosening. In other investigated prostheses, flat fretting zones have also been found on other areas of the stem. On stainless steel prostheses, this wear appears occasionally as slight fretting corrosion attack. One may, however, distinguish wear that took place after fracture of the stem.

A metallographic specimen was taken parallel to the stem surface and perpendicular through the fracture surface of the distal fragment. This section revealed a secondary crack that had originated at the lateral aspect of the stem. The top contour in Fig. 59(a) represents the fracture edge, where two crack openings along slip planes can be observed. On a transverse metallographic section (Fig. 59b), gas pores are apparent in the grain and at the grain boundaries.

Discussion. Figure 60(a) shows an overview of the fracture surface. The grain size is considerable. The plateau in the upper right-hand corner represents a single grain, which is identical to grain A in Fig. 61(a). It is the same grain through which the secondary crack shown in Fig. 59(a) runs, and it is where the fracture originated. Figure 60(b) shows a higher-magnification view of the section through the fracture surface. The stresses created through the fatigue process activated glide systems that serve the formation of secondary cracks along glide planes. On the section through the fracture surface, another secondary crack formation is found (Fig. 60c). At these cracks, multiple slip bands also formed in connection with the fracture surface, and the cracks follow along these structures. One of the cracks propagated through a larger gas pore.

Figures 61(a) to (d) show details of the fracture morphology by SEM. In Fig. 61(a), three distinct grains are marked. These grains are oriented differently with respect to the propagating crack and therefore exhibit different crystallographic fracture patterns. Grain A (Fig. 61b) has a relatively flat texture but also shows crystallographically oriented structures. Grain B (Fig. 61c) is characterized by a staircase pattern. Material separation occurred on preferred slip planes. The fine parallel line structures that run diagonally through the fractograph may be slip traces. Of special interest are the parallel microcracks that appear black and are superimposed on the other structures. On grain C (Fig. 61d), identical microcracks are found, although the grain is obviously oriented differently. A ruptured gas pore is visible in the center of Fig. 61(d). Typical fatigue striations were not found on the fracture surface. Glide systems appear to be activated at relatively low energies so that cracks can easily propagate along glide systems.

Conclusion. The failure of the cast cobalt-alloy stem involved fatigue and fretting wear and stem loosening due to bone resorption and bone cement degradation. Microstructural contributions to failure included a large grain size and the presence of a ruptured gas pore.

Fractures of Total Knee Joint Prostheses

Total knee prostheses are used to replace the articulating surface of diseased or damaged knee joints to restore as much natural function as possible. A typical knee prosthesis consists of a metal femoral component, generally made from a cobalt-chromium or titanium alloy, a polymeric wear surface made of ultrahigh molecular weight polyethylene (UHMWPE, ASTM F 648), and a metal tibial component to which the polyethylene is attached.

The femoral component articulates against the UHMWPE tibial cup, which in turn is anchored to the tibia by means of an alloy tibial tray. The tibial tray is anchored to the tibia either by a polymeric grouting agent known as acrylic bone cement (an admixture of polymethyl methacrylate/styrene copolymer beads,

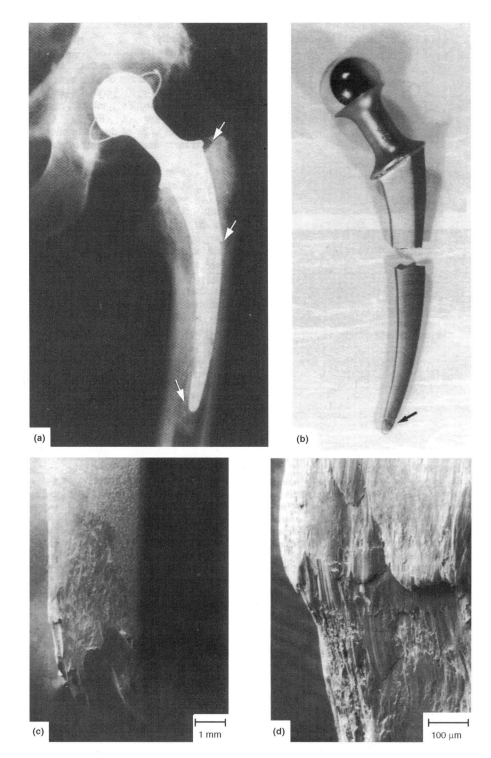

Fig. 58 Broken hip prosthesis of cast type ASTM F 75 Co-Cr-Mo alloy. (a) Radiograph of total hip prosthesis. Circular wire marks acetabulum component made from plastics. Arrows (from top to bottom) indicate the area where the prosthesis stem is loosening at the collar, a stem fracture, and a fracture of bone cement at the end of the stem, respectively. (b) Fracture of prosthesis stem. Wear at end of stem (arrow) indicates stem movement due to loosening. (c) Wear at end of stem. (d) Close-up view of stem end showing material transfer and layering from wear. Corrosion signs are not observed. See also Fig. 59 to 61.

methyl methacrylate monomer polymerized in place, and barium sulfate, which serves as a radiopacifier) or by the growth of bony tissue into the interstices of metal beads sintered onto the metal substrate. This porous structure allows bone tissue to grow into and mechanically lock the device in place. As described in the following example, failure of prosthetic knee components can occur due to fatigue overload as well as inadequate design and/or control during processing.

Example 19: Fatigue Fracture of Titanium Alloy Knee Prosthesis

Background. Total knee prostheses were retrieved from patients after radiographs revealed fracture of the Ti-6Al-4V (ELI) metal backing of the polyethylene tibial component. Porous-coated and uncoated tibial trays had failed.

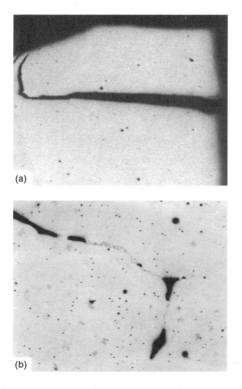

(a)

(b)

Fig. 59 Metallographic sections of failed hip prosthesis shown in Fig. 58. (a) Longitudinal section through fracture surface showing secondary fatigue crack parallel to fracture surface. 35×. (b) Cross section through prosthesis stem showing gas pores and second phase at grain boundaries and in grains. 105×

The prostheses were implanted into patients whose average age was 63.4 years and whose average weight was 90 kg (200 lb). These patients were active and fairly heavy. Typically, failure is observed in patients with poor underlying support for the tibial tray. Often, on implantation of the component, insufficient bone stock is present to adequately fix the device in place. In such cases, a bone graft is placed in the site to fill in the defect and provide support. If the graft resorbs or if one side of the tibia (usually the medial side, toward the centerline of the body) loses underlying support for the tibial component, then an asymmetric cantilever loading configuration results. This cantilever geometry results in tensile fatigue stresses on the superior (top) aspect of the metal tibial tray. Repeated loading caused by walking ultimately results in the formation of a fatigue crack that eventually propagates to failure.

A radiograph of a total knee prosthesis immediately after implantation is shown in Fig. 62(a). A radiograph taken after approximately 3.5 years, at which point failure of the tibial tray was observed, is shown in Fig. 62(b). Under the failed component are two bone-anchoring pins, which were used to support a bone graft. An average individual will cyclically load his or her leg approximately 1.5 million times per year; thus, 3.5 years represents a high-cycle fatigue regime.

ASTM F 136 and F 620 govern the compositional, microstructural, and mechanical properties of Ti-6Al-4V used in implant devices. Microstructurally, these specifications suggest that the alloy be used in the bimodal form obtained by thermomechanical treatment in the $\alpha + \beta$ phase field. According to these specifications, no coarse α platelets should be present.

Specimen Selection. Specimens were collected from patients after revision surgery was performed to replace the failed components. Those devices that best represented the nature and origin of the failure are discussed in this study. Some of the retrieved implants were severely damaged from postfracture abrasion and from removal.

Visual Examination. Failure of a tibial tray component (Fig. 63) occurs at or near the junction of the stem of the component, which extends into the tibia (coming out of the photograph), and the tray that is used to hold the polyethylene articulating surface (polyethylene is transparent to x-rays; see Fig. 62a). Also present in the tibial tray is a U-shaped notch. This recess is needed to preserve the posterior cruciate ligament of the knee in order to maintain stability of the joint and minimize the changes in anatomy required for implantation. These geometric features, besides being located at the maximum cantilever position, act as stress concentrations and were the sites of initiation for several of the failures observed. Figure 63 shows that the crack propagated to an elliptical hole in the tray. This site of fatigue-crack initiation was common in prostheses with cruciate-preserving notches.

The porous-coated components did not have a single stem; rather, they had three pegs that, along with the underside of the component, were coated with beads (Fig. 64). The device in Fig.

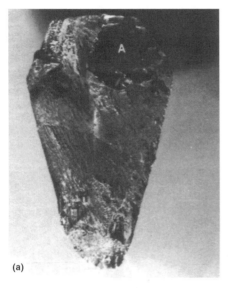

(a)

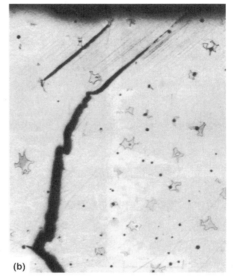

(b)

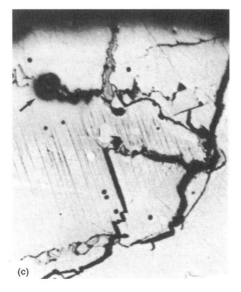

(c)

Fig. 60 Optical fracture analysis of the failed hip prosthesis shown in Fig. 58. (a) Fracture surface exhibiting large grains. The upper right grain is identical to grain A shown in Fig. 61(a). Crack originated at the lateral side of the stem. (b) Longitudinal section through fracture surface with glide systems activated by the fatigue process. Two cracks, one of which propagated through the grain, initiated along these glide systems. 195×. (c) Longitudinal section through fracture surface at the upper left area in Fig. 60(a). containing secondary cracks. Arrow indicates a gas pore. 270×

64 had several other features worthy of mention. Adjacent to the fatigue crack (right side of photograph) was another crack that did not quite propagate to failure. Again, the U-shaped cruciate-preserving notch influenced where the failure occurred (top of Fig. 64). The secondary fatigue crack can be seen emanating from this site.

The underside of the device in Fig. 64 was covered with beads of titanium sintered onto the metal substrate. In the vicinity of each fatigue crack, it was apparent that the beads had broken off the component. Once free, these beads migrated throughout the joint capsule and became embedded in the polyethylene articular cup. Figure 65 shows a severely worn polyeth-ylene cup with titanium beads embedded in the surface. The particulate debris resulting from this wear process can have a detrimental effect on the surrounding tissues.

Surface Examination of the Fracture Surfaces. Scanning electron microscopy was performed on several of the failed implants. Figure 66 is a low-power SEM micrograph of the initiation site for the fatigue fracture shown in Fig. 64 and 65. This was the region where the polyethylene cup was held in place. The right side of Fig. 66 shows the capture lip protruding from the raised rim of the tray.

A higher-magnification view (Fig. 67) shows that the initiation region consisted of several flat-faceted regions, where the initial fatigue

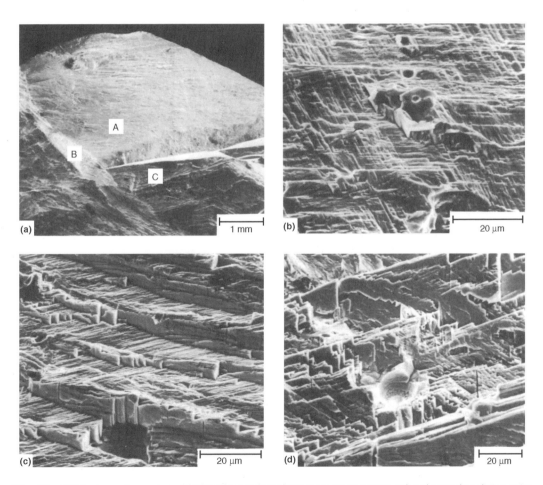

Fig. 61 SEM fracture-surface analysis of the failed hip prosthesis shown in Fig. 58. (a) Fracture surface showing three distinct grains labeled A, B, and C. (b) Grain A has a shallow, crystallographically oriented fracture structure. (c) Grain B has a crystallographically oriented fracture structure with slip traces. Note vertical cracks running in the same direction as some of the fracture planes. (d) Grain C has a crystallographically oriented fracture structure and small vertical cracks similar to those shown in (c). A ruptured gas hole is visible at the center of the fractograph.

damage occurred. These individual fracture sites grew and linked to form the final fracture surface. Figure 68 shows fatigue striations perpendicular to the direction of crack propagation, which occurred from the upper left to lower right. These striations were located in the base of the tray and clearly indicated the fatigue nature of the failure process.

Figure 69 shows another fractured tibial tray at the fatigue-initiation region. Again, this site was the polyethylene capture lip for the device. However, the initiation site was not at the top of the lip but rather at the base—as indicated by the convergence of the fracture lines to a point at the bottom of Fig. 69. At higher magnification (Fig. 70), the convergence of the fracture lines is more evident, indicating that the fracture initiated at the surface near the base of this region.

Figure 71 shows a higher-magnification view of the initiation region. A large prior-β grain was present, resulting in a large region of similar orientation that was favorable for the accumulation of fatigue damage. A secondary crack through the initiation site was also present.

Surface Examination of Bead-Tray Junctions. Porous coatings have been developed for orthopedic use primarily to provide a space into which bone can grow and mineralize, locking the device into place. This is termed biological fixation. During loading, however, this porous network is subjected to variable and nonintuitive stresses (that is, tensile stresses on a nominally compressive stress region), which may cause fracture or loss of the porous coating.

The beads used to create the interstitial space for bone ingrowth are sintered onto the surface of the tibial tray. This is accomplished by heating into the beta-phase field and holding for a sufficient time to allow for the formation of sinter necks between beads and between beads and tray. These sinter necks were observed by sectioning the bead-coated trays with a diamond saw, polishing, and imaging with backscattered electrons. The sinter necks resulting from this process are not always uniform or fully developed.

Figure 72, a micrograph of the tibial tray surface, shows where a bead was pulled out from

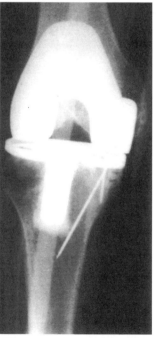

(a)

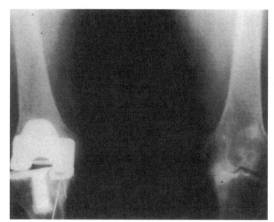

(b)

Fig. 62 X-ray radiographs. (a) Implanted total knee prosthesis. Femoral component is at top, tibial component is at bottom, and polyethylene, which cannot be seen with x-rays, is between the two components. (b) Failed tibial component after 3.5 years of implantation. Fracture is evident on the medial side.

the surface. The coarse beta microstructure resulting from the sintering heat treatment is just visible adjacent to this site. It is evident that the bead was not fully attached or incorporated onto the tray substrate but rather was attached only at local regions about the bead circumference.

Figure 73 shows a region of a bead where an adjacent bead has fractured off. Fractures are present on the circumference of this bead junction, which penetrate into the bead itself. The sintered neck junctions are regions of stress concentration and can give rise to notch-sensitive behavior of the beads.

Small fatigue fractures were noticed in several regions between the beads and the tray, as well as at interbead junctions. These fractures occurred away from the actual fatigue fracture and were sometimes present even in the case of "well-fixed" implants. Figure 74, a micrograph of a bead-tray junction, shows a fatigue crack propagating into the tray surface. Fracture of a bead-bead junction is shown in Fig. 75. Several cracks are present, traversing obliquely across the interbead junction. Fracture of the beads will result in their migration to regions where third-

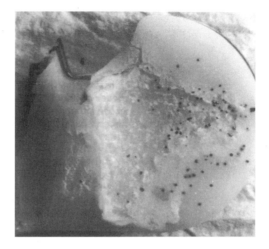

Fig. 65 Top surface of implant shown in Fig. 64. Note the severe wear pattern and the presence of beads in the polyethylene surface.

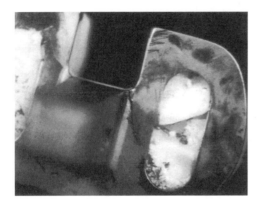

Fig. 63 Bottom of failed tibial tray. Fracture emanates from cruciate-preserving notch and propagates to elliptical hole used to lock implant to bone with bone cement.

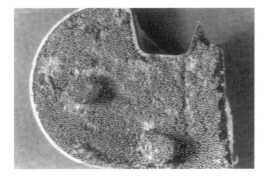

Fig. 64 Underside of porous-coated implant that failed by fatigue. Two fatigue cracks are present: the failure and a secondary crack parallel to the fracture surface. Porous beads fractured in the region adjacent to each fracture and migrated into the joint cavity.

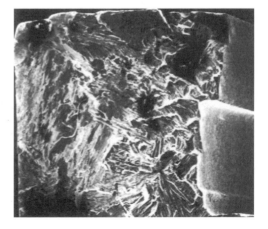

Fig. 66 SEM micrograph of polyethylene retaining lip of titanium tibial tray. Fatigue crack initiated at upper right region.

body wear and degradation processes can accelerate the failure of other components. Again, Fig. 74 and 75 show the coarse lamellar microstructure associated with a beta sintering heat treatment.

Discussion. The evidence was generally fractographic in nature. However, these knee prostheses revealed several aspects of materials failure. First, the metal backing used to support the polyethylene cup was subject to fatigue failure if there was incomplete support under one portion of the device. Fatigue cracks initiated on the superior aspect and propagated through the tray. If beads for porous ingrowth were present, the progressing tray fracture sometimes loosened and broke off the beads, which then mi-

grated to other parts of the joint and created severe wear problems.

Multiple fractures at bead-bead junctions and bead-tray junctions were observed in the porous-coated implants. The neck regions between beads and at bead-neck junctions resulted in severe stress-concentration effects, which can be detrimental because of the notch sensi-

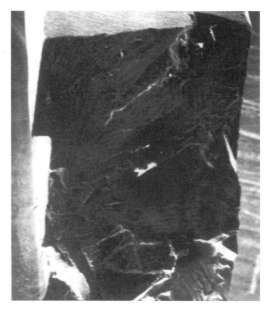

Fig. 69 Low-magnification micrograph of crack-initiation region at base of capture lip in a titanium-alloy tibial component

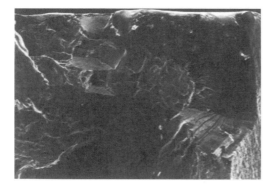

Fig. 67 Higher-magnification view of initiation region in Fig. 66. Localized fracture occurred at facets and eventually linked to form final fracture surface.

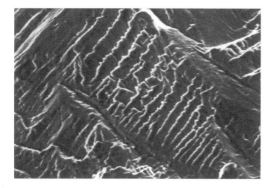

Fig. 68 Fatigue-crack-propagation region of device in Fig. 66. Crack propagated from upper left to lower right.

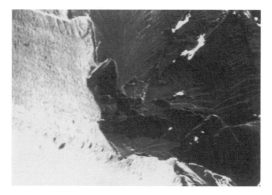

Fig. 70 Higher-magnification view of initiation region in Fig. 69

tivity of titanium in these implants. These fractures were present in regions remote from, as well as adjacent to, the macroscopic fatigue fractures and were sometimes present even in well-fixed implants. Also, the sintering process did not result in the complete formation of sinter necks, thus making these regions highly susceptible to fracture processes. The process of sintering transforms the α and β bimodal microstructure to a β microstructure that is known to be less resistant to fatigue initiation.

Conclusion and Recommendations. Porous-coated and uncoated tibial trays failed by a fatigue process in which cracks initiated on the superior aspects of the trays. The porous coating sintering method resulted in a microstructure that was not as fatigue-initiation resistant as the

bimodal microstructure recommended by ASTM F 136. Geometric constraints on the design, due to anatomic considerations, and asym-

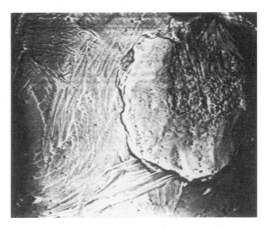

Fig. 73 Micrograph of sinter neck of titanium bead. Note appearance of fracture lines about the circumference of the bead neck.

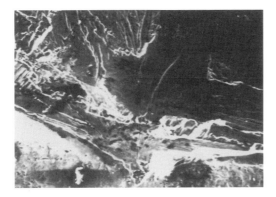

Fig. 71 Higher-magnification view of Fig. 70. Note appearance of large prior-β grain in initiation region.

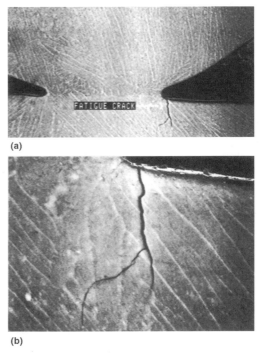

(a)

(b)

Fig. 74 (a) Micrograph of polished section of titanium tray-bead junction. Note fatigue crack penetrating into tray. (b) Higher-magnification view of (a)

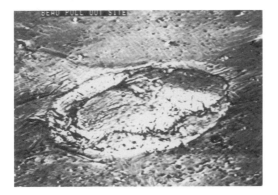

Fig. 72 Micrograph of surface of titanium-alloy tibial tray where a sintered bead has fractured off. Note incomplete fusing of the bead to the tray.

metric loading contributed to the ultimate failure of the components.

Because these components are subjected to high-cycle fatigue loading, a bimodal ($\alpha + \beta$) microstructure with equiaxed primary α should be used to resist fatigue-crack initiation. Porous coating processes or subsequent heat treatments that yield a coarse β microstructure should not be used. Also, better process control should be exerted to minimize the formation of incomplete sinter necks, which serve as stress-concentration sites and fracture-initiation regions.

Design modifications to minimize fatigue failure might include thickening the tray cross section in order to lower stresses or redesigning the cruciate-retaining "U" to minimize stress concentrations. Anatomical constraints limit the extent of modification. For instance, thickening of the tray can be accomplished either at the expense of polyethylene cup thickness or by the removal of greater amounts of bone. Alternative surgical techniques to inhibit asymmetric loading patterns might be employed, such as the use of metallic spacers or modular components instead of bone grafts to fill bone defects.

The sintering process appears to be highly variable in these devices, resulting in irregular sinter necks, which are highly susceptible to failure. Also, the sintering temperature is high enough to result in a β transformation of the microstructure. This microstructure decreases the fatigue-initiation resistance of the material and can degrade the high-cycle fatigue performance of the component. Alternate bonding techniques that do not result in a β transformation of the microstructure, such as diffusion bonding, should be explored.

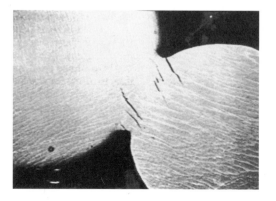

Fig. 75 Micrograph of interbead junction. Note fatigue cracks at oblique angle to neck.

ACKNOWLEDGMENTS

The information in this chapter is largely taken from:

- C. D'Antonio, Failure of a Stainless Steel Hip Fracture Fixation Device, *Handbook of Case Histories in Failure Analysis*, Vol 2, K.A. Esaklul, Ed., ASM International, 1993, p 439–441
- C. D'Antonio, Fracture of a Cast Stainless Steel Femoral Prosthesis, *Handbook of Case Histories in Failure Analysis*, Vol 2, K.A. Esaklul, Ed., ASM International, 1993, p 448–450
- J.L. Gilbert and S.D. Stulberg, Fatigue Fracture of Titanium Alloy Knee Prostheses, *Handbook of Case Histories in Failure Analysis*, Vol 2, K.A. Esaklul, Ed., ASM International, 1993, p 442–447
- O.E.M. Pohler, Failures of Metallic Orthopedic Implants, *Failure Analysis and Prevention*, Vol 11, *Metals Handbook*, 9th ed., ASM International, 1986, p 670–694
- E. Proverbio and L.M. Bonaccorsi, Microstructural Analysis of Failure of a Stainless Steel Bone Plate Implant, *Practical Failure Analysis*, Vol 1 (No. 4), Aug 2001, p 33–38
- H.J. Snyder and B.C. Snyder, Fatigue Fracture of 316L Stainless Steel Screws Employed for Surgical Implanting, *Handbook of Case Histories in Failure Analysis*, Vol 1, K.A. Esaklul, Ed., ASM International, 1992, p 315–317
- M.E. Stevenson, M.E. Barkey, and R.C. Bradt, Fatigue Failures of Austenitic Stainless Steel Orthopedic Fixation Devices, *Practical Failure Analysis*, Vol 2 (No. 3), June 2002, p 57–64

REFERENCES

1. D.C. Mears, *Materials and Orthopaedic Surgery*, The Williams & Wilkins Co., 1979
2. L.R. Rubin, Ed., Chapters 23–27, in *Biomaterials in Reconstructive Surgery*, The C.V. Mosby Co., 1983
3. M.E. Müller, M. Allgöwer, R. Schneider, and H. Willenegger, *Manual of Internal Fixation*, 2nd ed., Springer Verlag, 1979
4. H. Gerber et al., Quantitative Determination of Tissue Tolerance of Corrosion Products by Organ Culture, *Proceedings*

of the European Society for Artificial Organs, Vol 1, 1974, p 29–34

5. H. Gerber and S.M. Perren, Evaluation of Tissue Compatibility of In Vitro Cultures of Embryonic Bone, Evaluation of Biomaterials, G.D. Winter, et al., Ed., John Wiley & Sons, 1980

6. V. Geret, B.A. Rahn, R. Mathys, F. Straumann, and S.M. Perren, A Method for Testing Tissue Tolerance for Improved Quantitative Evaluation, Evaluation of Biomaterials, G.D. Winter et al., Ed., John Wiley & Sons, 1980

7. G.K. Smith, Systemic Aspects of Metallic Implant Degradation, Biomaterials in Reconstructive Surgery, L.R. Rubin, Ed., The C.V. Mosby Co., 1983

8. Medical Devices, Annual Book of ASTM Standards, Vol 13.01, ASTM, 1985

9. A.C. Guyten and J.E. Hall, Textbook of Medical Physiology, W.B. Saunders Co.

10. J.B. Park, Biomaterials: An Introduction, Plenum Press, 1979

11. P.G. Laing, Biocompatibility of Biomaterials, Orthopaedic Clinics of North America, Vol 4, C.M. Evarts, Ed., 1973

12. F. Pauwels, Der Schenkelhasbruch, Enke, Stuttgart, 1935

13. R. Schenk, Fracture Repair—Overview, Ninth European Symposium on Calcified Tissues, 1973

14. R. Schenk and H. Willenegger, Zur Histologie der primären Knochenheilung, Unfallheilkunde, Vol 80, 1977, p 155

15. S.M. Perren and M. Allgöwer, Nova Acta Leopoldina, Vol 44 (No. 223), 1976, p 61

16. S. Perren, R. Ganz, and A. Rüter, Mechanical Induction of Bone Resorption, Fourth International Osteol. Symposium, Prague, 1972

17. H. Yamada, Strength of Biological Materials, The Williams, & Wilkins Co., 1970

18. L.E. Sloter and H.R. Piehler, Corrosion-Fatigue Performance of Stainless Steel Hip Nails—Jewett Type, STP 684, ASTM, 1979, p 173

19. O.E.M. Pohler and F. Straumann, Fatigue and Corrosion Fatigue Studies on Stainless Steel Implant Material, Evaluation of Biomaterials, C.D. Winter et al., Ed., John Wiley & Sons, 1980

20. O.E.M. Pohler, "Study of the Initiation and Propagation Stages of Fatigue and Corrosion Fatigue of Orthopaedic Implant Materials," dissertation, Ohio State University, 1983

21. E. Powell, M.S. thesis, Ohio State University, 1983

22. R.W. Hertzberg, Deformation and Fracture Mechanics of Engineering Materials, John Wiley & Sons, 1976

23. O.E.M. Pohler, Degradation of Metallic Orthopaedic Implants, Biomaterials in Reconstructive Surgery, L.R. Rubin, Ed., The C.V. Mosby Co., 1983

24. B.C. Syrett and A. Acharya, Ed., Corrosion and Degradation of Implant Materials, STP 684, ASTM, 1979

25. A. Fraker and C.D. Griffin, Ed., Corrosion and Degradation of Implant Materials, STP 859, ASTM, 1985

26. J.O. Galante and W. Rostoker, Wear in Total Hip Prostheses, Acta Orthop. Scand. Suppl., Vol 145, 1973

27. M. Ungethüm, Technologische und Biomechanische Aspekte der Hüft- und Kniealloarthroplastik, Aktuelle Probleme in Chirurgie und Orthopaedie, Band 9, Verlag Hans Huber, Bern Stuttgart Wien, 1978

28. P. Griss et al., Ed., Findings on Total Hip Replacement for Ten Years, Aktuelle Probleme in Chirurgie und Orthopaedie, Band 21, Verlag Hans Huber, Bern Stuttgart Wien, 1982

29. R. Schneider, Die Totalprothese der Hüfte (Ein Biomechanisches Konzept und seine Konsequenzen), Aktuelle Probleme in Chirurgie und Orthopaedie, Band 24, Verlag Hans Huber, Bern Stuttgart Wien, 1982

30. M. Semlitsch and B. Panic, Corrosion Fatigue Testing of Femoral Head Prostheses Made of Implant Alloys of Different Fatigue Resistance, Evaluation of Biomaterials, G.D. Winter et al., Ed., John Wiley & Sons, 1980

31. M.F. Semlitsch, B. Panic, H. Weber, and R. Schoen, Comparison of the Fatigue Strength of Femoral Prothesis Stems Made of Forged Ti-Al-V and Cobalt-Base Alloys, STP 796, ASTM, 1983

32. M. Semlitsch and B. Panic, Ten Years of Experience with Test Criteria for Fracture-Proof Anchorage Stems of Artificial Hip Joints, Eng. Med., Vol 12, 1983, p 185

CHAPTER 6

Ceramic Materials

CERAMICS, GLASSES, AND GLASS-CERAMICS have been essential for a long time in the medical industry for eyeglasses, diagnostic instruments, chemical and laboratory ware, thermometers, tissue culture flasks, fiber optics, and so on. Insoluble porous glasses have been used as carriers for enzymes, antibodies, and antigens, offering the advantages of resistance to microbial attack, pH changes, solvent conditions, and temperature (Ref 1). Ceramics are also widely used in dentistry as restorative materials such as gold-porcelain crowns, glass- or silica-filled resin composites, dentures, and so forth. These applications are called dental ceramics and are discussed in Chapters 10, "Biomaterials for Dental Applications," and 12, "Friction and Wear of Dental Materials."

This chapter is limited to ceramics, glasses, and glass-ceramics used as biomedical implants. These materials are attractive as biological implants because bone bonds well to them, and they exhibit minimum foreign body reaction (implying inertness within the body), high stiffness, and low friction and wear as articulating surfaces. Their main drawback is their brittle nature and resultant low impact resistance.

Although dozens of compositions have been explored in the past, relatively few have achieved human clinical application. This chapter concentrates on these compositions, examines their differences in processing and structure, describes the chemical and microstructural basis for their differences in physical properties, and relates properties and hard tissue response to particular clinical applications. References 2 and 3 provide reviews of ceramic biomaterials.

Tissue Attachment Mechanisms

No one material is suitable for all biomaterial applications. As a class of biomaterials, ceramics, glasses, and glass-ceramics are generally used for repair or replacement of musculoskeletal hard connective tissues. Their use depends on achieving a stable attachment to connective tissue. Carbon-base ceramics are also used for replacement heart valves, where resistance to blood clotting and mechanical fatigue are essential characteristics.

The mechanism of tissue attachment is directly related to the type of tissue response at the implant interface. No material implanted in living tissues is inert: all materials elicit a response from living tissues. Four types of response are possible (Table 1). These types of tissue responses allow four different means of achieving attachment of prostheses to the musculoskeletal system. Table 2 summarizes the attachment mechanisms with examples.

A comparison of the relative chemical activity of the different types of bioceramics, glasses, and glass-ceramics is given in Fig. 1. Relative reactivity correlates very closely with the rate of formation of an interfacial bond of ceramic, glass, or glass-ceramic implants with bone (Fig. 2). Figure 2 is discussed in more detail in the section "Bioactive Glasses and Glass-Ceramics" in this chapter.

The relative level of reactivity of an implant influences the thickness of the interfacial zone or layer between the material and tissue. Analysis of failure of implant materials during the last 30 years generally shows failure originating from the biomaterial-tissue interface. When biomaterials are nearly inert (type 1 in Fig. 1) and the interface is not chemically or biologically bonded, there is relative movement and progressive development of a fibrous capsule in soft and hard tissues. The presence of movement at the biomaterial-tissue interface eventually leads to deterioration in function of the implant or the tissue at the interface or both. The thickness of the nonadherent capsule varies, depending on both material and extent of relative motion.

Inert and Nearly Inert Materials. The fibrous tissue at the interface of dense alumina (Al_2O_3) implants is very thin. Thus, if alumina devices are implanted with a very tight mechanical fit and are loaded primarily in compression, they are very successful. In contrast, if a nearly inert implant is loaded such that interfacial movement can occur, the fibrous capsule can become several hundred micrometers thick, and the implant can loosen very quickly.

The concept behind nearly inert microporous materials (type 2 in Fig. 1) is the ingrowth of tissue into pores on the surface or throughout the implant. The increased interfacial area between the implant and the tissues results in an increased inertial resistance to movement of the device in the tissue. The interface is established by the living tissue in the pores. Consequently, this method of attachment is often termed *biological fixation.* It is capable of withstanding more complex stress states than implants with morphological fixation. The limitation associated with type 2 porous implants, however, is that for the tissue to remain viable and healthy, it is necessary for the pores to be greater than 50 to 150 μm (Fig. 3). The large interfacial area required for the porosity is due to the need to provide a blood supply to the ingrown connective tissue; vascular tissue does not appear in pores less than 100 μm in size. If micromovement occurs at the interface of a porous implant, tissue is damaged, the blood supply may be cut off, the tissues will die, inflammation ensues, and interfacial stability can be destroyed. When the material is a metal, the large increase in surface area can provide a focus for corrosion of the implant and loss of metal ions into the tissues. This can be mediated by using a bioactive ceramic material such as hydroxylapatite (HA) as a coating on the porous metal. The fraction of

Table 1 Possible tissue responses to biomedical implants

Implant material characteristics	Tissue response
Toxic	Surrounding tissue dies
Nontoxic, biologically inactive	Fibrous tissue of variable thickness forms
Nontoxic, bioactive	Interfacial bond forms
Nontoxic, dissolves	Surrounding tissue replaces material

Table 2 Tissue attachment mechanisms for bioceramic implants

Type of attachment	Example
Dense, nonporous, nearly inert ceramics attached by bone growth into surface irregularities by cementing the device into the tissues, by press-fitting into a defect, or attachment via a sewing ring (morphological fixation)	Al_2O_3 (single-crystal and polycrystalline) LTI (low-temperature isotropic carbon)
For porous inert implants, bone ingrowth occurs, which mechanically attaches the bone to the materials (biological fixation)	Al_2O_3 (polycrystalline) Hydroxylapatite-coated porous metals
Dense, nonporous, surface-reactive ceramics, glasses, and glass-ceramics attach directly by chemical bonding with the bone (bioactive fixation)	Bioactive glasses Bioactive glass-ceramics Hydroxylapatite
Dense, nonporous (or porous), resorbable ceramics are designed to be slowly replaced by bone	Calcium sulfate (plaster of paris) Tricalcium phosphate Calcium phosphate salts

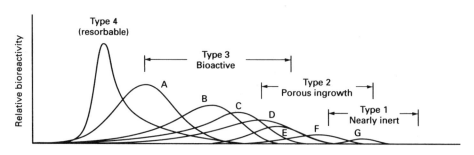

Fig. 1 Relative rates of bioreactivity for ceramic implant materials. A, 45S5 Bioglass; B, KGS Ceravital; C, 55S4.3 Bioglass; D, A/W glass-ceramic (GC); E, hydroxylapatite (HA); F, KGX Ceravital; G, Al_2O_3, silicon nitride (see Table 6 for compositions)

large porosity in any material also degrades the strength of the material proportional to the volume fraction of porosity. Consequently, this approach to solving interfacial stability is best when used as coatings or when used as unloaded space fillers in tissues.

Resorbable biomaterials (type 4 in Fig. 1) are designed to degrade gradually over a period of time and be replaced by the natural host tissue. This leads to a very thin interfacial thickness. This is the optimal solution to the biomaterials problem, if the requirements of strength

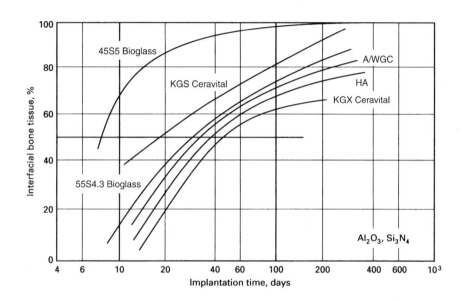

Fig. 2   Time dependence of formation of bone bonding for the materials shown in Fig. 1

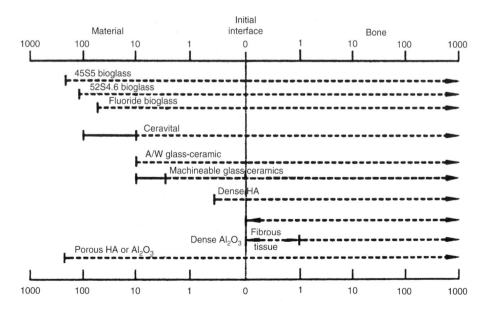

Fig. 3   Comparison of interfacial thickness (μm) of reaction layers of bioactive implants, of fibrous tissue, and inactive bioceramics in bone. Source: Ref 2

and short-term performance can be met. Natural tissues can repair themselves and are gradually replaced throughout life. Thus, resorbable biomaterials are based on the same principles of repair that have evolved over millions of years. Complications in the development of resorbable bioceramics are:

- Maintenance of strength and the stability of the interface during the degradation period and replacement by the natural host tissue
- Matching resorption rates to the repair rates of body tissues

Some materials dissolve too rapidly and some too slowly. Because large quantities of material may be replaced, it is also essential that a resorbable biomaterial consists only of metabolically acceptable substances. Porous or particulate calcium phosphate ceramic materials such as tricalcium phosphate (TCP) are successful materials for resorbable hard tissue replacements when low loads are applied to the material.

Bioactive Materials. Another approach to solving problems of interfacial attachment is the use of bioactive materials (type 3 in Fig. 1). The concept of bioactive materials is intermediate between resorbable and bioinert. A bioactive material is one that elicits a specific biological response at the interface, which results in the formation of a bond between the tissues and the material. This concept has now been expanded to include a large number of bioactive materials with a wide range of rates of bonding and thicknesses of interfacial bonding layers (Fig. 1 to 3). They include bioactive glasses such as Bioglass (University of Florida), bioactive glass-ceramics such as Ceravital (E. Leitz Wetzlar GmBh), A/W glass-ceramic, or machinable glass-ceramics; dense HA such as Durapatite (Sterling Winthrop) or Calcitite (Calcitek) or bioactive composites such as Palavital (E. Leitz Co.) or stainless steel fiber-reinforced Bioglass. All of the aforementioned bioactive materials form an interfacial bond with adjacent tissue. However, the time dependence of bonding, the strength of bond, the mechanism of bonding, and the thickness of the bonding zone differ for the various materials.

Relatively small changes in the composition of a biomaterial can dramatically affect whether it is bioinert, resorbable, or bioactive. These compositional effects on surface reactions are discussed in the section "Bioactive Glasses and Glass-Ceramics" in this chapter.

Nearly Inert Crystalline Ceramics

Alumina. High-density, high-purity (>99.5%) Al_2O_3 is used in load-bearing hip prostheses and dental implants because of its combination of excellent corrosion resistance, good biocompatibility, high wear resistance, and high strength (Ref 3–5). Although some dental implants are single-crystal sapphire, most Al_2O_3 devices are very fine-grained polycrystalline α-Al_2O_3 produced by pressing and sintering at temperatures of 1600 to 1700 °C (2910 to 3090 °F). A very small amount (<0.5%) of magnesia (MgO) is used as an aid to sintering and to limit grain growth during sintering.

Strength, fatigue resistance, and fracture toughness of polycrystalline α-Al_2O_3 are functions of grain size and purity. Alumina with an average grain size of <4 μm and >99.7% purity exhibits good flexural strength and excellent compressive strength. These and other physical properties are summarized in Table 3, along with the International Standards Organization (ISO) requirements for Al_2O_3 implants. Similar ASTM International requirements are listed in Table 4. Extensive testing has shown that Al_2O_3 implants that meet or exceed ISO and/or ASTM standards have excellent resistance to dynamic and impact fatigue and also resist subcritical crack growth (Ref 6). An increase in average grain size to >7 μm can decrease mechanical properties by approximately 20%. High concentrations of sintering aids must be avoided, because they remain in the grain boundaries and degrade fatigue resistance.

Methods exist for lifetime predictions and statistical design of proof tests for load-bearing ceramics. Applications of these techniques

Table 3 Physical characteristics of Al_2O_3 bioceramics

	High-alumina ceramics	ISO 6474
Alumina content, %	<99.8	≥99.50
Density, g/cm³	>3.93	≥3.90
Average grain size, μm	3–6	<7
Surface roughness (R_a), μm	0.02	. . .
Vickers hardness	2300	>2000
Compressive strength, MPa (ksi)	4500 (653)	. . .
Bending strength, MPa (ksi) (after testing in Ringer's solution)	550 (80)	400 (58)
Young's modulus, GPa (psi × 10⁶)	380 (55.2)	. . .
Fracture toughness (K_{Ic}), Mpa $\sqrt{m}$ (ksi $\sqrt{in.}$)	5–6 (4.5–5.5)	. . .

show that specific prosthesis load limits can be set for an Al_2O_3 device based on the flexural strength of the material and its use environment. Load-bearing lifetimes of 30 years at 12,000 N (2700 lbf) loads have been predicted (Ref 5). Results from aging and fatigue studies show that it is essential that Al_2O_3 implants be produced at the highest possible standards of quality assurance, especially if they are to be used as orthopedic prostheses in younger patients

Alumina has been used in orthopedic surgery for nearly 30 years, motivated largely by two factors:

- Excellent biocompatibility and very thin capsule formation, which permits cementless fixation of prostheses
- Exceptionally low coefficients of friction and wear rates

The superb tribologic properties (friction and wear) of Al_2O_3 occur only when the grains are very small (<4 μm) and have a very narrow size distribution. These conditions lead to very low surface roughness values ($R_a \leq 0.02$ μm, see

Table 3). If large grains are present, they can pull out and lead to very rapid wear of bearing surfaces due to local dry friction.

Alumina-on-alumina load-bearing wearing surfaces, such as in hip prostheses, must have a very high degree of sphericity produced by grinding and polishing the two mating surfaces together. An Al_2O_3 ball and socket in a hip prosthesis are polished together and used as a pair. The long-term coefficient of friction of an Al_2O-Al_2O_3 joint decreases with time and approaches the values of a normal joint. This leads to wear of Al_2O_3-on-Al_2O_3 articulating surfaces being nearly 10 times lower than the metal-polyethylene surfaces (Fig. 4).

Low wear rates have led to widespread use in Europe of Al_2O_3 noncemented cups press-fitted into the acetabulum of the hip. The cups are stabilized by bone growth into grooves or around pegs. The mating femoral ball surface is also of Al_2O_3, which is bonded to a metallic stem. Long-term results in general are excellent, especially for younger patients. However, stress shielding due to the high elastic modulus of Al_2O_3 may be responsible for cancellous bone atrophy and loosening of the acetabular cup in older patients with senile osteoporosis or rheumatoid arthritis (Ref 5). Consequently, it is essential that the age of the patient, nature of the disease of the joint, and biomechanics of the repair be considered carefully before any prosthesis is used, including Al_2O_3 ceramics.

Other clinical applications of Al_2O_3 include knee prostheses, bone screws, alveolar ridge and maxillofacial reconstruction, ossicular bond substitutes, keratoprostheses (corneal replacements), segmental bone replacements, and blade and screw and postdental implants.

Table 4 Minimum physical characteristics of Al_2O_3 bioceramics in accordance with ASTM F 603

Alumina content, %	≥99.5
Density, g/cm³	3.94
Median grain size, μm	≤4.5
Vickers hardness, GPa (10^6 psi)	18 (2.56)
Compressive strength, GPa (ksi)	4 (580)
Flexural strength, MPa (ksi)	400 (58)
Elastic modulus, GPa (ksi)	380 (55,100)
Weibull modulus	8

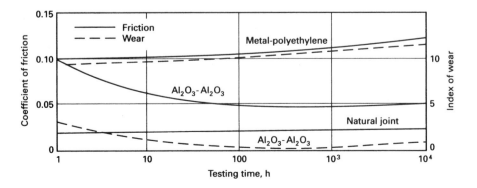

Fig. 4 Friction and wear of Al_2O_3-Al_2O_3 hip joint compared to a metal-polyethylene prosthesis and a natural joint in in-vitro tests

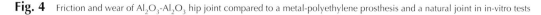

High-purity dense yttria-stabilized tetragonal zirconia polycrystal (Y-TZP) is also used as the articulating ball in total hip prostheses. This is a fine-grain, high-strength, moderate-high fracture toughness material. Properties of Y-TZP are listed in Table 5. High-strength Y-TZPs are manufactured by sintering at relatively low sintering temperatures (1400 °C, or 2550 °F). Nearly 100% of the zirconia is in the tetragonal symmetry, and the average grain size is approximately 0.4 to 0.8 μm. The tetragonal phase in this microstructure is very stable. Higher firing temperatures (1550 °C, or 2800 °F) result in a high-strength (800 MPa, or 116 ksi), high fracture toughness (8.5 MPa$\sqrt{m}$, or 7.7 ksi$\sqrt{in.}$), fine-grain material with excellent wear resistance. The microstructure (Fig. 5) consists of a mixture of 1 to 2 μm tetragonal grains (90 to 95%) and 4 to 8 μm cubic grains (5 to 10%).

Porous Ceramics

The potential advantage offered by a porous ceramic implant (type 2 in Fig. 1) is its inertness combined with the mechanical stability of the highly convoluted interface developed when bone grows into the pores of the ceramic. Mechanical requirements of prostheses, however, severely restrict the use of low-strength porous ceramics to nonload-bearing applications. Studies reviewed in Ref 1 and 3 have shown that when load bearing is not a primary requirement, nearly inert porous ceramics can provide a functional implant. When pore sizes exceed 100 μm, bone will grow within the interconnecting pore channels near the surface and maintain its vascularity and long-term viability. In this manner, the implant serves as a structural bridge and model or scaffold for bone formation.

The microstructures of certain corals make an almost ideal investment material for the casting of structures with highly controlled pores sizes. White et al. (Ref 7) developed the replamineform process to duplicate the porous microstructure of corals that have a high degree of uniform pore size and interconnection. The first step is to machine the coral with proper microstructure into the desired shape. The most promising coral genus, *Porites,* has pores with a size range of 140 to 160 μm with all the pores interconnected. Another interesting coral genus, *Goniopora,* has a larger pore size, ranging from 200 to 1000 μm. The machined coral shape is fired to drive off carbon dioxide from the limestone ($CaCO_3$), forming calcia (CaO) while maintaining the microstructure of the original coral. The CaO structure serves as an investment material for forming the porous material. After the desired material is cast into the pores, the CaO is easily removed from the material by dissolving in dilute HCl.

The primary advantages of the replamineform process are that the pore size and microstructure are uniform and controlled, and there is complete interconnection of the pores. Replamineform porous materials of α-Al_2O_3, titanium dioxide (TiO_2), calcium phosphates,

Table 5 Minimum physical characteristics of yttria-stabilized tetragonal zirconia polycrystal bioceramics in accordance with ASTM F 1873

Zirconia content, %	≥93.2
Yttria content, %	4.5 to 5.4
Density, g/cm³	≥6.0
Median grain size, μm	≤0.6
Vickers hardness	1200 HV
Flexural strength, MPa (ksi)	800 (116)
Weibull modulus	10
Elastic modulus GPa (10⁶ psi)	200 (29)

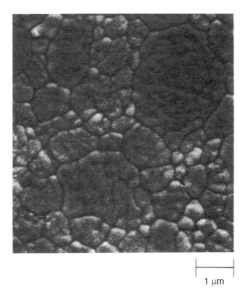

Fig. 5 Scanning electron micrograph of a yttria-stabilized tetragonal zirconia polycrystal sample. The larger 3 to 5 μm grains are cubic (~5%); the smaller 1 to 2 μm grains are tetragonal (~95%).

polyurethane, silicone rubber, polymethyl methacrylate, and cobalt-base alloys have been used as bone implants, with the calcium phosphates being the most acceptable (Ref 7, 8).

Porous ceramic surfaces can also be prepared by mixing soluble metal or salt particles into the surface or using a foaming agent such as $CaCO_3$, which evolves gases during heating. Pore size and structure is determined by the size and shape of the soluble particles that are subsequently removed with a suitable etchant. The porous surface layer produced by this technique is an integral part of the underlying dense ceramic phase. Porous materials are weaker than the equivalent bulk form in proportion to the percentage of porosity. Much surface area is also exposed, so that the effects of the environment on decreasing the strength become much more important than for dense, nonporous materials. The environmental sensitivity of the high-strength ceramics and the loss of strength of porous ceramics with aging are reviewed in Ref 1.

Bioactive Glasses and Glass-Ceramics

Certain compositions of glasses, ceramics, glass-ceramics, and composites have been shown to bond to bone (Ref 1, 9–11). These materials have become known as bioactive ceramics. Some even more specialized compositions of bioactive glasses will bond to soft tissues as well as bone. A common characteristic of bioactive glasses and bioactive ceramics is a time-dependent, kinetic modification of the surface that occurs on implantation. The surface forms a biologically active HA layer that provides the bonding interface with tissues.

Materials that are bioactive develop an adherent interface with tissues that resists substantial mechanical forces. In many cases, the interfacial strength of adhesion is equivalent or greater than the cohesive strength of the implant material or the tissue bonded to the bioactive implant.

Glasses. Bonding to bone was first demonstrated for a certain compositional range of bioactive glasses that contained silica (SiO_2), soda (Na_2O), calcia, and phosphorus oxide (P_2O_5). There were three key compositional features to these glasses that distinguished them from traditional soda-lime-silica glasses: (1) less than 60 mol% SiO_2, (2) high Na_2O and CaO content, and (3) high CaO/P_2O_5 ratio. These

compositional features make the surface highly reactive when exposed to an aqueous medium.

Many bioactive silica glasses are based on the formula called 45S5, signifying 45 wt% SiO_2 (S = the network former) and 5 to 1 molar ratio of CaO to P_2O_5. Glasses with lower molar ratios of CaO to P_2O_5 do not bond to bone. However, substitutions in the 45S5 formula of 5 to 15 wt% boron oxide (B_2O_3) for SiO_2 or 12.5 wt% calcium fluoride (CaF_2) for CaO, or ceraming the various bioactive glass compositions to form glass-ceramics, has no measurable effect on the ability of the material to form a bone bond. However, addition of as little as 3 wt% Al_2O_3 to the 45S5 formula prevents bonding.

The compositional dependence of bone and soft tissue bonding on the Na_2O-CaO-P_2O_5-SiO_2 glasses is illustrated in Fig. 6. All the glasses in Fig. 6 contain a constant 6 wt% of P_2O_5. Compositions in the middle of the diagram (region A) form a bond with bone. Consequently, region A is termed the bioactive bone-bonding boundary. Silicate glasses within region B (e.g., window or bottle glass, or microscope slides) behave as nearly inert materials and elicit a fibrous capsule at the implant-tissue interface. Glasses within region C are resorbable and disappear within 10 to 30 days of implantation. Glasses within region D are not technically practical and therefore have not been tested as implants.

Glass-Ceramics. Gross et al. (Ref 10) have shown that a range of low-alkali (0 to 5 wt%)

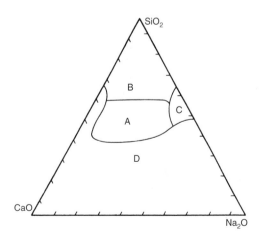

Fig. 6 Bioglass compositional range for bonding to rat bone. A, bonding at less than 31 days; B, nonbonding, reactivity is too low; C, nonbonding, reactivity is too high; D, nonbonding, nonglass-forming. Source: Ref 2

bioactive silica glass-ceramics (Ceravital) also bonds to bone. They find that small additions of Al_2O_3, tantalum, titanium, or zirconium inhibit bone bonding. A two-phase silica-phosphate glass-ceramic composed of apatite [$Ca_{10}(PO_4)_6$ (OH_1F_2)] and wollastonite ($CaO \cdot SiO_2$) crystals and a residual silica glassy matrix termed A/W glass-ceramic (Ref 11) also bonds with bone. Addition of Al_2O_3 or TiO_2 to the A/W glass-ceramic inhibits bone bonding, whereas incorporation of a second phosphate phase, B-whitlockite ($3CaO \cdot P_2O_5$), does not.

Another multiphase bioactive phosphosilicate containing phlogopite [$(Na,K)Mg_3 (AlSi_3 O_{10})F_2$] and apatite crystals bonds to bone even though Al_2O_3 is present in the composition (Ref 12). However, the Al^{3+} ions are incorporated within the crystal phase and do not alter the surface reaction kinetics of the material. Compositions of these various bioactive glasses and glass-ceramics are compared in Table 6.

Surfaces characteristic of bioactive glasses and glass-ceramics form a dual protective film rich in CaO and P_2O_5 on top of an alkali-depleted SiO_2-rich film. When multivalent cations such as Al^{3+}, Fe^{3+}, or Ti^{4+} are present in the glass or in the solution, multiple layers form on the glass as the saturation of each cationic complex is exceeded. This leads to a surface that does not bond to tissue.

A general equation describes the overall rate of change of glass surfaces and gives rise to the interfacial reaction rates and time dependence of bone-bonding profiles shown in Fig. 2. The reaction rate, R, depends on at least five terms (for a single-phase glass). For polycrystalline ceramics, or glass-ceramics, which have several phases in their microstructures, each phase will have a characteristic reaction rate, R_i, which must be multiplied times its areal fraction exposed to tissue in order to describe overall kinetics of bonding:

$$R = -k_1 t^{0.5} - k_2 t^{1.0} + k_3 t^{1.0} + k_4 t^y + t_5 \quad \text{(Eq 1)}$$

Stage 1   Stage 2   Stage 3   Stage 4   Stage 5

The first term describes the rate of alkali extraction from the glass and is called a stage 1 reaction.

In stage 1, the initial or primary stage of attack is a process that involves ion exchange between alkali ions from the glass and hydrogen ions from the solution, during which the remaining constituents of the glass are not altered. During stage 1, the rate of alkali extraction from the glass is parabolic in character.

Stage 2 is interfacial network dissolution whereby siloxane bonds are broken, forming a large concentration of surface silanol groups. Stage 2 kinetics are linear. A resorbable glass experiences a combination of stage 1 and stage 2 attacks.

Stages 3 and 4 result in a glass surface with a dual protective film. The thickness of the secondary films can vary considerably, from as little as 0.01 mm for Al_2O_3-SiO_2-rich layers on inactive glasses to as much as 30 mm for CaO-P_2O_5-rich layers on bioactive glasses. The for-

Table 6 Compositions and structures of bioactive glasses and glass-ceramics

All compositions in wt%

	Material										
Constituent	45S5 Bioglass	45S5F Bioglass	45S5.4F Bioglass	40S5B5 Bioglass	52S4.6 Bioglass	55S4.3 Bioglass	KGC Ceravital	KGS Ceravital	KGy213 Ceravital	A/W-GC	MB-GC
SiO_2	45	45	45	40	52	55	46.2	46	38	34.2	19–52
P_2O_5	6	6	6	6	6	6	...	...	...	16.3	4–24
CaO	24.5	12.25	14.7	24.5	21	19.5	20.2	33	31	44.9	9–3
$Ca(PO_3)_2$	...	...	...	...	...	...	25.5	16	13.5	...	...
CaF_2	...	12.25	9.8	...	...	...	...	...	...	0.5	...
MgO	...	...	...	...	...	...	2.9	...	...	4.6	5–15
MgF_2	...	...	...	...	...	...	...	...	...	...	...
Na_2O	24.5	24.5	24.5	24.5	21	19.5	4.8	5	4	...	3–5
K_2O	...	...	...	...	...	...	0.4	...	...	...	3–5
Al_2O_3	...	...	...	...	...	...	...	...	7	...	12–33
B_2O_3	...	...	...	5	...	...	...	...	...	...	...
Ta_2O_5/TiO_2	...	...	...	...	...	...	...	...	6.5	...	...
Structure	Glass	Glass	Glass	Glass	Glass	...	Glass-ceramic	Glass-ceramic	...	Glass-ceramic	Glass-ceramic

mation of the dual films is due to a combination of the repolymerization of SiO_2 on the glass surface (stage 3) by the condensation of the silanols (Si–OH) formed from the stage 1 and 2 reactions, for example:

$$Si\text{–}OH + OH\text{–}Si \rightarrow Si\text{–}O\text{–}Si + H_2O \qquad (Eq\ 2)$$

Stage 3 protects the glass surface. The SiO_2 polymerization reaction contributes to the enrichment of surface SiO_2 characteristic of bone-bonding glasses. It is described by the third term in Eq 1. This reaction is interface controlled with a time dependence of $+k_3t^{1.0}$. The interfacial thickness of the most reactive bioactive glasses is largely due to this reaction. The fourth term in Eq 1, $+k_4t^y$ (stage 4) describes the precipitation of an amorphous calcium phosphate film, which is characteristic of bioactive glasses.

In stage 5, the amorphous calcium phosphate film crystallizes to form HA crystals. The calcium and phosphate ions in the glass or glass-ceramic provide the nucleation sites for crystallization. Carbonate anions (CO_3^{2-}) substitute for OH^- in the apatite crystal structure to form a hydroxyl-carbonate apatite (HCA) similar to that found in living bone. Incorporation of calcium fluoride (CaF_2) in the glass results in incorporation of fluoride ions in the apatite, resulting in a hydroxyl carbonate fluorapatite that matches dental enamel. Crystallization of HCA occurs around collagen fibrils present at the implant interface and results in interface bonding.

In order for the material to be bioactive and form an interfacial bond, the kinetics of reaction in Eq 1, and especially the rates of stages 4 and 5, must match the rate of biomineralization that normally occurs in vivo. If the rates in Eq 1 are too rapid, the implant is resorbable; if the rates are too slow, the implant is not bioactive.

By changing the compositionally controlled reaction kinetics (Eq 1), the rates of formation of hard tissue at a bioactive implant interface can be altered, as shown in Fig. 2. Thus, the level of bioactivity of a material, $t_{0.5bb}$, can be related to the time for more than 50% of the interface to be bonded: index of bioactivity, I_B, $= (100/t_{0.5bb})$. It is necessary to impose a 50% bonding criterion for an index of bioactivity, because the interface between an implant and bone is irregular (Ref 10). The initial concentration of cell at the interface varies as a function of the frit of the implant and the condition of the

bony defect. Consequently, all bioactive implants require an incubation period before bone proliferates and bonds, with the length of the incubation period varying over a wide range, depending on composition.

Bioactive implants with intermediate I_B values do not develop a stable soft tissue bond; instead, the fibrous interface progressively mineralizes to form bone. Consequently, there appears to be a critical boundary beyond which bioactivity is restricted to stable bone bonding. Inside the critical boundary, the bioactivity includes both stable bone and soft tissue bonding, depending on the progenitor stem cells in contact with the implant.

The thickness of the bonding zone between a bioactive implant and bone is proportional to its index of bioactivity, I_B. The failure strength of a bioactively fixed bond appears to be inversely dependent on the thickness of the bonding zone. For example, 45S5 Bioglass with a very high I_B develops a gel bonding layer 200 μm thick that has a relatively low shear strength. In contrast, A/W glass-ceramic, with an intermediate I_B value, has a bonding interface in the range of 10 to 20 μm and a very high resistance to shear. Thus, the interfacial bonding strength appears to be optimal for I_B values of ~4. However, it is important to recognize that the interfacial area for bonding is time-dependent. Therefore, interfacial strength is time-dependent and is a function of morphological factors such as the change in interfacial area with time, progressive mineralization of the interfacial tissues, and resulting increase of elastic modulus of the interfacial bond as well as shear strength per unit of bonded area. A comparison of the increase in interfacial bond strength of bioactive fixation of implants bonded to bone with other types of fixation is given in Fig. 7.

Clinical applications of bioactive glasses and glass-ceramics are reviewed in Ref 9 to 11 and shown in Table 7. The successful use of Ceravital glass-ceramics in middle ear surgery (Ref 11) is especially encouraging, as is the use of A-W glass-ceramic in vertebral surgery (Ref 11) and the use of 45S5 Bioglass in endosseous ridge maintenance.

Calcium Phosphate Ceramics

Calcium-phosphate-base bioceramics have been in use in medicine and dentistry for nearly thirty years, as reviewed in Ref 14 to 16. Applications include dental implants, periodontal treatment, alveolar ridge augmentation, orthopedics, maxillofacial surgery, and otolaryngology (Table 7). Different phases of calcium phosphate ceramics are used depending on whether a resorbable or bioactive material is desired.

The stable phases of calcium phosphate ceramics depend considerably on temperature and the presence of water, either during processing or in the use environment. At body temperature, only two calcium phosphates are stable in contact with aqueous media, such as body fluids; at pH < 4.2, the stable phase is $CaHPO_4 \cdot 2H_2O$ (dicalciumphosphate or brushite), while at pH $\geq$ 4.2, the stable phase is $Ca_{10}(PO_4)_6(OH)_2$ (hydroxylapatite, HA). At higher temperatures, other phases, such as $Ca_3(PO_4)_2$ (β-tricalciumphosphate, C_3P, or TCP) and $Ca_4P_2O_9$ (tetracalcium phosphate, C_4P), are present. The unhydrated high-temperature calcium phosphate phases interact with water, or body fluids, at 37 °C (98.6 °F) to form HA. The HA forms on exposed surfaces of TCP by the following reaction:

$$4Ca_3(PO_4)_2 + 2H_2O \rightarrow$$
(Solid)

$$Ca_{10}(PO_4)_6(OH) + 2Ca^{2+} + 2HPO_4^{2-} \quad \text{(Eq 3)}$$
(Surface)

Thus, the solubility of a TCP surface approaches the solubility of HA and decreases the pH of the solution, which further increases the solubility of TCP and enhances resorption. The presence of micropores in the sintered material can increase the solubility of these phases.

Sintering of calcium phosphate ceramics usually occurs in the range of 1000 to 1500 °C (1830 to 2730 °F) following compaction of the powder into the desired shape. The phases formed at high temperature depend not only on temperature but also the partial pressure of water in the sintering atmosphere. This is because with water present, HA can be formed and is a stable phase up to 1360 °C (2480 °F). Without water, C_4P and C_3P are the stable phases. The temperature range of stability of HA increases with the partial pressure of water, as does the rate of phase transitions of C_3P or C_4P to HA. Due to kinetics barriers that affect the rates of formation of the stable calcium phosphate phases, it is often difficult to predict the volume fraction of high-temperature phases that are formed during sintering and their relative stability when cooled to room temperature.

Starting powders can be made by mixing in an aqueous solution the appropriate molar ratios of calcium nitrate and ammonium phosphate, which yields a precipitate of stoichiometric HA.

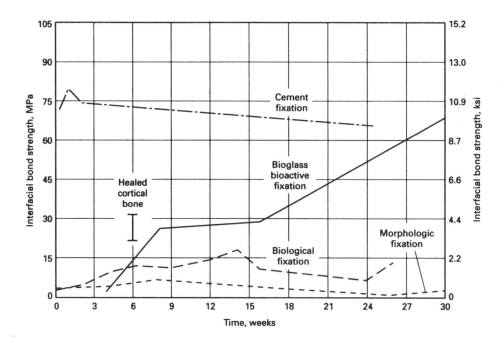

Fig. 7 Time-dependence of interfacial bond strength of various fixation systems in bone. Source: Ref 13

The Ca^{2+}, PO_4^{3-} and OH^- ions can be replaced by other ions during processing or in physiological surroundings; for example, fluorapatite, $Ca_{10}(PO_4)_6(OH)_{2-x}$ with $0 < x < 2$; and carbonate apatite, $Ca_{10}(PO_4)_6(OH)_{2-2x}(CO_3)_x$ or $Ca_{10-x+y}(PO_4)_{6-x}(OH)_{2-x}-2y$, where $0 < x < 2$ and $0 < y < \frac{1}{2}x$, can be formed. Fluorapatite is found in dental enamel, and hydroxyl-carbonate apatite is present in bone. For discussion of the structure of these complex crystals, see Ref 16.

The mechanical behavior of calcium phosphate ceramics strongly influences their application as implants. Tensile and compressive strength and fatigue resistance depend on the total volume of porosity. Porosity can be in the form of micropores (<1 µm in diameter, due to incomplete sintering) or macropores (>100 µm in diameter, created to permit bone growth). The dependence of compressive strength, σ_c, and total pore volume, V_p, is described in megapascals (Ref 17):

$$\sigma_c = 700 \exp - 5V_p \qquad \text{(Eq 4)}$$

Table 7 Present uses of bioceramics

Application	Material(s) used
Orthopedic load-bearing applications	Al_2O_3
Coatings for chemical bonding (orthopedic, dental and maxillary prosthetics)	HA, surface-active glasses and glass-ceramics
Dental implants	Al_2O_3, HA, surface-active glasses
Alveolar ridge augmentations	Al_2O_3, HA, HA-autogenous bone composite, HA-PLA composite, surface-active glasses
Otolaryngological applications	Al_2O_3, HA, surface-active glasses and glass-ceramics
Artificial tendons and ligaments	PLA-carbon-fiber composites
Coatings for tissue ingrowth (cardiovascular, orthopedic, dental, and maxillofacial prosthetics)	Al_2O_3
Temporary bone space fillers	Trisodium phosphate, calcium and phosphate salts
Periodontal pocket obliteration	HA, HA-PLA composites, trisodium phosphate, calcium and phosphate salts, surface-active glasses
Maxillofacial reconstruction	Al_2O_3, HA, HA-PLA composites, surface-active glasses
Percutaneous access devices	Bioactive glass-ceramics
Orthopedic fixation devices	PLA-carbon fibers, PLA-calcium/phosphorus-base glass fibers

HA, hydroxylapatite

where V_p is between 0 and 0.5. Tensile strength, σ_t (in megapascals), depends greatly on the volume fraction of microporosity, V_m:

$$\sigma_t = 220 \exp - 20V_m \qquad \text{(Eq 5)}$$

The Weibull factor, n, of HA implants is low ($n = 12$) in physiological solutions, which indicates low reliability under tensile loads. Consequently, in clinical practice, calcium phosphate bioceramics should be used as:

- Powders
- Small, unloaded implants, such as in the middle ear
- With reinforcing metal posts, as in dental implants
- As coatings (for example, composites)
- As low-loaded porous implants where bone growth acts as a reinforcing phase

The bonding mechanisms of dense HA implants appear to be very different from that described previously for bioactive glasses. Evidence for the bonding process for HA implants is described in Ref 15. A cellular bone matrix from differentiated osteoblasts appears at the surface, producing a narrow, amorphous, electron-dense band only 3 to 5 µm wide. Between this area and the cells, collagen bundles are seen. Bone mineral crystals have been identified in this amorphous area. As the site matures, the bonding zone shrinks to a depth of only 0.05 to 0.2 µm. The result is normal bone attached through a thin epitaxial bonding layer to the bulk implant. Transmission electron microscope image analysis of dense HA bone interfaces has shown an almost perfect epitaxial alignment of the growing bone crystallites with the apatite crystals in the implant.

A consequence of this ultrathin bonding zone is a very high gradient in elastic modulus at the bonding interface between HA and bone. This is one of the major differences between the bioactive apatites and the bioactive glasses and glass-ceramics. The implications of this difference on the implant interfacial response is discussed in Ref 1.

Resorbable Calcium Phosphates

Resorption or biodegradation of calcium phosphate ceramics is caused by: physiochemical dissolution, which depends on the solubility product of the material and local pH of its environment; physical disintegration into small particles due to preferential chemical attack of grain boundaries; and biological factors, such as phagocytosis, which causes a decrease in local pH concentrations.

All calcium phosphate ceramics biodegrade at increasing rates in the following order: α-TCP > β-TCP $\gg$ HA. The rate of biodegradation increases as:

- Surface area increases (powders > porous solid > dense solid)
- Crystallinity decreases
- Crystal perfection decreases
- Crystal and grain size decrease
- Ionic substitutions of CO_3^{2-} Mg^{2+}, and Sr^{2+} in Ha increase

Factors that tend to decrease rate of biodegradation include:

- F^- substitution in HA
- Mg^{2+} substitution in β-TCP
- Lower β-TCP/HA ratios in biphasic calcium phosphates

Carbon-Base Implant Materials

Primarily three types of carbon are used in biomedical devices: the low-temperature isotropic (LTI) variety of pyrolytic carbon, glassy (vitreous) carbon, and the ultralow-temperature isotropic (ULTI) form of vapor-deposited carbon (Ref 18, 19).

These carbon materials in use are integral and monolithic materials (glassy carbon and LTI carbon) or impermeable thin coatings (ULTI carbon). These three forms do not suffer from the integrity problems typical of the other available carbon materials. With the exception of the LTI carbons codeposited with silicon, all the clinical carbon materials are pure elemental carbon. Up to 20 wt% Si has been added to LTI carbon without significantly affecting the biocompatibility of the material. The composition, structure, and fabrication of the three clinically relevant carbons are uniquely compared with the more common naturally occurring form of carbon (graphite) and other industrial forms produced from pure elemental carbon.

Subcrystalline Forms. The LTI, ULTI, and glassy carbons are subcrystalline forms and represent a lower degree of crystal perfection. There is no order between the layers as there is in graphite, so the crystal structure of these carbons is two-dimensional.

The densities of these carbons range between approximately 1.4 and 2.1 g/cm^3. High-density LTI carbons are the strongest bulk forms of carbon, and their strength can be further increased by adding silicon. ULTI carbon can also be produced with high densities and strengths, but it is available only as a thin coating (0.1 to 1 μm) of pure carbon. Glassy carbon is inherently a low-density material and as such is weak. Its strength cannot be increased through processing. Processing of all three types of medical carbons is discussed in Ref 19.

The mechanical properties of the various carbons are intimately related to their microstructures. In an isotropic carbon, it is possible to generate materials with low (20 GPa, or 2.9×10^6 psi) elastic moduli and high flexural strength (275 to 620 MPa, or 40 to 90 ksi). There are many benefits as a result of this combination of properties. Large strains (~2%) are possible without fracture.

Carbon materials are extremely tough compared with ceramics such as Al_2O_3. The energy to fracture for LTI carbon is approximately 5.5 MJ/m^3 (115×10^3 ft · lbf/ft^3) compared with 0.18 MJ/m^3 (3.8×10^3 ft · lbf/ft^3) for Al_2O_3; that is, the carbon is more than 25 times as tough. The strain to fracture for the vapor-deposited carbons is greater than 5.0%, making it feasible to coat highly flexible polymeric materials such as polyethylene, polyesters, and nylon without fear of fracturing the coating when the substrate is flexed. For comparison, the strain to failure of Al_2O_3 is approximately 0.1%, approximately one fiftieth that of the ULTI carbons.

These carbon materials have extremely good wear resistance, some of which can be attributed to their toughness—that is, their capacity to sustain large local elastic strains under concentrated or point loading without galling or incurring surface damage.

The bond strength of the ULTI carbon to stainless steel and to Ti-6Al-4V exceeds 70 MPa (10.2 ksi) as measured with a thin-film adhesion tester. This excellent bond is, in part, achieved through the formation of interfacial carbides. The ULTI carbon coating generally has a lower bond strength with materials that do not form carbides.

Another unique characteristic of the carbons is that they do not fail in fatigue; unlike metals, ultimate strength does not degrade with cyclical

Table 8 Properties of biomedical carbons

Property	Material		
	Low- to high-density LTI carbon	Silicon-alloyed LTI carbon	ULTI carbon
Density, g/cm^3	1.5–2.2	2–2.2	1.5–2.2
Crystallite size (L_c), nm	3–4	3–4	0.8–1.5
Flexural strength, MPa (ksi)	275–550 (40–80)	550–620 (80–90)	345 to >690 (50 to >100)
Young's modulus, GPa (psi × 10^6)	17–28 (2.5–4.1)	28–41 (4.1–5.9)	14–21 (2–3)
Fatigue limit/flexural strength ratio	1	1	1
Poisson's ratio	0.2	0.2	. . .
Diamond pyramid hardness	150–250	230–370	150–250
Thermal expansion coefficient, 10^{-6}/K	4–6	5	. . .
Silicon content, wt%	0	5–12	0
Strain energy to fracture, MJ/m^3 (ft · lbf × 10^3/ft^3)	2.7–5.5 (56.4–115)	5.5 (115)	9.9 (207)
Strain to fracture, %	1.6–2.1	2.0	>5.0
Impurity level, ppm	<100	<100	<100

LTI, low-temperature isotropic; ULTI, ultralow-temperature isotropic

loading. The fatigue strength of these carbon structures is equal to the single-cycle fracture strength. It appears that unlike other crystalline solids, these forms of carbon do not contain mobile defects that, at normal temperatures, can move and provide a mechanism for the initiation of a fatigue crack.

Some of the more important known properties of biomedical carbons are listed in Table 8.

Biocompatability. Carbon surfaces are not only thromboresistant but also compatible with the cellular elements of blood. The materials do not influence plasma proteins or alter the activity of plasma enzymes. In fact, one of the proposed explanations for the blood compatibility of these materials is that they adsorb blood proteins on their surface without altering them.

Applications. The most important biomedical application is the cardiovascular area, such as in heart valves, the first of which was implanted in 1969. Since then, more than 600,000 pyrolytic carbon valve components have been produced for implantation. The cardiovascular application is particularly demanding. Early attempts at producing successful heart valves failed because the materials used were either thrombogenic or suffered from high wear and mechanical failure. Thrombus, wear, distortion, and biodegradation have been virtually eliminated because of the biocompatibility and mechanical durability of pyrolytic carbon, clearly establishing it as the material of choice for heart valves.

Table 9 summarizes the successful uses of glassy, LTI, and ULTI carbons in various medical areas.

Table 9 Successful applications of glassy, low-temperature isotropic (LTI), and vapor-deposited ultralow-temperature isotropic (ULTI) carbons

Application	Material
Mitral and aortic heart valves	LTI
Dacron and Teflon heart valve sewing rings	ULTI
Blood access device	LTI/titanium
Dacron and Teflon vascul grafts	ULTI
Dacron, Teflon, and polypropylene septum and aneurism patches	ULTI
Pacemaker electrodes	Porous glassy carbon-ULTI-coated porous titanium
Blood oxygenator microporous membranes	ULTI
Otologic vent tubes	LTI
Subperiosteal dental implant frames	ULTI
Dental endosseous root form and blade implants	LTI
Dacron-reinforced polyurethane aloplastic trays for alveolar ridge augmentation	ULTI
Percutaneous electrical connectors	LTI
Hand joints	LTI

Dacron, Teflon, E.I. DuPont de Nemours & Co., Inc.. Source: Ref 17

ACKNOWLEDGMENT

The information in this chapter was largely taken from:

• L.L. Hench, Medical and Scientific Products, *Ceramics and Glasses,* Vol 4, *Engineered Materials Handbook,* ASM International, 1991, p 1007–1013

REFERENCES

1. L.L. Hench and E.C. Ethridge, *Biomaterials: An Interfacial Approach,* Academic Press, 1982
2. L.L. Hench, Ceramics, Glasses, and Glass-Ceramics, *An Introduction to Materials in Medicine,* B.D. Ratner, A.S. Hoffman, F.J. Schoen, and J.E. Lemons, Ed., Academic Press, 1996, p 73–84
3. R.H. Doremus, Review: Bioceramics, *J. Mater. Sci.,* Vol 27, 1992, p 285–297
4. P.M. Boutin, *Ceramics in Clinical Applications,* P. Vincenzini, Ed., Elsevier, 1987, p 297
5. P. Christel, A. Meunier, J.M. Dorlot, J.M. Crolet, J. Witvolet, L. Sedel, and P. Boritin, Biomechanical Compatibility and Design of Ceramic Implants for Orthopedic Surgery, *Bioceramics: Material Characteristics Versus In-Vivo Behavior,* P. Ducheyne and J. Lemons, Ed., Vol 523, *Annals of NY Academy of Science,* 1988, p 234
6. E. Dörre and W. Dawihl, Ceramic Hip Endoprostheses, *Mechanical Properties of Biomaterials,* G.W. Hastings and D.F. Williams, Ed., John Wiley & Sons, 1980, p 113–127
7. E.W. White, J.N. Webber, D.M. Roy, E.L. Owen, R.T. Chiroff, and R.A. White, *J. Biomed. Mater. Res. Symp.,* Vol 6, 1975, p 23–27
8. R.T. Chiroff, E.W. White, J.N. Webber, and D. Roy, *J. Biomed. Mater. Res. Symp.,* Vol 6 (No. 29), 1975, p 45
9. L.L. Hench and J.W. Wilson, Surface-Active Biomaterials, *Science,* Vol 226, 1984, p 630
10. V. Gross, R. Kinne, H.J. Schmitz, and V. Strunz, *CRC Crit. Rev. Biocompatibility,* Vol 4 (No. 2), 1988
11. T. Yamamuro, L.L. Hench, and J. Wilson, *Handbook on Bioactive Ceramics,* Vol I, *Bioactive Glasses and Glass-Ceramics,* Vol II, *Calcium-Phosphate Ceramics,* CRC Press, 1990
12. W. Hohland, W. Vogel, K. Naurnann, and J. Gummel, Interface Reactions between Machinable Bioactive Glass-Ceramics and Bond, *J. Biomed. Mater. Res.,* Vol 19, 1985, p 303
13. L.L. Hench, Bioactive Ceramics, *Bioceramics: Materials Characteristics Versus In-Vivo Behavior,* P. Ducheyne and J. Lemons, Ed., Vol 523, *Annals of NY Academy of Science,* 1988, p 54
14. K. de Groot, *Bioceramics of Calcium-Phosphate,* CRC Press, 1983
15. M. Jarcho, Calcium Phosphate Ceramics as Hard Tissue Prosthetics, *Clin. Orthop. Relat. Res.,* Vol 157, 1981, p 259
16. R.Z. Le Geros, Calcium Phosphate Materials in Restorative Dentistry: A Review, *Adv. Dent. Res.,* Vol 2, 1988, p 164–180
17. K. de Groot, C.P.A.T. Klein, J.G.C. Wolke, and J. de Blieck-Hogervorst, Chap. 1, *Handbook on Bioactive Ceramics: Vol II,* CRC Press, 1990
18. J.C. Bokros, Carbon Biomedical Devices, *Carbon,* Vol 15, 1977, p 355–371
19. A.D. Haubold, R.A. Yapp, and J.C. Bokros, *Concise Encyclopedia of Medical and Dental Materials,* D. Williams, Ed., Pergamon Press, 1990

CHAPTER 7

Polymeric Materials

POLYMER-BASED MATERIALS offer the greatest versatility in properties and processing among all biomaterials. They have addressed neurological, cardiovascular, ophthalmic, and reconstructive pathologies with implantable devices designed to sustain or enhance life. They have also been found useful in temporary therapies such as hemodialysis, coronary angioplasty, blood oxygenation, electrosurgery, and wound treatment. In addition to these nondental applications, polymers are also used extensively in dentistry as composite (resin-ceramic) restorative materials, implants, dental cements, and denture bases and teeth. Polymers used for dental applications are discussed in Chapter 10, "Biomaterials for Dental Applications," in this handbook.

Characteristics and Classification of Polymers

This section provides a brief overview of polymers, including how they compare with metals and ceramics, their structural characteristics, their classification scheme, and some important application areas. More detailed information on polymer chemistry, processing, and properties can be found in the Selected References listed at the conclusion of this chapter.

Structure. Polymers do not have crystal structures as do metals and ceramics. The main feature that sets polymers apart from other materials is that polymers are made of long molecules. They contain a chain of atoms held together by covalent bonds, with carbon normally being in a high proportion. The carbon atoms are connected to form long chains and extensive networks, which form a backbone for the structure. Attached to this backbone are hydrogen atoms in organic and inorganic groups. Geometrically, the long polymer molecules can be linear, branched, or a three-dimensional network. The molecular architecture of a polymer determines the properties of the material. Polymers have strength properties inferior to metals and ceramics but are lighter in weight, more easily formed, and, theoretically, can be modified for maximum biocompatibility and acceptable mechanical properties.

Classification. Polymers are typically classified into three groups: thermoplastics, thermosets, and elastomers (or rubbers). Although all three groups are used for medical applications, the thermoplastics are the most widely used.

Thermoplastics are linear or branched polymers that can be melted upon the application of heat; they can be molded and remolded using conventional techniques. The processing characteristics of thermoplastics are analogous to those of paraffin wax, which is heated until it softens and liquefies, poured into a mold, and allowed to cool. The wax takes the shape of the mold. If reheated, the wax can be molded into a different shape.

Thermosets are heavily cross-linked polymers that are normally rigid and intractable. They consist of a dense, three-dimensional molecular network. Thermosets cannot be remelted; they degrade rather than melt upon heating. The processing characteristics of thermosets are analogous to those of concrete. Once the slurry consisting of cement, aggregate, and water hardens, it cannot return to its original semisolid state.

Rubbers are materials that exhibit elastomeric properties (i.e., they can be stretched easily to high extensions and will spring back rapidly when the stress is released) and are described as cross-linkable linear polymers. Like thermosets, rubbers or elastomers also degrade rather than melt upon heating.

Table 1 lists a number of common polymers used for medical applications. Most of these are thermoplastics, the exceptions being functionally terminated polydimethylsiloxanes, described as silicones, and thermosetting polyurethanes. Figure 1 illustrates the variety of clinical applications for polymeric biomaterials.

Table 1   Common polymers and their medical uses

Polymer	Typical use
Polyethylene	Tubing, connectors and bottles, plastic surgery implants
Polypropylene	Disposable syringe, membrane for membrane oxygenator, connectors, finger-joint prostheses, nonabsorbable sutures
Polytetrafluoroethylene, polydifluoromethylene	Vascular graft prostheses, heart patch, stapes prosthesis, retinal detachment treatment
Polystyrene	Disposable laboratory articles (e.g., test tubes)
Polymethyl methacrylate	Bone cement, artificial teeth, implanted teeth, denture materials, dental fillings, intraocular lens, membrane for dialysis or ultrafiltration
Polyvinyl chloride	Disposable medical articles, hemodialysis or hemoperfusion, blood tubing line, cardiac catheters, blood bags, artificial limb materials
Polydimethylsiloxanes (silicone rubber, silastic)	Plastic surgery implants, artificial heart, heart-assist pump materials, atrioventricular shunts, finger-joint repair, impressing material, heart pacemaker leads
Polyacrylonitrile	Membrane for dialysis
Polyurethane	Artificial heart pump materials and heart assists, balloon for intraaortic balloon pump, heart-valve prostheses, vascular graft prostheses, tubing, coating for blood compatibility
Polyvinyl alcohol	Drug-delivery system
Polyamides (nylons)	Nonabsorbable sutures, tendon prosthesis, drug-delivery system, tracheal tubes
Polyethylene terephthalates	Nonabsorbable sutures, tendon and ligament reconstruction, heart-valve and vascular graft, tracheal replacement, surgical mesh fabrics
Hydrogels	Contact lenses, wound dressings, ophthalmic implants, drug delivery system

Source: Ref 1

Biodegradation of Medical Polymers. It has long been considered that polymers have a significant advantage over metals in the context of medical applications, because the isotonic saline solution that comprises the body's extracellular fluid is extremely hostile to metals but is not normally associated with the degradation of many synthetic high-molecular-weight polymers (Ref 3). It should be possible to select polymers that will be stable under the conditions found in the body, taking into consideration that the circumstances under which polymers are most susceptible, including those of elevated temperature, electromagnetic radiation, and atmospheric oxygen, are not operative here. The fact is, however, that polymers do break down in the body, although they are not necessarily subjected to what is normally defined as corrosion, which is one of the primary forms of metallic degradation. The result can be tissue interaction with residual monomers remaining after polymerization, chemical degradation of molecular structure of the polymer, and leaching of additives such as plasticizers, fillers, and colorants (Ref 4). Some polymers are designed to degrade (resorb) in the body (see the subsequent section, "Biodegradable Polymers," in this chapter); others degrade but are not intentionally designed to do so. The deterioration of polymers can affect the main polymer chain, cross links, and side groups. Sometimes, undesirable cross linking can occur and degrade a linear polymer, while in other cases, a desired cross link is broken by interaction of thermal energy or other elements (e.g., oxygen) with the polymer. Some polymers absorb lipids or interact with proteins; hydrolysis occasionally can occur.

The body environment is quite hostile to man-made materials, and polymers will start to degrade as soon as they are implanted. Hydroxyl (OH^-) ion attack or interactions with dissolved oxygen are the principal chemical sources of polymer degradation. The degradation of polymers in the body is much more complex than the attack of metals and ceramics. Excellent reviews of the chemical and biochemical degradation of medical polymers can be found in Ref 3 and 5.

Table 2 lists mechanisms of physical and chemical deterioration that may occur alone or in concert at various stages of a polymer history. Moreover, the treatment of a material prior to implant may predispose it to stable or unstable end-use behavior. A prominent example of biomaterial degradation caused by preimplant processing is the gamma irradiation sterilization of ultrahigh molecular weight polyethylene used in total joint prostheses. The process generates free radicals within the material that react with oxygen to produce undesirable oxidation products. Chain oxidation and scission can occur for periods of months to years, causing loss of strength and embrittlement, with limited shelf life. Similarly, some adhesives used in medical-device assembly cannot undergo autoclave steam sterilization because of the high temperatures involved (see Chapter 8, "Adhesives," in this handbook for details).

Biodegradable Polymers. One of the leading areas of research in the biomaterials science field is that of the development of biodegradable or bioresorbable polymers. These materials are designed to interact with and, in time, are integrated into the biological environment. They do not have to be removed surgically. The popularity of biodegradable polymers as biomaterials has been steadily increasing in the past 25 years.

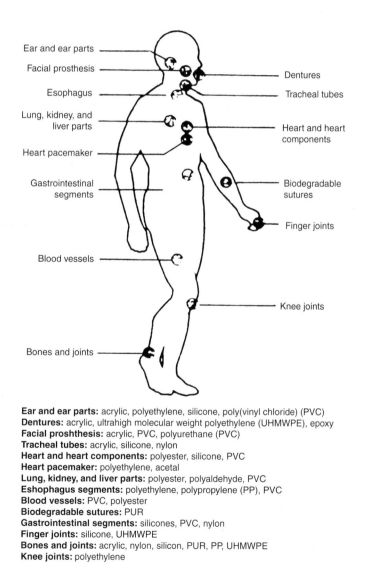

Ear and ear parts: acrylic, polyethylene, silicone, poly(vinyl chloride) (PVC)
Dentures: acrylic, ultrahigh molecular weight polyethylene (UHMWPE), epoxy
Facial proshthesis: acrylic, PVC, polyurethane (PVC)
Tracheal tubes: acrylic, silicone, nylon
Heart and heart components: polyester, silicone, PVC
Heart pacemaker: polyethylene, acetal
Lung, kidney, and liver parts: polyester, polyaldehyde, PVC
Eshophagus segments: polyethylene, polypropylene (PP), PVC
Blood vessels: PVC, polyester
Biodegradable sutures: PUR
Gastrointestinal segments: silicones, PVC, nylon
Finger joints: silicone, UHMWPE
Bones and joints: acrylic, nylon, silicon, PUR, PP, UHMWPE
Knee joints: polyethylene

Fig. 1   Common clinical applications and types of polymers used in medicine. Source: Ref 2

The attractiveness of these materials is that they can be designed as temporary implants that stay intact until the healing process in the body is complete, whereupon they degrade by hydrolytic or enzymatic action and are excreted from the body as waste products (Ref 6). Another advantage of biodegradable implants is that they circumvent some of the problems related to long-term safety of permanently implanted devices. Clinically, they are used primarily as sutures and drug-delivery devices, although other applications have been realized (Table 3).

Table 2 Mechanisms leading to degradation of polymer properties

Physical	Chemical
Sorption	Thermolysis
Swelling	Radical scission
Softening	Depolymerization
Dissolution	Oxidation
Mineralization	Chemical
Extraction	Thermooxidative
Crystallization	Solvolysis
Decrystallization	Hydrolysis
Stress cracking	Alcoholysis
Fatigue fracture	Aminolysis, etc.
Impact fracture	Photolysis
	Visible
	Ultraviolet
	Radiolysis
	Gamma rays
	X-rays
	Electron beam
	Fracture-induced radical reactions

Note: Some degradation processes may involve combinations of two or more individual mechanisms. Source: Ref 5

Table 3 Some short-term medical applications of degradable polymeric biomaterials

Application	Comments
Sutures	The earliest successful application of synthetic degradable polymers in human medicine
Drug-delivery devices	One of the most widely investigated medical applications for degradable polymers
Orthopedic fixation devices	Requires polymers of exceptionally high mechanical strength and stiffness
Adhesion prevention	Requires polymers that can form soft membranes or films
Temporary vascular grafts and stents	Only investigational devices are presently available. Blood compatibility is a major concern.

Source: Ref 7

Additional information on these materials can be found subsequently in the sections "Drug-Delivery Systems" and "Suture Materials" in this chapter, and in Ref 7.

Historical Development of Polymeric Biomaterials (Ref 1)

Synthetic materials became available in the 1920s, making the creative concepts of medical-device pioneers possible. From the 1930s into the 1950s, polymethyl methacrylate was the most widely used polymer for biomaterials, because its biocompatibility and versatility made it the material of choice when rigidity was required in medical devices. As described subsequently in the section "Applications Overview" in this chapter, it is still being used today for bone cements and intraocular lenses. Table 4 lists some significant developments that were achieved by medical-device manufacturers from the 1930s through the 1990s.

In the 1940s, polyvinyl chloride and polydimethylsiloxane (silicone) became available. The flexibility of silicones has allowed the development of flexible-device components. Polyvinyl chloride is now the most widely used material for blood bags and medical tubing, and silicone has been the premier implantable elastomer since the hydrocephalus shunt was first implanted in 1955.

1940–1960. Between 1940 and 1960, tremendous advances took place in the medical-device industry, establishing the era of biomaterials. This was the era of pacemakers, dialysis systems, blood pumps, heart-lung machines, angioplasty devices, and vascular prostheses. Mammary prostheses, dental restoratives, contact lenses, intraocular lenses, occlusive wound dressings, and tissue adhesives (cyanoacrylates and hydrocolloids) were also developed during this period. Significant experimentation also occurred in which many commercial polyurethanes, epoxy thermosets, silicones, and thermoplastics were evaluated and used in medical devices.

1960–1980. Early polyurethane implants were orthopedic-fixation devices intended for use on chronic ailments. Because they were based on polyester polyols, they degraded within a few months. Polyurethane, developed in the 1960s and 1970s, provided the necessary

Table 4 Historical development of polymeric biomaterials

Year	Device	Biomaterials
1930s–1950s		
1930s	Tooth fillings	Polymethyl methacrylate
1943	Artificial kidney	Cellophane tubing wrapped around a horizontal aluminum rotating drum(a)
1946	Femoral head prosthesis	Polymethyl methacrylate
1945–1949	Polymeric vascular prosthesis	Polymethyl methacrylate, polyethylene tubing
Late 1940s–early 1950s	Ocular reconstructive and restorative devices	Polyamides, polyurethanes, polyethylene, polymethyl acrylate and methacrylate, polyvinyl chloride
1950	Bubble-type blood oxygenator	Polydimethylsiloxane-coated glass, polyethylene, polymethyl methacrylate
1950s	Hard contact lenses	Polymethyl methacrylate
1951	Acrylic bone cement	Polymethyl methacrylate
1951	Keratoprostheses (artificial cornea)	Polymethyl methacrylate
1951	Intraocular lens	Polymethyl methacrylate
Early 1950s	Pump-oxygenator (heart-lung) machine for open-heart surgery	Polyvinyl chloride tubing, polymethyl methacrylate machined parts, stainless steel discs and sponge (polydimethylsiloxane antifoam coated), pump components of polyethylene and rubber
1952	Cage-ball heart valve (descending thoracic aorta position)	Polymethyl methacrylate
1952	Synthetic vascular prosthesis	Vinyon N (polyvinyl chloride polyacrylonitrile copolymer) textile
1955	Hydrocephalus shunt	Polydimethylsiloxane
1958	Artificial cells	Synthetic polymer (e.g., collodion-silicone, polyacrylonitrile-polymer-lipid-lipid membranes) encapsulating bioactive molecules (polyhemoglobin)
1958	Implantable artificial heart	Polyvinyl chloride plastisol bladder
1958	Tissue adhesives	Alkyl cyanoacrylates
1958–1959	Implantable cardiac pacemaker	Silicone-coated, epoxy-encased pulse generator with polytetrafluoroethylene-insulated stainless steel wire leads
1959	Denture, skin adhesive	Hydrocolloid (pectin, gelatin, sodium carboxymethyl cellulose, polyisobutylene)
1959	Bone-fixation implants	Polyester urethane rigid foam
Late 1950s	Synthetic vascular prosthesis	Nylon polyamide, Dacron polyethylene terephthalate, Orlon polyacrylonitrile, Teflon polytetrafluoroethylene textile, and Ivalon polyvinyl alcohol sponge tubes(b)
Late 1950s	Soft contact lenses	Poly(hydroxyethyl methacrylate) hydrogel
1960s		
1960s	Tooth restoratives	Glycidyl dimethacrylates, bisphenol dimethacrylates, polyurethanes
1960	Vascular access for hemodialysis	Polytetrafluoroethylene and polydimethylsiloxane tubing and tips
1961	Intraaortic balloon pump	Latex rubber on polyethylene catheter, polyvinyl chloride, polydimethylsiloxane
1962	Occlusive wound dressing	Polyethylene
1962	Mammary prosthesis	Polydimethylsiloxane
1962	Artificial graft	Bovine cartoid artery cross linked with dialdehyde starch
1962	Starr-Edwards ball-and-cage heart valve	Polydimethylsiloxane ball, Stellite alloy cage, and knitted sewing ring
1962	Artificial hip	Stainless steel/ultrahigh molecular weight polyethylene
1963	Antithrombogenic-coated cardiovascular devices	Benzalkonium chloride, graphite, heparin
1965	Synthetic biodegradable sutures, surgery implants	Polyhydroxy acids
1965	Velour-lined blood-pump diaphragms and vascular patches	Polyethylene terephthalate, polyamide, polymethylsiloxane
1967	Blood-pump devices	Avcothane polyetherurethane/polydimethyl-siloxane copolymer
1970s		
1970	Cardiovascular devices	Segmented polyetherurethane urea, biomer composed of methylene dianiline diisocyanate, polytetramethylene, ether glycol, and aliphatic diamines
1970	Foam-covered-gel breast prosthesis	Polyesterurethane foam over silicone-gel-filled polydimethyl-siloxane bag
1972	Implantable drug-delivery device	Polydimethylsiloxane-coated titanium and bellows with polydimethylsiloxane septum and catheter

(a) Cellophane, VCB Films, Inc. (b) Dacron and Teflon, E.I. DuPont de Nemours & Co., Inc.; Ivalon, Ivalon, Inc. Source: Ref 1

(continued)

biodurability that was important for long-term applications. Early silicone-cage heart valves failed because of lipid absorption by the silicone due to inadequate curing of the silicone. Nylon fabric-based implants did not exhibit long-term durability because of chemical breakdown.

Through the 1960s, advances in orthopedic devices led to the development of routine artificial hip and knee replacements. New tissue-fixation techniques produced durable prosthetic valves from animals. Bioabsorbable sutures and reconstructive surgery implants were introduced (see the section "Suture Materials" later in this chapter).

The 1970s brought refinement and greater complexity to the devices developed earlier. Mammary prostheses were coated with foam for better tissue attachment. Techniques for coating

Table 4 (continued)

Year	Device	Biomaterials
1972	Transdermal drug device	Ethylene vinylacetate matrix for scopolamine
1974	Ligament replacement device	Ultrahigh molecular weight polyethylene
1975	Artificial skin	Polydimethylsiloxane-coated collagen-glycosaminoglycan film, with or without seeded skin cells
1978	Stimulation-sensing electrodes with conductive hydrogel adhesives	Poly(2-acrylamido-2-methyl propane-sulfonic acid) and copolymers
1980s		
1980	Silicone contact lenses	Polydimethylsiloxane, modified to produce surface hydroxyl groups
1980	Flexible hip-joint prosthesis	Fiber-reinforced polysulfone
1982	Trileaflet heart valve	Polyether urethane urea tricuspid valve
1983	Cardiovascular devices with durable nonthrombogenic surfaces	End-point covalently attached heparin
1987	Clinical bioartificial liver	Hepatocytes in polypropylene-supported cellulosic membrane
Late 1980s	Flexible hip-joint prosthesis	Carbon-fiber-reinforced polyetherketone
Late 1980s	Cloth barrier for postsurgical adhesions	Oxidized, regenerated cellulose woven fiber
Late 1980s	Orthopedic-fixation plates	Polymeric composites of polyhydroxy acid fibers and matrices (self-reinforced)
Late 1980s	High-lubricity silicone pacing leads	Plasma-surface-treated polydimethylsiloxane insulation
1990s		
1990	Hydrogel films for prevention of arterial restenosis	Copolymer of polyethylene glycol and polylactic acid endcapped with acrylate ester, photopolymerized to bioabsorbable hydrogel
1990	Biodurable polyurethane for implantable devices (e.g., vascular prosthesis)	Aliphatic and aromatic polycarbonate urethane
1990	Cell membrane mimetic	Polymeric coatings from methacryloyloxyethyl phosphorylcholine
1990	Artificial hip or knee implant bearing surfaces with enhanced properties	Ultralight molecular weight polyethylene recrystallized under high-temperature/pressure conditions
1990	Smallest programmable cardiac pacemaker	Lithium-powered device in poly-chloro-paraxylylene-coated titanium case with polyurethane polydimethylsiloxane
1990	Clinical subcutaneous glucose sensor	Teflon polytetrafluoroethylene-coated platinum electrode to which glucose oxidase is bonded and covered with a polyurethane membrane
1990	Cardiovascular-device components	Aliphatic polyurethane with hydrocarbon backbone based on dimerized fatty acid derivatives with high biostability
1990	Implantable female contraceptive drug delivery	Polydimethylsiloxane matrix for Levonorgestrel
1993	Clinical-hybrid bioartificial pancreas	Human islet cells encapsulated in alginate-polylysine-alginate immunoprotective membrane
1993	Bone-repair scaffold	Bone marrow on collagen/sea coral derivative
1993	Sealants for blood vessel punctures	Collagen plugs; collagen sponge bioabsorbable anchor and suture
1994	Hybrid bioartificial cartilage	Autologous chondrocytes grown in polyglycolic acid bioabsorbable scaffolds with adhesion (RGD) peptides
1994	Clinical surgical-adhesions-preventive coating	Bioabsorbable hydrogel from photopolymerized macromer of acrylated polyethylene glycopolyactic acid copolymer
1994	Hydrocarbon-base polyurethane for blood-pump sac	Copolyurethane urea of polyisobutylene diol, methylene dianiline diisocyanate, and ethylene diamine
1994	Hybrid bioartificial adrenal cortex	Adrenal cortical cells encapsulated in sodium alginate/poly-L-lysine to secrete cortisol

(a) Cellophane, VCB Films, Inc. (b) Dacron and Teflon, E.I. DuPont de Nemours & Co., Inc.; Ivalon, Ivalon, Inc. Source: Ref 1

synthetic blood vessels with endothelial cells were developed. The balloon catheter was introduced as an improvement over the technique of sequentially applying catheters of increasing diameter in percutaneous transluminal coronary angioplasty. Polyetherurethanes were introduced for cardiac pacemaker lead insulation, allowing thinner catheters to be used. Expanded polytetrafluoroethylene was introduced for medium-diameter vascular prostheses. New devices, such as implantable drug pumps, artificial finger joints, biodegradable artificial skin, and artificial ligaments, were introduced.

The most successful concepts included the first transdermal drug-delivery device, which was commercialized in the early 1970s. Later in the 1970s, the first synthetic conductive-hydrogel skin adhesive was developed for stimulation and sensing electrodes. This solid-hydrogel design served to effectively replace earlier electrodes that used a paste electrolyte core and a hydrophobic peripheral adhesive.

1980–1990. The 1980s were characterized by tremendous improvements in several clinical devices. Artificial-ligament replacement and augmentation devices were improved. Pacemaker lead wires were modified with steroid tips for lower pacing thresholds, and their silicone insulators were plasma treated for greater lubricity. Blood oxygenators received durable heparin coatings to provide reduced thrombogenicity and to permit the use of less systemic heparinization. Silicone contact lenses allowed extended wear.

Perhaps the highest technical achievement of biomaterials technology in the 1980s was the polyurethane heart developed at the University of Utah. The polyurethane heart provided total circulatory support to patients for up to 620 days without showing sign of failure. However, attempts at using the same polyetherurethane urea to make durable trileaflet heart valves were less successful, because they were susceptible to severe mineralization in chronic animal studies. Engineers and scientists began to turn their focus increasingly toward the interactions of the body with biomaterials, between the host and the device. It was recognized that all biomaterials are affected by the physiological response; there was no such thing as an inert implant.

1990s–Present. The trend in the 1990s involved devices that were designed to intervene in cellular or biochemical processes. For example, clinical-hybrid bioartificial pancreas and adrenal therapies delivered insulin and pain-relief drugs from cells across semipermeable membranes. Devices and tissues such as blood vessels and surgical wounds were coated with barrier films or bioactive molecules to modulate biological responses, including adhesion formation after coronary angioplasty. Implantable sensors with increased sophistication were developed to monitor physiological processes.

Researchers are now exploring intelligent biomaterials that can change characteristics in response to environmental stimuli. Indeed, some polymers are sensitive to physical and chemical stimuli, generally yielding a physical response. For example, hydrogel polymers, such as poly-N-isopropylacrylamide, polyethyloxazoline, and poly-2-acrylamido-2-methyl-propane-sulfonic acid, respond to thermal, pH, or electrical stimuli by swelling, contracting, or eroding. By incorporating enzymes or other bioactive molecules into hydrogel backbones, they can be directed to specific sites for delivery or can respond to changes in metabolic components (e.g., glucose) within the host. Polyurethane wound dressings can self-adjust their moisture-vapor transmission rates in response to wetness changes in the wound.

The Future (Ref 8). One area of intense research activity is the use of biodegradable polymers for tissue engineering (see the discussion of tissue engineering in the section "Applications Overview" in this chapter). Tissue engineering is at an early but promising stage of development.

Combinatorial chemistry is an emerging discipline of tremendous potential for biomaterials development and the entire realm of polymer science. Combinatorial chemistry is the product of advances in molecular biology, microfabrication, and information technology. This new approach to the synthesis of materials and the characterization of their properties uses multi-component screening, high-throughput chemical synthesis, and advanced computational techniques to produce and analyze a large number of novel monomeric and polymeric entities.

In a combinatorial synthesis, automated methods are used to process a relatively small number of ingredients in a parallel fashion so as to generate a large library of elemental combinations on a microscopic scale. Such incrementally controllable, permutationally designed systems hold out the promise of precise structure/property correlations to determine which specific materials will fulfill specific performance needs. One of the first reported examples of a combinatorially prepared library of biomaterials involved A-B-type copolymers in which one monomer was a diphenol and the second a diacid. A total of 14 different diphenols were copolymerized in all combinations with eight different diacids to produce 112 (14 × 8) structurally related polyarylate copolymers. The characteristics of this series of new materials—properties such as wettability, glass transition temperature, and cellular response—were then analyzed in a systematic manner to identify the relationship between polymer structure, properties, and performance.

Another new field of great promise is supramolecular chemistry, which is concerned with developing molecular assemblies for biological applications based on macromolecular architectures that mimic nanoscale systems or mechanisms in nature. Novel synthesis methods based on supramolecular chemistry have been used to create branched, cyclic, cross-linked, star, and dendritic polymer structures. Examples of the ability of supramolecular polymer systems that can meet complex performance requirements and function similar to natural chemomechanical materials can be seen in recent studies using polyrotaxanes—polymers comprising cyclic compounds that are threaded onto linear polymeric chains capped with bulky end groups. Biodegradable polyrotaxanes are being developed for use in two-stage drug-delivery systems.

Other new formulations currently being studied include:

- Phospholipids for vascular grafts, implantable glucose sensors, hemodialyzer filters, and as a rinsing agent to protect contact lenses from protein deposition
- Polymers for gene therapy
- Novel families of silicon-urethane copolymers that offer improved biostability, thromboresistance, abrasion resistance, thermal stability, and surface stability when compared with traditional polyurethane biomaterials
- Protein-based polymers for temporary replacement implants, scaffolds for tissue engineering, and drug-delivery systems

Applications Overview

The biocompatibility of a medical implant will be influenced by a number of factors, including the toxicity of the materials employed, the form and design of the implant, the skill of the surgeon inserting the device, the dynamics of movement of the device in situ, the resistance of the device to chemical or structural degradation (biostability), and the nature of the reactions that occur at the biological interface (Ref 8). These factors vary significantly depending on whether the implant is deployed, for example, in soft tissue, hard tissue, or the cardiovascular system. Among the prominent applications for polymeric biomaterials are:

- *Orthopedics:* joint replacements (hip, knee), bone cements, bone defect fillers, fracture-fixation plates, and artificial tendons and ligaments
- *Cardiovascular:* vascular grafts, heart valves, pacemakers, artificial heart and ventricular-assist-device components, stents, balloons, and blood substitutes
- *Ophthalmics:* contact lenses, corneal implants and artificial corneas, and intraocular lenses
- *Other applications:* dental implants, cochlear implants, tissue screws and tacks, tissue adhesives and sealants, drug-delivery systems, matrices for cell encapsulation and tissue engineering, and sutures

As indicated in Fig. 1 and Tables 1 and 4, a wide range of synthetic and natural polymers are used for these applications. This section presents an overview of some of the more important applications for polymers.

Orthopedics

There are two specific applications in orthopedics in which polymers have proved useful. First, they are used for fixation as a structural interface between implant component and bone tissue. The cement adheres mechanically to the bone and the alloy implant, but no metallurgical bond is formed on the alloy. Second, polymers are used for one of the articulating surface components in a joint prosthesis. These polymers must have a low coefficient of friction and low wear rate when they are in contact with the opposing surface, which is usually made of metal (e.g., cobalt-chromium alloys) or ceramic (e.g., alumina).

Bone Cements. Polymethyl methacrylate (PMMA) is a linear-chain polymer that is sold under trade names such as Plexiglas (Atofina Chemicals, Inc.) and Lucite (INEOS Acrylics, Inc.). As a biomaterial, it is used extensively as a bone cement, which is primarily used to support the stems of total hip-joint prostheses in the medullary cavity of bone. Bone cement is also used sometimes to fill defects in bone. Because this material is radiolucent, it is not visible on x-rays films; thus, barium sulfate is added to it to render it radiopaque. The name *bone cement* is a misnomer, because the primary purpose of the material is to fill the space between the prostheses and bone to achieve more uniform stress distribution, and bone cements do not serve as adhesives.

For surgery, bone cement is provided as a kit with two separate components that have to be mixed together in the operating room. The first part is a dry powder that contains a PMMA powder, barium sulfate, and a free-radical source such as benzoyl peroxide. The second component is a liquid that comprises methyl methacrylate monomer, an initiator, and a stabilizer. On mixing the two components, a polymerization reaction ensues, and the monomer turns into PMMA polymer, interpenetrating and binding the existing PMMA particles. This curing process takes a few minutes, during which the surgeon can pack the doughlike material in place. To ensure long-lasting and useful function of the bone cement, it is important to remove air pockets from the material and pack it tightly. Oftentimes, centrifuging and vacuum techniques are used for reducing microporosity and improving the strength of bone cements. Fillers or fibers can also be used to reinforce the cement. Studies have shown that adding hydroxyapatite (HA) to the PMMA matrix can improve mechanical and biological activity. If the HA is treated with a coupling agent, the tensile and fatigue properties of the reinforced cements have been found to improve. Ion beam processing has also been used to improve the bond properties of PMMA bone cements.

The physical requirements of both the powder and liquid components of bone cements are covered by ASTM F 451. This specification calls for a minimum compressive strength of 70 MPa (10 ksi) for the cured polymer after setting.

Joint Prostheses (Ref 6). Ultrahigh molecular weight polyethylene (UHMWPE) is used as a bearing material in total joint prostheses (hip, knee, shoulder, wrist, finger, or toe joints). In the 1960s, John Charnley, an orthopedic sur-geon, used polytetrafluoroethylene (PTFE, or Teflon) as a bearing material in hip prostheses. Although this material afforded good frictional characteristics, it exhibited rapid wear in the body and elicited a severe foreign-body reaction to the wear debris. Charnley then substituted UHMWPE for PTFE with great success.

The bearing material in a total joint prosthesis is subjected to a very demanding environment due to repeated loading under high forces. For a hip replacement, the bearing couple consists of a metallic femoral head articulating against an UHMWPE acetabular cup (Fig. 2). Strength requirements for fabricated-form UHMWPE are listed in Table 5.

Any use of a joint, such as walking, in the case of hips or knees, results in cyclic articulation of the polymer cup against the metal or ceramic ball. Due to significant localized contact stresses at the ball/socket interface, small regions of UHMWPE tend to adhere to the metal or ceramic ball. During the reciprocating motion of normal joint use, fibrils will be drawn from the adherent regions on the polymer surface and break off to form submicrometer-sized wear debris. This adhesive wear mechanism, coupled with fatigue-related delamination of the UHMWPE (most prevalent in knee joints), results in billions of tiny polymer particles being shed into the surrounding synovial fluid and tissues. The biological interaction with small particles in the body then becomes critical. The

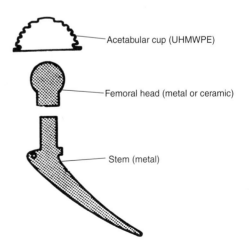

Fig. 2 Example of a total hip replacement showing the articulating ultrahigh molecular weight polyethylene (UHMWPE) cup and the metal or ceramic femoral head

body's immune system attempts, unsuccessfully, to digest the wear particles (as it would a bacterium or virus). Enzymes are released that eventually result in the death of adjacent bone cells, or osteolysis. Over time, sufficient bone is resorbed around the implant to cause mechanical loosening, which necessitates a costly and painful implant replacement, or revision.

It is not clear whether it is the sheer number of these particles that triggers the aggressive adverse response in the body or if the particle size and morphology are responsible. Research has shown that contact conditions and material parameters significantly influence the size and shape of the UHMWPE wear particles.

Efforts are underway in both academia and industry to reduce the wear by using improved sterilization and manufacturing techniques in concert with materials modification and development. The use of polymer-on-ceramic and ceramic-on-ceramic systems is also being explored. The wear rate of UHMWPE against well-polished alumina does appear to be lower than that against the metals currently used in orthopedic implants.

The wear of UHMWPE is a major problem in orthopedics because every year, several hundred thousand total joints are implanted in the United States alone. However, it should be borne in mind that the majority of patients with total joint prostheses do well, regain function of their affected limb, and benefit from a significant decrease in pain.

Cardiovascular Applications (Ref 9)

Cardiovascular devices that employ polymeric materials include mechanical heart valves, vascular grafts, pacemakers, blood oxygenators, and heart-assist systems (intraaortic balloon pumps, ventricular-assist devices, and total artificial hearts). Advances in the design and materials for these devices are ongoing.

Heart Valves. Prosthetic (mechanical or tissue) heart valves are used to replace the natural heart valves (mitral, tricuspid, aortic, and pulmonic) when these no longer perform their normal functions because of disease. Prosthetic heart valves were first used in humans in 1960. Mechanical valves are constructed entirely from synthetic materials. Tissue valves are made entirely or partly of materials of biologic origin.

The mechanical heart valves using polymers come in caged ball, tilting disc, and bi- and trileaflet designs. The materials most widely used in mechanical valves are cobalt-chromium alloys, titanium, pyrolytic carbon, and silicone elastomer. Silicone elastomer has been used for the poppet or ball in caged valves. All prostheses have a fabric sewing ring that surrounds the valve orifice at the base and is used for suturing the device into the surgically prepared implantation site. Sewing rings are made from expanded polytetrafluoroethylene (ePTFE, or Teflon) or polyethylene terephthalate (PET, or Dacron). Figure 3 shows a polymeric sewing ring on a mechanical heart valve.

Dacron cloth-covered flexible polypropylene struts are used in tissue valves. Dacron is also used as a covering for designs incorporating titanium frames.

A polyaromatic, semicrystalline (30 to 35% crystallinity) thermoplastic has been developed for the frame of a synthetic trileaflet heart valve. A polyaryletherketone, it can be readily

---

Table 5 Requirements for ultrahigh molecular weight polyethylene fabricated forms used in total joint prostheses

Property	Test method	Requirement		
		Type 1	Type 2	Type 3
Density, kg/m^3	ASTM D 792 or D 1505	930–940	927–938	927–944
Ash, mg/kg (maximum)	ISO 3451-1	150	150	300
Tensile strength, 23 °C, MPa, (minimum)	ASTM D 638, type IV, 5.08 cm/min			
Ultimate		35	27	27
Yield		21	19	19
Elongation, % (minimum)	ASTM D 638, type IV, 5.08 cm/min	300	300	250
Impact strength, kJ/m^2 (minimum)	ASTM F 648, annex A1	140	73	30
Deformation under load, maximum % after 90 min recovery	ASTM D 621 (A) (7 MPa for 24 h)	2	2	2
Hardness, shore D, (minimum)	ASTM D 2240 (shore D)	60	60	60

Source: ASTM F 648

processed by injection molding, machining, and extrusion. These valves are designed to overcome the problems with both mechanical and tissue valves. Mechanical valves require patients to undergo daily anticoagulant treatments, while tissue valves have a limited life span. The semicrystalline material has a tailor-made combination of excellent biocompatibility and long-term tribological and mechanical properties.

Vascular grafts, like heart valves, are of either biologic (natural materials such as veins harvested from the patient's body) or synthetic origin. Biologic vascular grafts are used for small-vessel replacement such as coronary artery bypass grafting, lower-extremity bypass procedures, and for hemodialysis access. Synthetic vascular grafts are usually made of Dacron or ePTFE. These materials work well for large-diameter vascular grafts (>5 or 6 mm, or >0.20 or 0.24 in.). At present, Dacron fabric is still the major constituent of vascular prostheses (80% of synthetic graft applications). Dacron vascular grafts can be constructed in woven and conventional knit and velour (cloth) configurations. Expanded PTFE has proved to

be the most satisfactory in terms of requisite tensile strength and low incidence of occlusion caused by thrombosis or excessive hyperplasia. Different types of microporous polyurethanes have also been studied for vascular prostheses.

As the incidence and frequency of vascular procedures increase from year to year, researchers are increasingly looking to modified natural materials as a compromise between biologic grafts and synthetic grafts. One possible solution is to use natural materials such as collagen, either modified or combined with a synthetic material, to form a graft that more closely mimics the body's natural function and has low thrombogenicity and low incidence of stenosis.

Pacemakers were developed to overcome abnormalities in heart rhythm. Approximately 500,000 persons in the United States are living with these devices. A pacemaker system consists of a pulse generator with lead connector, electrodes, and a lead wire connecting the two. Polymeric materials used in pacemakers include polyurethane, silicone elastomer, and silicone medical adhesives. The structure and materials of cardiac pacemakers are described in more detail in Chapter 1, "Overview of Biomaterials and Their Use in Medical Devices," in this handbook.

Blood oxygenators (cardiopulmonary bypass, or CPB, systems) are designed to pump unoxygenated blood from the right side of the heart through a synthetic oxygenator, rather than through the lungs, and to return oxygenated blood to the systemic arterial circulation. Developed in the 1950s, these devices have enabled the extraordinary advances in open-heart surgery that have been made over the past 40 to 50 years. Hollow-fiber membrane oxygenators consist of microporous polypropylene. Blood passes along the outside surface of the fibers, which are embedded in a cast polyurethane casing and emerge with open lumens from the casting of the case. Inside the container, also in contact with blood, is a series of epoxy-resin-coated aluminum tubes that act as heat exchangers. Other materials used in various components of CPB systems include silicone elastomer as a material for fabricating oxygenator membranes, polyester (mesh in filter), acrylonitrile-styrene polymers, polyurethane, and polycarbonate.

Ventricular-Assist Devices and Total Artificial Hearts. Both ventricular-assist devices (VADs) and total artificial hearts (TAHs) are

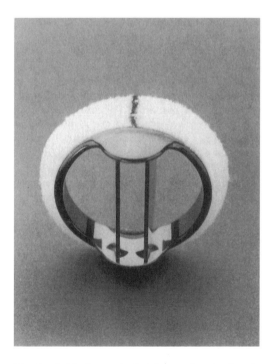

Fig. 3 A bileaflet mechanical heart valve showing the sewing (outer) ring of polymeric fabric. Source: Ref 9

used to replace the mechanical functions of part or all of the heart when those functions have failed irreversibly. These devices are implanted for short-term use (days to weeks) to support the patient until a donor heart becomes available for transplant. Improved design and better modes of antithrombotic and antibacterial therapy may allow these devices to be used for longer time periods.

Beyond the totally implantable artificial heart, an implantable VAD is the most complex cardiovascular device to be implanted in humans. Figure 4 shows an example of a VAD. Table 6 lists typical biomaterials used in a VAD. The biomaterials of the blood-pumping chamber represent a substantial challenge to the bioengineer. The blood pumping must: (1) be biocompatible (an objective not yet fully realized), (2) possess necessary mechanical properties (structure, flex pattern), (3) be impermeable to water, (4) allow gas transfer for barometric and altitude equilibration, (5) prevent bacteria adhesion (not yet achieved), and (6) not degrade during the useful life of the implant.

Other design factors consist of possible local tissue response to biomaterial extractables and erosion caused by device motion or vibration. Continuous relative motion between the VAD and the surrounding tissue produces inflammation and a thick, fibrous encapsulation of the implant. This can lead to a site of pocket infection that is untreatable, because oral antibiotics are walled off from the implant.

Ophthalmic Applications (Ref 10)

Diverse polymeric devices, such as eyeglasses, contact lenses, and intraocular implants, are used to correct the optical function of the eye. The materials used in eyeglass lenses are beyond the scope of this chapter. Contact lenses, however, being in intimate contact with the tissues of the eye, are subject to the same regulations that govern the use of implant materials.

Soft contact lenses are made from hydrogels. A hydrogel is a polymeric, water-swollen network. Hydrogels swell in water to an "equilibrium water content" value but are not soluble in water (Ref 11). Hydrogels have a large number of biomedical applications, and their bulk and interfacial properties have been the subject of intensive research.

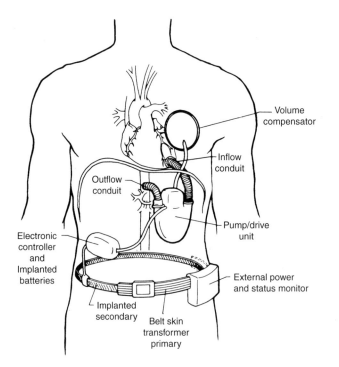

Fig. 4   Implantable ventricular-assist device. See Table 6 for materials of construction. Source: Ref 9

The soft hydrogel contact lenses (SCLs) are supple and fit snugly on the corneal surface. Because there is little tear exchange under these lenses, most of the oxygen that reaches the cornea must permeate through the lens. The oxygen permeability coefficient of hydrogel materials increases exponentially with water content.

The hydrogel lenses are made of slightly cross-linked hydrophilic polymers and copolymers. The original hydrogel contact lens material was poly(2-hydroxyethyl methacrylate), or poly-HEMA, which was developed in the late 1950s (refer to Table 4). At equilibrium swelling in physiological saline solution, it contains approximately 40% water of hydration (hydration of hydrogel contact lenses is customarily given as a percentage of water by weight, on a wet basis). Soon, improved formulations were developed for SCLs. New fabrication techniques were also developed to make ultra-thin SCLs. Other hydrogel contact lens materials include HEMA copolymers with other monomers, such as methacrylic acid, acetone acrylamide, and vinyl pyrrolidone. Commonly used also are copolymers of vinyl pyrrolidone and methyl methacrylate, and of glyceryl methacrylate and methyl methacrylate. A variety of other monomers as well as a variety of cross-linking agents are used as minor ingredients in hydrogel contact lenses (Table 7).

Rigid contact lenses fit loosely on the cornea and move with the blink more or less freely over the tear film that separates the lens from the corneal surface. The mechanical properties of rigid contact lenses must be such that any flex on the lens provoked by blinking must recover instantaneously at the end of the blink.

The first widely available contact lenses were made of PMMA, which is an excellent optical

Table 6 Materials of construction for the ventricular-assist device shown in Fig. 4

Device component	Device subcomponent	Biomaterial
Blood-contacting materials (inner surface)		
Pump/drive unit	Blood-pump sac	Segmented polyether, polyurethane (Biomer)
	Inflow and outflow valves	Porcine valve (with silicone flange)
Inflow and outflow conduits	Luminal surface	Urethane elastomer (Adiprene L-100)
		Dacron vascular graft
Tissue-contacting materials (outer surface)		
Pump/drive unit	Encapsulation shell	Titanium (CP-1)
		Medical-grade adhesive A (silicone)
		Expoxy (polyamine)
Inflow and outflow conduits	Outer surface (graft)	Dacron vascular graft
Variable volume compensator	External reinforcement	Polypropylene
	Flexing diaphragm, connecting tube	Segmented polyether, polyurethane (Biomer), Dacron velour fabric
	Rigid housing	Titanium (Ti-6Al-4V)
Energy control and power unit	Hermetic encapsulation shell	Titanium (CP-1)
Belt skin transformer	Belt body	Silicone
		Medical-grade adhesive A (silicone), silver contacts
Interconnecting leads	Outer encapsulation	Silicone, medical-grade adhesive A (silicone)
Special structural materials		
Pump/drive unit	Solenoid energy converter	Titanium decoupling spring (Ti-6Al-4V), vanadium Permendur (2V-49Co-49Fe), magnetic core, copper coils
	Blood pump	Lightweight structural composite
Variable volume compensator	Gas-filled (replenishable) reservoir	. . .
Energy control and power unit	Hybrids	. . .
	Application-specific integrated circuits, rechargeable batteries	Nickel-cadmium
Belt skin transformer (secondary)	Multistrand wire	Silver, copper

Source: Ref 9

biomaterial in almost all respects except for its virtual impermeability to oxygen. Several materials that were specially developed for the manufacture of rigid gas-permeable (RGP) contact lenses are copolymers of methyl methacrylate with siloxanylalkyl methacrylates. To compensate for the hydrophobic character imparted to the polymer by the high siloxane content of these copolymers (required for oxygen permeability), the copolymer also contains some hydrophilic comonomers. The most commonly used hydrophilic comonomer in rigid lenses is methacrylic acid. There are also minor ingredients and cross-linking agents. A diversity of RGP contact lenses, consisting of different but closely related comonomers used in a variety of proportions to obtain the most desirable properties, are commercially available. Examples include:

- Cellulose acetate dibutyrate
- 3-[3,3,5,5,5-pentamethyl-1,1-bis[pentamethyldisiloxanyl)oxy] trisiloxanyl]propyl methacrylate with methyl methacrylate (MMA), methacrylic acid (MMA), and tetraethyleneglycol dimethacrylate (TEGDMA)
- MMA with MAA, ethyleneglycol dimethacrylate (EGDMA), 3-[3,3,3,-trimethyl-1,1-bis(trimethylsiloxy)disiloxanyl] propyl methacrylate (TRIS), and N-(1,1-dimethyl-3-oxybutyl)acrylamide
- 1-vinyl-2-pyrrolidone (VP) with 2-hydroxyethyl methacrylate (HEMA), TRIS, allyl methacrylate, and α-methacryloyl-ω-(methacryloxy) poly(oxyethylene-co-oxy(dimethylsilylene)-co-oxyethylene

Table 7   Chemical constituents in hydrogels used for soft contact lenses

Polymer	Percent H$_2$O
2-hydroxyethyl methacrylate (HEMA) with ethyleneglycol dimethacrylate (EGDM)	38
HEMA with methacrylic acid (MAA) and EGDM	44, 55
HEMA with sodium methacrylate and 2-ethyl-2-(hydroxymethyl)-1,3-propanediol trimethacrylate	58
HEMA with divinyl benzene, methyl methacrylate (MMA), and 1-vinyl-2-pyrrolidone (VP)	43
HEMA with VP and MAA	71
HEMA with N-(1,1-dimethyl-3-oxobutyl) acrylamide and 2-ethyl-2-(hydroxymethyl)-1,3-propanediol trimethacrylate	45, 55
2,3-dihydroxypropyl methacrylate with MMA	39
VP with MMA, allyl methacrylate, and EGDM	70, 79
MAA with HEMA, VP, and EGDM	55

Source: Ref 10

- TRIS with MMA, dimethyl itaconate, MAA, and TEGDMA
- TRIS with 2,2,2,-trifluoro-1-(trifluoromethyl) ethyl methacrylate, VP, MAA, and EGDMA
- TRIS with 2,2,2-trifluoroethyl methacrylate, MAA, MMA, VP with EGDMA

The development of the fluorine-containing contact lenses and the realization that the fluoroderivatives may improve oxygen permeability and resistance to deposit formation caused contact lens chemists to include a fluoroalkyl methacrylate or a similar fluorine-content monomer as an additional ingredient in the siloxanylalkyl methacrylate/comethyl methacrylate RGP contact lens materials. These perfluoroalkyl-siloxanylalkyl-methyl methacrylate contact lenses have high oxygen permeability and, supposedly, better surface properties than the non-fluorine-containing rigid contact lenses.

Other copolymers useful as contact lens materials are isobutyl and isopropyl styrene, with hydrophilic comonomers of the HEMA or vinyl pyrrolidone type.

Intraocular Lens Implants. Intraocular lenses (IOLs) are used after cataract extraction to replace the opaque crystalline lens of the eye. Intraocular lenses consist of an optical portion and the haptics that support the optical portion in its proper place in the eye (Fig. 5). Intraocular lenses may be placed in the anterior chamber, in the pupil, or in the posterior chamber, as shown in Fig. 6. Intraocular lens placement in the posterior chamber is most commonly used; IOLs are usually placed within the posterior capsule of the crystalline lens, which remains in the eye after the lens contents have been surgically removed.

The requirements of IOL materials are good optical properties and biocompatibility with the surrounding tissues. Most IOLs are made of PMMA, and the haptics are made of the same material. Soft IOLs have been made of poly-HEMA or other hydrogels, which can be inserted into the eye fully hydrated or in the dehydrated state; in the latter case, they will swell in situ to their equilibrium hydration. Flexible IOLs are also made of silicone rubber and of alkyl acrylate copolymers.

Biopolymers in the form of a viscoelastic solution are also used in IOL implantation. The corneal endothelium is an extremely delicate cell layer and can be irreversibly damaged on contact with an IOL, during or after insertion. The surgeon must be extremely careful not to touch the corneal endothelium with the IOL or with any instrument used during surgery. Highly viscous, and preferably viscoelastic, solutions of biopolymers, such as sodium

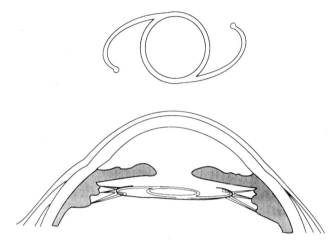

Fig. 5 (Top) Schematic representation of a typical intraocular lens implant with a central optical portion and the haptics, or side-arms, that hold the lens in the eye. (Bottom) A schematic representation of the anterior segment of the eye with an intraocular lens placed into the empty crystalline lens bag. Source: Ref 10

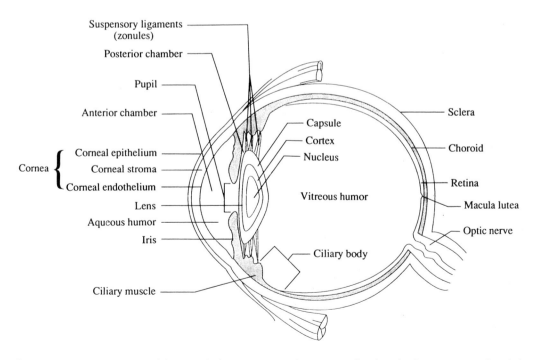

Fig. 6 Schematic representation of the eye. Light that penetrates into the eye is partially refracted in the cornea, passes through the aqueous humor and the pupil (the opening in the center of the iris), is further refracted in the crystalline lens, passes through the vitreous humor, and converges on the retina. Source: Ref 10

hyaluronate, chondroitin sulfate, or hydroxypropyl methylcelluose, are useful adjuncts in IOL implant surgery for maintaining anterior chamber depth during introduction of the implant and for preserving the corneal endothelium. Other important developments may be the surface modification of IOLs with permanent hydrophilic or hydrophobic coatings.

Drug-Delivery Systems (Ref 6, 12, and 13)

Since the late 1960s, there has been a rapid development of innovative techniques for the controlled delivery of drugs (Ref 12). This has been a result of the growing awareness that efficient therapy of an ailment with minimal adverse effects requires optimal delivery of drugs through proper design of the dosage form. The increased concern of pharmaceutical scientists over the daily administration of high doses of conventional drugs, as well as the increased cost of developing newer drug moieties, has been the impetus toward the development of rate-controlled drug-delivery systems. A rate-controlled drug-delivery system is a system that can regulate or control the release of a therapeutic agent. Such systems are advantageous over their conventional counterparts in that they deliver the drug at a predetermined rate, through which they maintain the steady-state drug concentration within a narrow therapeutic range, for a prolonged period of time. Table 8 lists some of the polymers that have use in the construction of rate-controlled drug-delivery systems.

Implantable Systems Using Biodegradable Polymers (Ref 6). Biodegradable polymers also function well as implantable drug-delivery systems. The drug is incorporated in a matrix of a biodegradable polymer, which is then implanted in the body. As the polymer matrix biodegrades over a period of time, the drug is gradually released. Such systems are especially useful when a specific site or lesion within the body has to be treated and the treatment drug can result in complications if administered systemically through injections or pills. Implantation of the delivery system at the site of a disease, such as cancer, can reduce the effects the drug might have on other parts of the body.

The most popular biodegradable polymers are polylactic acid (PLA), polyglycolic acid (PGA), and their copolymers; other biodegradable materials of interest include polyorthoesters, poly-

caprolactones, and polyanhydrides. The degradation by-products of PLA and PGA enter the tricarboxylic acid cycle in the body and are finally excreted as water and carbon dioxide. The mechanical properties of these materials are highly susceptible to variations in the starting virgin material, the fabrication process, and any postfabrication treatments. For example, the elastic modulus of PLA can vary from 0.5 to 10 GPa (0.07 to 1.45×10^6 psi).

Transdermal Drug Delivery (Ref 13). Diffusional delivery of drugs through the skin has advanced more than other fields of controlled drug delivery. This is apparent from the number

Table 8   Some polymers used in rate-controlled drug-delivery systems

Natural polymers

Cellulose acetate phthalate
Hydroxypropyl cellulose
Carboxymethyl cellulose
Ethyl cellulose
Methyl cellulose
Collagen
Zein
Gelatin
Natural rubber
Guar gum
Gum agar
Albumin

Synthetic polymers

Elastomers
  Silicone rubber
  Polysiloxane
  Polybutadiene
  Polyisoprene
Hydrogels
  Polyhydroxyalkyl methacrylates
  Polyvinyl alcohol
  Polyvinyl pyrrolidone
  Alginates
  Polyacrylamide
Biodegradable
  Polylactic acid
  Polyglycolic acid
  Polyalkyl 2-cyanoacrylates
  Polyurethanes
  Polyanhydrides
  Polyorthoesters
Adhesives
  Polyisobutylenes
  Polyacrylates
  Silicones
Others
  Polyvinyl chloride
  Polyvinyl acetate
  Ethylene-vinyl acetate
  Polyethylene
  Polyurethanes

Source: Ref 12

of drug-delivery systems that have been marketed (Table 9). In transdermal devices, a polymeric delivery system is held on the skin by an adhesive. The device contains the drug either in a reservoir with a rate-controlling membrane (typically made of ethylene-vinyl acetate) or dispersed in a rate-controlling matrix made from either a lipophilic or a hydrophilic polymer. A schematic of a membrane-controlled device is shown in Fig. 7. The drug is released from these devices through the skin and is taken up by systemic circulation.

Suture Materials (Ref 14)

Suture Categories. Sutures are broadly categorized according to:

- The type of material from which they are made (natural or synthetic)
- The permanence of the material (absorbable or nonabsorbable)
- The construction process (braided, twisted, or monofilament)

Table 10 lists both natural and synthetic suture materials. Approximately half of today's sutures are nonabsorbable and remain indefinitely intact when placed in the body. Common engineering polymers such as polypropylene, nylon, polyethylene terephthalate, and polyethylene are used as nonabsorbable sutures. Absorbable sutures include PGA, copolymers of glycolide and lactide, polydioxanone, and poly(glycolide-co-trimethylene carbonate).

Properties. Regardless of whether a suture is made from a natural or synthetic material, or if it is absorbable or permanent, it must meet the strength requirements necessary to close a wound under a given clinical circumstance. In addition to tensile strength and knot pull strength (Table 11), there are a number of characteristics that must be considered when selecting a suture for the patient. As listed in Table 12, these parameters range from objective issues, such as suture diameter, strength retention, and tissue response, to the subjective issues, such as how does the suture "feel" in the surgeon's hands.

Tissue Engineering (Ref 6)

Polymeric biomaterials play a significant role in the multidisciplinary and rapidly growing field of tissue engineering. Tissue engineering can be defined as an interdisciplinary field in which the principles of engineering and the life sciences are applied toward the generation of biologic substitutes aimed at the creation, preservation, or restoration of lost organ function. The impetus to this area is provided by the shortage of available transplant organs and tissue. Additionally, the spread of presently incurable diseases, such as AIDS, has raised concerns regarding tissue transplant. The ultimate goal of tissue engineering is to either grow tissue and organs on biomaterials outside the body and then implant them or to provide the body with the appropriate biomaterial scaffolds and biological ingredients so that it can regenerate the diseased or missing tissue.

Biomaterial Scaffold Requirements. One of the key components in successful tissue engineering is the production of the correct scaffold using biomaterials. Although the complete list

Table 9 Examples of transdermal drug-delivery systems that have been marketed

Drug administered	Developing company
Clonidine	Boehringer-Ingelheim
Estradiol	Ciba-Geigy
	Besins-Iscovesco
Etofenamate	Bayer
Fentanyl	Janssen
Isosorbide dinitrate	Yamanouchi
Nicotine	Parke-Davis
	Ciba-Geigy
	Marion
	Lederle
Nitroglycerine	Several companies:
	Key Pharmaceuticals
	G.D. Searle
	Ciba-Geigy
	Wyeth
	Bolar, others
	Nippon Kayaku/Taiho
	3M Riker
Progesterone	Besins-Iscovesco
Scopolamine	Ciba-Geigy
	Myum Moon Pharm

Source: Ref 13

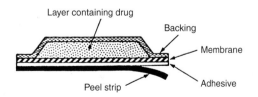

Fig. 7 Schematic of membrane-controlled transdermal device

Table 10 Major commercially available polymeric sutures

Suture type	Construction(a)	Sterilization method(b)	Major clinical use
Natural materials			
Catgut(c)	Tw	EtO/rad.	Ob/gyn, urology
Silk	B	EtO/rad.	Cardiovascular, vascular
Synthetic absorbable			
Polyglycolic acid	B	EtO	General, ob/gyn
Poly(glycolide-co-lactide)	B	EtO	General, ob/gyn
Poly(p-dioxanone)	M	EtO	General, ob/gyn
Poly(glycolide-co-trimethylene carbonate)	M	EtO	General, ob/gyn
Synthetic nonabsorbable			
Polybutylene terephthalate	B, M	EtO/rad.	Cardiovascular, orthopedics
Polyethylene terephthalate	B, M	EtO/rad.	Cardiovascular, orthopedics
Poly[p(tetramethylene ether) terephthalate-co-tetramethylene]	M	EtO/rad.	Plastic/cuticular
Polypropylene	M	EtO	Cardiovascular, vascular
Nylon 66	B, M	EtO/rad.	Plastic/cuticular, ophthalmic

(a) Construction: Tw, twisted; B, braided; M, monofilament. (b) Sterilization method: EtO, ethylene oxide; rad., gamma radiation. (c) Catgut is derived from animal intestines. Source: Ref 14

Table 11 Representative mechanical properties of commercial sutures

Suture type	Tensile strength		Knot pull strength		Elongation to break, %	Subjective flexibility
	MPa	ksi	MPa	ksi		
Natural materials						
Catgut	370	54	160	23	25	Stiff
Silk	470	68	265	38	21	Very supple
Synthetic absorbable						
Polyglycolic acid	840	122	480	70	22	Supple
Poly(glycolide-co-lactide)	740	107	350	51	22	Supple
Poly(p-dioxanone)	505	73	290	42	34	Moderately stiff
Poly(glycolide-co-trimethylene carbonate)	575	83	380	55	32	Moderately stiff
Synthetic nonabsorbable						
Polybutylene terephthalate	520	75	340	49	20	Supple
Polyethylene terephthalate	735	107	345	50	25	Supple
Poly[p(tetramethylene ether) terephthalate-co-tetramethylene terephthalate]	515	75	330	48	34	Supple
Polypropylene	435	63	300	44	43	Stiff
Nylon 66	585	85	315	46	41	Stiff
Steel	660	96	565	82	45	Rigid

Source: Ref 14

of characteristics an ideal scaffold should possess is still being developed by scientists, the scaffold should be biocompatible, bioabsorbable, highly porous, and extremely permeable. Additionally, the scaffold should provide the correct biomechanical environment, degrade in tune with tissue growth, and possess a surface that encourages cell attachment and growth. Thus, the ideal scaffold should provide cells not only with a structural framework but also with the appropriate mechanical and biochemical conditions so that these cells can proliferate and produce extracellular matrix to form tissue.

Table 12   Suture characteristics

Objective	Subjective
Tensile strength	Suppleness
Knot security	Ease of tying
Diameter	Ease on hands
Strength retention	
Flexibility	
Memory out of the package	
Tissue drag	
Infection potentiation (wicking)	

Source: Ref 14

Areas of research in tissue engineering include the repair or regeneration of skin, blood vessels, nerves, liver, bone, and articular cartilage. Several new start-up biotechnology companies are pursuing these goals with the assistance of multinational corporations. The repair or regeneration of articular cartilage is of particular interest because, unlike other tissues, cartilage does not heal itself and, if damaged by trauma or age, leads to osteoarthritis. Several hundred million people around the world suffer the painful and debilitating effects of arthritis.

Laboratories are experimenting with different types of biodegradable scaffolds to achieve cartilage healing. Different techniques include implanting these scaffolds in their bare form or in conjunction with cells or growth proteins that stimulate tissue growth. PLA and PGA are prime candidates for such scaffolds because they are biocompatible, provide the appropriate mechanical environment, can be easily fabricated, and, moreover, are biodegradable. Collagen sponges are also under investigation.

It is conceivable that in the future it will be possible to custom-produce or grow organs and tissues to replace those damaged by disease or trauma. People will no longer succumb to death due to the nonavailability of transplant organs, burn victims will have access to artificially grown skin, congenital deformities in children will be correctable, and the elderly will not have to suffer the pain of arthritis.

REFERENCES

1. M. Moukwa, The Development of Polymer-Based Biomaterials Since the 1920s, *JOM*, Feb 1997, p 46–50

2. S.A. Visser, R.W. Hergenrother, and S.L. Cooper, Polymers, *Biomaterials Science: An Introduction to Materials in Medicine*, B.D. Ratner, A.S. Hoffman, F.J. Schoen, and J.E. Lemons, Ed., Academic Press, 1996, p 50–60

3. D.F. Williams, Biodegradation of Medical Polymers, *Concise Encyclopedia of Medical and Dental Materials*, D.F. Williams, Ed., Pergamon Press and The MIT Press, 1990, p 69–74

4. M. Donachie, Biomaterials, *Metals Handbook Desk Edition*, 2nd ed., J.R. Davis, Ed., ASM International, 1998, p 702–709

5. A.J. Coury, Chemical and Biomechanical Degradation of Polymers, *Biomaterials Science: An Introduction to Materials in Medicine*, B.D. Ratner, A.S. Hoffman, F.J. Schoen, and J.E. Lemons, Ed., Academic Press, 1996, p 243–260

6. C.M. Agrawal, Reconstructing the Human Body Using Biomaterials, *JOM*, Jan 1998, p 31–35

7. J. Kohn and R. Langer, Bioresorbable and Biodegradable Materials, *Biomaterials Science: An Introduction to Materials in Medicine*, B.D. Ratner, A.S. Hoffman, F.J. Schoen, and J.E. Lemons, Ed., Academic Press, 1996, p 64–73

8. J. Katz, Developments in Medical Polymers for Biomaterials Applications, *Med. Device Diagnostic Ind.*, Jan 2001, p 122

9. P. Didisheim and J.T. Watson, Cardiovascular Applications, *Biomaterials Science: An Introduction to Materials in Medicine*, B.D. Ratner, A.S. Hoffman, F.J. Schoen, and J.E. Lemons, Ed., Academic Press, 1996, p 283–297

10. M.F. Refojo, Ophthalmologic Applications, *Biomaterials Science: An Introduction to Materials in Medicine*, B.D. Ratner, A.S. Hoffman, F.J. Schoen, and J.E. Lemons, Ed., Academic Press, 1996, p 328–335

11. M.J. Lydon, Wound Dressing Materials, *Concise Encyclopedia of Medical and Dental Materials*, D.F. Williams, Ed., Pergamon Press and The MIT Press, 1990, p 367–371

12. R. Toddywala and Y.W. Chien, Polymers for Controlled Drug Delivery, *Concise Encyclopedia of Medical and Dental Materials*, D.F. Williams, Ed., Pergamon

Press and The MIT Press, 1990, p 280–289

13. J. Heller, Drug Delivery Systems, *Biomaterials Science: An Introduction to Materials in Medicine,* B.D. Ratner, A.S. Hoffman, F.J. Schoen, and J.E. Lemons, Ed., Academic Press, 1996, p 346–356

14. D. Goupil, Sutures, *Biomaterials Science: An Introduction to Materials in Medicine,* B.D. Ratner, A.S. Hoffman, F.J. Schoen, and J.E. Lemons, Ed., Academic Press, 1996, p 356–360

SELECTED REFERENCES

- F.W. Billmeyer, Jr., *Textbook of Polymer Science,* 3rd ed., Wiley-Interscience, 1984
- L.L. Clements, Polymer Science for Engineers, *Engineering Plastics,* Vol 2, *Engineered Materials Handbook,* ASM International, 1988, p 48–62
- P.J. Flory, *Principles of Polymer Chemistry,* Cornell University Press, 1953
- C. Hall, *Polymeric Materials: An Introduction for Technologists and Scientists,* Macmillan, 1981
- F. Rodrigues, *Principles of Polymer Systems,* 2nd ed., McGraw-Hill, 1982
- R.B. Seymour and C.E. Carraker, Jr., *Polymer Chemistry: An Introduction,* 2nd ed., Wiley-Interscience, 1988
- L.H. Sperling, *Introduction to Physical Polymer Science,* Wiley-Interscience, 1986
- M. Szycher, Ed., *Biocompatible Polymers, Metals, and Composites,* Technomic Publishing, 1983

CHAPTER 8

Adhesives

AN ADHESIVE, as defined by ASTM International, is a "substance capable of holding materials together by surface attachment." Inherent in the concept of adhesion is the fact that a bond that resists separation is formed between substrates or surfaces (adherends) comprising the joint, and force is required to separate them.

"Adhesive" is a general term that covers designations such as cement, glue, paste, fixative, and bonding agent used in various areas of adhesive technology. Adhesive systems may comprise one- or two-part organic and/or inorganic formulations that set or harden (i.e., cure) by several mechanisms. The curing of polymeric adhesives can be achieved using moisture or catalysts in the presence or absence of air at room temperature; thermally, at elevated temperature; or photochemically, using irradiation (e.g., ultraviolet, UV, or visible light).

Applications for adhesive biomaterials fall into three primary areas:

- Medical device assembly, which includes the manufacture of life-support equipment, sterile disposable items (e.g., syringes, catheters, and blood oxygenators), sterile reusable items (e.g., endoscopes and laparoscopes), and sensing/monitoring/reporting devices
- Hard tissue attachment in the fields of orthopedics and dentistry
- Soft tissue attachment such as wound closure

Of these, the assembly and manufacture of medical devices is the principal application area and is the emphasis of this chapter. Materials for hard tissue attachment include polymethyl methacrylate used for orthopedic implant fixation and dental cements used for securing crowns, fixed partial dentures (bridges), and restorations. These materials are discussed in Chapters 7, "Polymeric Materials," and 10, "Biomaterials for Dental Applications," respectively. Adhesives for soft tissue are not discussed extensively in this chapter, but information pertaining to this subject can be found in various medical texts such as Ref 1.

Adhesives used for medical device assembly must pass U.S. Pharmacopoeia (USP) class VI tests to prove they are compatible with human tissue and blood. The life-support equipment and sterile disposable/reusable medical goods sectors are based on plastics, glass, and metallic (primarily stainless steel) substrates. These substrates require unique adhesive properties to withstand sterilization processing (steam autoclaving, gamma radiation, or ethylene oxide, EtO, exposure) and have a zero-defect quality level.

The plastics used in the medical device business are some of the most difficult to bond, including polyethylene, polypropylene, fluoropolymer, and acetal homopolymer. Adhesives and other joining methods used with these plastics and other inert, noncorroding substrates are often required to provide a seal as well as a structurally strong bond. When adhesives have been used, acrylics, cyanoacrylates, epoxies, urethanes, and silicones have been the most popular.

Adhesive Bonding Criteria (Ref 2)

Conditions that call for adhesive bonding include:

- Bonding of dissimilar materials or materials with poor mechanical property matches
- Joining to promote maximum stress distribution or to promote impact resistance

- Joining of materials that are too thin to be welded
- Joining of premanufactured subassemblies
- Bonding to augment the performance of a mechanical joint (bolts, screws, rivets, spot welds)

Properties of Importance. Choosing an adhesive for a medical application follows the same general protocol as choosing an adhesive for any other purpose. Criteria include the particular substrates to be joined, strength requirements, type of loading, impact resistance, temperature resistance, humidity resistance, chemical resistance, electrical resistance, and processing requirements. The choice of substrates often disqualifies many generic adhesive classes and establishes the basic adhesive chemistry. Strength and loading requirements will also disqualify certain types of adhesives. Because impact and temperature resistance are correlated, the softening of an adhesive to improve its toughness will most likely reduce its temperature resistance. Characteristics such as humidity, chemical, and electrical resistance are intrinsic properties of the adhesive material. The manner of processing is dictated by the choice of adhesive and its performance requirements in the application. Table 1 summarizes the properties of common adhesives.

Failures. An adhesive is not a substrate—its job is not to be load bearing, but rather to transmit load from one component to another. The goal of any proper bond is to be strong enough to achieve substrate failure, in which the bond is stronger than the materials themselves. The next-best expectation is cohesive failure, wherein the adhesive splits in failure but remains firmly attached to both substrates. Adhesive failure, in which the adhesive releases from one surface or the other, is generally considered unacceptable.

Loading and Joint Design. Careful attention must be paid to joint design. Adhesives work best in compression, and anything that promotes compressive loading is useful. Pure tension and shear are good loading modes for structural adhesives. The difficulty comes in avoiding peel (unsymmetrical tension) and cleavage (splitting). Adhesives that load well in tension may fail easily in peel. Thin joint gaps are typically preferred over thick gaps: a bond thickness range of 0.05 to 0.4 mm (0.002 to 0.015 in.) is a good target. The thicker the bond line, the more likely the adhesive will fail cohesively.

Surface Pretreatment

Successful material-joining adhesives normally require suitable surface treatment of the adherends prior to bonding (Ref 3). The selection and application of an appropriate surface treatment is one of the major factors for achieving good wettability and improved long-term durability in adhesively bonded joints. Inadequate or unsuitable surface treatment is one of the most common causes of premature degrada-

Table 1 Properties and characteristics of common adhesives used for medical bonding applications

Property	Acrylic	Epoxy	Urethane	Phenolics	Silicones	Polyolefins (vinylics)	High performance thermoplastic
Shear strength	Good	Best	Average	Very good/best	Lower	Lower	Good/very good
Multimode loading	Average	Best	Average	Average	Watch creep	Average	Average
Impact resistance	Average	Average	Very good	Lower	Best	Lower	Good
Substrate choice	Good	Good/best	Best	Lower	Good	Average	Lower
Chemical resistance	Average	Very good	Average	Best	Average	Good	Very good
Humidity resistance	Average	Lower	Average	Very good	Best	Average	Average
Electrical resistance	Average	Very good	Average	Best	Very good	Average	Very good
Temperature resistance	150 °C (300 °F)	230 °C (445 °F)	100 °C (212 °F)	230 °C (445 °F)	−40 to 250 °C (−40 to 480 °F)	100 °C (212 °F)	200 °C (390 °F)
Application form	L1, 2; W1	L1, 2; P1, 2; F	L, P, W; 1, 2; HM	L2, F	L1, 2; P, 2	L1 (>150 °C, or 300 °F); F	L1 (>260°C, or 500 °F); F
Curing speed	Best	Lower	Very good/best	Lower	Average	Very good	Very good
Curing method	HT, RT, UV	HT, RT, (UV)	HT, RT, HM, UV	HT, (RT)	HT, RT, UV	HM	HM
Storage (months)	6	6	6	1–3	6	12	12

L, liquid; P, paste; W, waterbase; 1, one part; 2, two part; F, film; HT, heat; RT, ambient; UV, ultraviolet; HM, hot melt. Source: Ref 2

tion and failure. The function of surface treatment includes the removal of contaminants or weak boundary layers and the alteration of surface chemistry, topography, and morphology to enhance adhesion and durability.

Surface preparation techniques are generally divided into mechanical or chemical methods. Mechanical methods include abrasion, grit blasting, and shot blasting. A laser technique has also been tried (Ref 3). Chemical methods include degreasing, etching, and anodizing; the use of adhesion promoters (accelerators and primers); and flame, corona, and plasma treatments. Table 2 lists recommended surface pretreatments for various polymer and metal substrates. Additional information on surface treatments for plastics and metals can be found in Ref 4 and 5.

Effect of Surface Characteristics on Bonding.
Most materials rated as "difficult to bond" have poor adhesion chemistry or low surface energy (Ref 2). For an adhesive to function, it must wet the surface. Wetting is a function of the surface energy of both the adhesive and the substrates, the viscosity of the adhesive, and the surface tension of the adhesive.

The best way to improve adhesive bonding is to improve surface polarity and the stability of the surface chemistry. This usually requires an oxidative process for plastics (to increase polarity) and an etching or anodizing process for metals (to stabilize surface chemistry).

Surface Preparation of Polymers (Ref 2).
Plastics have naturally low surface energies, ranging from about 15 dyne level for fluoropolymers to 55 dyne level for polyesters. Corona treatment is a quick and inexpensive method for improving surface energy on plastics. This process involves the atmospheric generation of ozone in an electrical discharge, which induces oxidation of the surface. An alternative is oxygen plasma treatment, which requires a closed chamber but leads to more reliable oxidation. Strong plasma treatment can damage subsurface layers, so it is essential to use correct power and exposure times. Flame treatment is effective and inexpensive, but requires good process control to prevent scorching.

Strong oxidizing acids, such as chromic acid, can also be used to oxidize a substrate surface, though acid oxidation carries the drawback of hazardous material handling and waste. Grit blasting or scuff sanding (abrasion) can be useful on some plastics, although these methods merely increase surface area and do not improve surface energy. Thus, if the surface energy is poor, one has simply increased the amount of poorly bonded surface.

Primers can be used to form a modification layer on the surface that provides an interactive

Table 2 Surface preparation and adhesive alternatives for various types of materials

Adherend	Surface preparation						Adhesive				
	Abrade	Corona	Plasma	Acid	Anodize	Primer	Acrylic	Cyanoacrylate	Epoxy	Urethane	Hot melt
Polymer											
ABS	(X)	...	...	...	...	...	X	X	...	X	X
Polyamide	X	X	...	...	...	...	X	(X)	(X)	X	X
Polycarbonate	X	(X)	...	...	...	...	X	X	X	X	...
Polyethylene	...	X	...	X	X	...	X	...		X	X
Polymethyl methacrylate	X	(X)	...	...	...	...	...	X	X	X	X
Polyphenylene sulfide	X	X	X	X	...	...	(X)	...	X	...	...
Polypropylene	...	X	X	X	...	X	X	(X)	(X)	X	X
Polyvinyl chloride	X	...	...	...	...	...	X	X	X	X	X
Fluoropolymers	(X)	...	X	X	...	...	...	...	X	X	(X)
Silicones	X	...	X	...	X	...	...	...	...	(X)	...
Metal											
Aluminum	...	...	X	X	X	X	X	X	X	...	...
Nickel, platinum	...	...	...	X	...	X	...	...	X	...	...
Stainless steel	X	...	...	X	...	X	X	X	X	...	(X)
Titanium	...	...	...	X	X	X	...	...	X	...	...

An "(X)" indicates combinations that are feasible but not advisable. Source: Ref 2

surface chemistry for the adhesive. Primers are best used in very small amounts, typically resulting in a surface coating thickness of less than 10 mm (0.5 mils). Priming can be combined with other methods such as surface abrading or etching, as is frequently the case with metals bonding. Figure 1 shows the effect of primers on the bond strength of various plastic adherends.

Differing preparation methods produce varying results on different materials. This is particularly evident with widely diverse plastics. For example, although they are chemically similar, polyethylene and polypropylene show different responses to the same surface treatments. On polar plastics, such as polyesters or epoxies, simple abrasion can work well.

Fluoropolymers represent a special situation. The very low surface energies of fluoropolymers (18 to 28 dyne level) require extensive surface preparation for most adhesives. Sodium naphthenate and potassium hydroxide etches are effective, and some methods for direct priming have been developed using molten materials to chemically modify the surface. Interestingly, copolymers of fluoropolymer with other materials allow surface preparation specific to either species. For example, a copolymer of fluoropolymer and polyethylene can be treated either at the fluorinated sites or the polyethylene sites using a chosen method such as naphthenate etch or flame treatment, respectively.

Surface Preparation of Metals (Ref 2). Metals are acid etched or anodized using sulfuric, phosphoric, or chromic acids. Stainless steels, nickel, platinum, and titanium all require some type of surface etch or anodization for proper bonding. This may be followed by application of a primer. Etching acts almost as a deep cleaner, but does not give a high surface profile. Anodization produces a deeper profile, but is most effective with low-viscosity primers and adhesives. Otherwise, the deep profile remains unfilled and the mechanical advantage is lost.

Problems arise when the oxide layers rehydrate, forming unstable phases or friable hydroxides that can promote failure at the interface of the oxide and the metal, not at the adhesive-surface interface. The function of a surface preparation such as anodization on a metal is to provide a stable oxide layer that will remain constant, even following inevitable rehydration.

Adhesives for Device Assembly (Ref 2 and 7)

The types of adhesives commonly used for medical device assembly include acrylics, cyanoacrylates, epoxies, urethanes, and silicones. Their relative properties are presented in Table 1. Recommended adhesives for various types of materials are listed in Table 2. Ideally, the surface energy of the adhesive will match that of the substrate. Urethanes, which work exceptionally well for bonding of many plastics, have a surface energy in the 40 to 45 dyne level range, while epoxies are at about the 45 dyne level. Cyanoacrylates have surface energies that range from low-viscosity types (20 dyne level) to high-viscosity levels (900 dyne level). Like cyanoacrylates, acrylics range from low-viscosity formulations (~50 dyne level) to thixotropic gels. Metals have naturally high surface energies provided by their oxide layers.

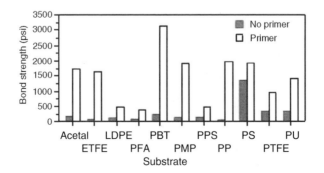

Fig. 1 Effect of polyolefin primers on bond strength of ethyl cyanoacrylate to plastics. All assemblies tested in accordance with ASTM D 4501 (block shear method). ETFE, ethylene tetrafluoroethylene copolymer; LDPE, low-density polyethylene; PFA, polyperfluoroalkoxyethylene; PBT, polybutylene terephthalate; PMP, polymethylpentene; PPS, polyphenylene sulfide; PP, polypropylene; PS, polystyrene; PTFE, polytetrafluoroethylene; PU, polyurethane. Source: Ref 6

Acrylics are among the fastest-curing adhesives, with excellent substrate versatility, good strength and humidity resistance, and a wide formulating range. Gap filling is modest, with joint thicknesses of 0.25 mm (0.010 in.) or less being favored. Maximum use temperature is approximately 150 °C (300 °F).

Among the numerous medical applications involving acrylic adhesives are:

• Needle assembly, including lancets, syringes, injectors, hypodermics, blood collection sets, and introducer catheters
• Anesthesia-mask bonding
• Polycarbonate component assembly (e.g., filters, blood oxygenators, blood-pressure transducers, surgical pumps, heat exchangers, arteriograph manifolds, and cardiotomy reservoirs)
• Blood and drug delivery sets and suction and intravenous (IV) tubes
• Wound closure tapes

Cyanoacrylates. A derivative of acrylic chemistry, cyanoacrylates are sometimes referred to as the "superglues." These materials fix rapidly to polar surfaces, especially those that have hydroxyl groups or residual moisture. Full cure requires about one day. Maximum temperature limit is approximately 105 °C (220 °F), which means that these adhesives are not autoclavable. Some are highly flexible and quite impact resistant, whereas others can be brittle.

In the late 1970s, the addition of rubber to standard ethyl cyanoacrylate formulations resulted in significant improvements in peel and impact strengths. A standard ethyl cyanoacrylate tested in peel mode provides an average strength of less than 3 lb per width inch (pwi) according to ASTM D 1876 on degreased steel. In comparison, a rubber-modified cyanoacrylate exhibits peel strength of approximately 40 pwi.

Cyanoacrylates are used for joining latex balloons onto polyvinyl chloride (PVC), urethane, and multilumen tubes for balloon catheters for angioplasty. They are also used for the assembly of stainless steel tips for catheters and the assembly of tube sets. The polypropylene moldings of drug-administration guns are often bonded together using cyanoacrylate adhesives.

Epoxies are among the most common structural adhesives for use with processing temperatures more than 150 °C (300 °F), and they bond well to many materials. Their major positive attributes are high strength in many loading modes and excellent chemical and electrical resistance. The principal drawbacks of epoxies are relatively slow cure times and susceptibility to long-term moisture pickup in very humid atmospheres.

The fact that epoxies can bond a variety of substrates and fill large gaps makes them useful for deep-section potting of medical components and needle assembly. Epoxies are also used for joining polycarbonate filter components.

Urethanes are extremely versatile in bonding to many substrates and are the first general adhesive of choice to use when joining plastics or difficult surfaces. They can cure rapidly and have good impact resistance. Their temperature limit maximizes at about 120 °C (250 °F), which makes them borderline candidates for autoclaving. They also display relatively poor bonding with metals under humid conditions.

Although urethane adhesives can be applied to a range of substrates, they occasionally mandate the use of a primer to increase the reactivity of the surface to be bonded. Many of these primers require long on-part times in order to effectively prepare the surface for the adhesive.

Common uses of urethanes in the medical device market include bonding tips on catheters and optical scopes, sealing oxygenators and heat exchangers, and assembling components that require significant flexibility. Newer urethane adhesive formulations based on carbonate polyols show promise for implantable device bonding.

Silicones display a wide range of temperature applicability, being useful at temperatures as high as 260 °C (500 °F) and as low as –50 °C (–60 °F). They mechanically adhere to many different surfaces, but their tensile strengths and surface peel strengths are low, suggesting they are more useful as a structural sealant than as a structural adhesive. Silicones have excellent chemical and electrical resistance. Fluorinated silicones have shown benefits in bonding to fluoropolymers by virtue of both their low surface energy and the fluorination.

Typical silicone applications involve bonding and sealing of silicone-based assemblies, coating of components to minimize rough edges or burrs, and coating of highly flexible assemblies such as endotracheal and tracheotomy tubes.

Pressure-Sensitive Adhesives for Medical Applications (Ref 3)

Pressure-sensitive adhesives are used in medical tapes and labels. The adhesive is permanently in tacky form at room temperature and can be used to join various materials with the application of moderate pressure. Pressure-sensitive adhesives are not normally used in sustained-load-bearing applications and can often be removed without leaving a residue.

Most pressure-sensitive adhesives are based on elastomers (e.g., natural or synthetic rubbers), acrylics or hot-melt thermoplastics, tackifiers, or antioxidants. Single- or double-coated pressure-sensitive adhesives are employed in many medical applications. These tapes are available as woven, nonwoven, or elastic materials; they are compatible with skin and can be easily removed with minimal residue. There are medical tapes and transfer adhesives available that can withstand both gamma and EtO sterilization.

Pressure-sensitive adhesives have also been used in transdermal drug-delivery systems. This type of system offers many advantages over conventional oral medications, mainly because it delivers less drug to achieve the same therapeutic effects. The transdermal method delivers drugs directly into the bloodstream via skin and then the liver, rather than by absorption in the gastrointestinal system. A transdermal drug-delivery system usually consists of a patch with drug formulations, an adhesive to maintain contact with the skin, a release liner to protect the patch during storage, and a backing layer that protects the patch from external factors during use.

Other medical applications of pressure-sensitive adhesives include wound coverings and closures, surgical drapes, electrosurgical grounding pads, ostomy mounts, and electrocardiograph electrode mounts.

Adhesives in Medical Electronics (Ref 3)

In the area of electronic components for medical devices, there a wide range of polymeric materials available. They are used variously as attachments, substrates, and interconnections, and for encapsulation or protection.

In recent years, the use of adhesives and encapsulants in medical electronics and implantable devices has increased considerably. This is due to the availability of a wide range of materials that offer different properties, better adhesion, improved durability, suitability for automated dispensing, and rapid curing.

Typical examples include the use of electrically conductive adhesives in pacemakers and ultrasound imaging devices. A two-part silver-filled epoxy is used for bonding critical components in hybrid circuits within pacemakers. In another application, a silver-loaded electrically conductive adhesive is used to join a piezoelectric transducer (PZT) ring to a tungsten carbide tube. The ring and tube are two components of a cardiac catheter tip, which functions as part of an ultrasound imaging device for the quantitative and diagnostic analysis of coronary arteries.

Regulatory Issues (Ref 3 and 7)

In addition to performance issues, medical device manufacturers must also consider regulatory requirements. Device manufacturers rely on their component suppliers for assurance that neither the substrate nor the adhesive will cause problems with the biocompatibility of the device. In an effort to address such issues, both raw material suppliers and adhesive manufacturers now test their components using procedures similar to those used to qualify end-use devices. Tests to determine biological reactivity of polymeric materials and devices are described in the USP and in the ISO 10993 standard.

According to the injection and implantation testing requirements specified under the USP biological reactivity tests, in vivo polymers are classified on a scale of I to VI. To test a polymer, extracts of the material are generated in various media. The extracts are then injected systemically and intracutaneously into rabbits or mice to evaluate their biocompatibility including:

- Their effect on cells (cytotoxicity)
- Their effect on blood constituents (hemolysis)
- Their effect on adjacent tissues following implantations
- Their overall systemic effect

Classes I, II, III, and V polymers do not require implantation testing; Classes IV and VI polymers do require such testing.

ISO Standard 10993 consists of 16 parts. Each part describes specific tests that include a variety of toxicity tests. For example, the tests in part 10 are used for the identification and quantification of degradation products from polymers.

Many polymeric adhesives may be qualified as USP class IV and class VI materials. These materials can pass the relevant incutaneous-toxicity (in vivo), acute-systemic toxicity (in vivo), and implantation (in vivo) testing requirements. Merely passing USP class VI standards does not guarantee that an adhesive will meet Federal Drug Administration (FDA) requirements in a particular application; however, passing the test is a strong indication of the nontoxicity of an adhesive.

Certain types of medical-grade epoxy adhesives are capable of being sterilized by autoclaving, ethylene oxide (EtO), and chemical methods. These epoxy resins can be used in medical devices that require sterilization prior to use.

REFERENCES

1. D.C. Smith, Adhesives and Sealants, *Biomaterials Science: An Introduction to Materials in Medicine,* B.D. Ratner, A.S. Hoffman, F.J. Schoen, and J.E. Lemons, Ed., Academic Press, 1996, p 319–328
2. G.W. Ritter, Using Adhesives Effectively in Medical Devices, *Med. Device Diagnost. Ind.,* Nov 2000, p 52
3. M. Tavakoli, The Adhesive Bonding of Medical Devices, *Med. Device Diagnost. Ind.,* June 2001, p 58
4. Surface Preparation of Plastics, *Adhesives and Sealants,* Vol 3, *Engineered Materials Handbook,* ASM International, 1990, p 276–280
5. H.M. Clearfield, D.K. McNamara, and G.D. Davis, Surface Preparation of Metals, *Adhesives and Sealants,* Vol 3, *Engineered Materials Handbook,* ASM International, 1990, p 259–275
6. P.J. Courtney and C. Verosky, Advances in Cyanoacrylate Technology for Device Assembly, *Med. Device Diagnost. Ind.,* Sept 1999, p 62
7. C. Salerni, Selecting Engineering Adhesives for Medical Device Assembly, *Med. Device Diagnost. Ind.,* June 2000, p 90

CHAPTER 9

Coatings

COATINGS are applied to orthopedic components and other medical devices for a variety of reasons. Porous metal and ceramic coatings deposited on implants facilitate implant fixation and bone ingrowth. Implant surfaces modified by ion implantation or physical vapor deposition exhibit superior hardness and wear resistance. Polymeric coating formulations are used to enhance biocompatibility and biostability, thromboresistance, antimicrobial action, dielectric strength, and lubricity; make medical devices used within the body more visible to ultrasound; and for delivery of drugs.

This chapter reviews some of the more important application areas for coatings, with emphasis placed on enhanced orthopedic implant performance. It should be noted that this is one of the fastest-growing areas in the field of biomaterials and that many developments are anticipated over the next decade. The technical status of biomedical coatings has been the focus of a number of recently published market research studies (see, for example, Ref 1 and 2).

Porous Coatings for Orthopedic Implants

Secure tissue-prosthesis attachment is a necessary requirement for the successful performance of most surgical implants. Load-bearing orthopedic implants for bone and joint replacement are effective only if they can be firmly fixed with the host bone.

Until the 1970s, polymethyl methacrylate (PMMA) bone cement was the predominant means of fixing a joint-replacement implant to the skeletal system. This surgical technique involves preparing sized cavities within the bone, placing PMMA in a viscous, partially cured state within the prepared site, and inserting the implant. The PMMA then cures and fixes the implant in place. This fixation is primarily mechanical.

Cement penetrates into the cancellous bone and locks onto small surface irregularities on the implant. Shrinkage of the cement during curing also locks the cement onto the stem of the device. However, over time the implant may become loose within the cement. This is particularly true for younger, more physically active patients. In some cases, this loosening may either cause pain or increased stress on the implant and subsequent implant failure. Both of these effects may necessitate reoperation.

Porous Metal-Coated Implants

Problems with the loosening of conventional (cemented) joint-replacement implants resulted in studies of alternative approaches for implant fixation to bone including the use of porous-coated implants. Metal, polymer (porous polysulfone and polyethylene), and polymer-based composites (carbon-fiber-filled polytetrafluoroethylene, PTFE) were investigated, and this led to the current widespread use of porous-coated joint replacement implants, principally porous metal-coated hip- and knee-joint implants. Porous metal-coated implants provide enhanced fixation through either cement interlocks with the porous structure or fixation via ingrowth of bone tissue.

Effect of Pore Size. For mineralized bone to grow into the porous coating, certain minimum pore sizes must be achieved. If these minimums are not met, either soft tissue will form or ingrowth will not occur at all. Studies have shown that the *minimum* pore size for load-bearing implants, such as artificial hips and knees, should be approximately 100 to 150 μm (4 to 6 mils) (Ref 3). The pore size of cancellous bone ranges from 400 to 500 μm (16 to 20 mils). Most porous coatings have pore sizes that range from 100 to 400 μm (4 to 16 mils).

Forms and Fabrication Techniques. The porous coatings can take various forms and require different technologies. Cobalt-chromium and titanium porous coatings can be produced from:

- Spherical metal powders made by gas atomization (Fig. 1a). The tiny spheres, or beads as they are frequently referred to in the medical field, are 175 to 250 μm (7 to 10 mils) in

diameter. Porous coatings produced from spherical powders are most frequently used on cobalt-chromium implant materials.
- Wires or fibers that are formed into porous pads

In the case of alloy beads, the manufacturer will apply the coating material using binders over specific regions of the implant surface (e.g., on the proximal portion of the femoral stem as shown in Fig. 2) and then attach the coating to the substrate by various high-temperature sintering stages. Generally, sintering involves heating the implant to about one-half or more of the melting temperature of the alloy to enable

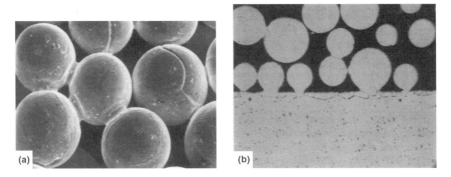

Fig. 1 Porous Co-Cr-Mo coating produced by sintering. (a) Scanning electron micrograph of gas-atomized spheres (beads). (b) Metallographic cross section. Note the necking between the beads. Bead-to-bead bonding is also evident in the cross-sectional view.

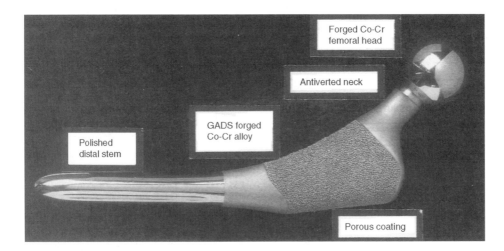

Fig. 2 Porous coated cobalt alloy total hip replacement implant. GADS, gas-atomized dispersion-strengthened alloy

diffusion mechanisms to form necks that join the beads to one another and to the surface of the implant (Fig. 1b). The porous coatings so formed (35 to 50 vol% porosity) are typically 500 to 1000 μm (20 to 40 mils) thick and consist of a regular three-dimensional interconnected porous structure (Ref 3). Tissue ingrowth into this three-dimensional porous results in resistance to shear, compressive, and tensile forces at the tissue/implant interface. Figure 3 shows a section from a cobalt-chromium powder-coated canine femoral knee implant after an implantation of 9 months (Ref 4). The pores have been filled with well-developed bone.

Titanium wire- and fiber-made coatings are used on Ti-6Al-4V. They are attached by a lower-temperature pressure sintering (diffusion-bonding) process. These coatings have very high pore volumes (up to about 65 to 70%).

An alternative surface treatment to sintering is plasma spraying a metal (most often commercially pure, CP, titanium) onto the surface of an implant (Ti-6Al-4V). In this application, the spraying parameters are adjusted such that the metal powder or wire being injected into the plasma is only partially melted as it is being accelerated toward the substrate. Plasma sprayed coatings, like sintered coatings, are 500 to 1000 μm (20 to 40 mils) thick, but they do not form a regular three-dimensional interconnected array of pores. The plasma sprayed coatings essentially form irregular surfaces with very little interconnected porosity throughout the thickness of the coating. Bone tissue will integrate onto the textured coating, providing some degree of implant fixation. Figure 4 shows the rough surface of a plasma sprayed titanium implant (Ref 5).

Fatigue Strength of Porous Metal-Coated Implants. A major concern with the use of porous-coated implants in highly loaded applications is the effect the porous surface layer might have on the mechanical properties of the implants, particularly fatigue strength. Studies have shown that titanium alloy implants, in particular, experience drastic reductions in fatigue strengths following porous coating treatments. For example, a consequence of the use of sinter-processed powder or chopped-wire porous coatings on a Ti-6Al-4V substrate is a reduction of the high-cycle fatigue (HCF) strength from >600 to <200 MPa (>87 to <29 ksi) (Ref 6). Plasma spray processing also leads to a reduction in HCF, but not as drastic as for sinter processing (HCF ≈370 MPa, or 54 ksi, for plasma spray porous coating compared with >600 MPa, or 87 ksi, for nonporous-coated Ti-6Al-4V) (Ref 6). The addition of post plasma spray heat treatment to improve coating bond strength results in further reductions in HCF. The cause of this loss in properties has been attributed to easier fatigue crack initiations at the regions of particle-substrate bonding (Ref 3). The contact zones present regions of high stress concentrations and, possibly, altered composition (higher interstitial levels) and microstructure. Titanium is known to be notch sensitive, so that the topology alone could cause the much lower fatigue strengths. The current practice in designing porous-coated titanium alloy implants is to avoid porous coatings on surfaces that might be subjected to substantial tensile stresses in service (Ref 3). This limitation is unfortunate because titanium alloys offer significant advantages over other metals in terms of corrosion resistance, metal ion release, and biocompatibility.

Bond Failure of Sintered Porous Coatings. The metallurgical process to adhere the coating to the implant is a complex high-temperature treatment that requires a series of steps. The challenge is to provide strong bonds between each of the powder spheres (beads) and between the coating and the implant without significantly degrading the strength and corrosion resistance of the component. Proper processing prior to applying the porous coating is also critical for adequate bonding.

Figure 5 shows a cast cobalt alloy (ASTM F 75) femoral knee implant that was returned to

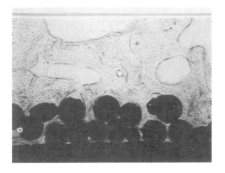

Fig. 3 Histological section of a porous coated canine femoral knee component after implantation of 9 months. Well-developed bone is observed within the pores. Source: Ref 4

the casting vendor for analysis after exhibiting poor bond strength between the cast substrate and the sintered porous coating. Metallographic analysis indicated that a decarburized layer existed on all surfaces of the casting (Fig. 6). It was determined that the decarburized layer resulted from improper casting and machining (grinding) practices (Ref 7). The decarburized layer prevented bonding during the sintering thermal cycle. Bead-to-bead bonding within the coating was sufficient (Fig. 7), and no decarburized layer was present on the bead surfaces.

The effect of a decarburized layer on bond strength after porous coating can be understood by referring to the carbon-cobalt phase diagram shown in Fig. 8. The lower-carbon-content surface layer effectively increases the solidus temperature from approximately 1425 °C (2600 °F) for a 0.30% C alloy to up to 1495 °C (2720 °F) for pure cobalt. Because the rate of diffusion and consequently the rate of diffusion bonding are functions of the homologous temperature

$(T/T_{melting})$, the lower-carbon surface layer can be expected to inhibit diffusion and significantly reduce the effectiveness of the sintering cycle (Ref 7). This is consistent with the absence of decarburization observed metallographically in castings that exhibited sufficient bond strength.

Hydroxyapatite Porous Coatings

Coating calcium hydroxyapatite (HA), $Ca_{10}(PO_4)_6(OH)_2$, on a bioinert metallic implant surface is an effective method of using this bioactive calcium phosphate compound in the human body (Ref 8). Some biological advantages of HA coatings are enhancement of bone formation, accelerated bonding between the implant surface and surrounding tissues, and the reduction of potentially harmful metallic ion release. Hydroxyapatite has been used to coat many types of implants such as hip and dental implants. Hydroxyapatite also establishes

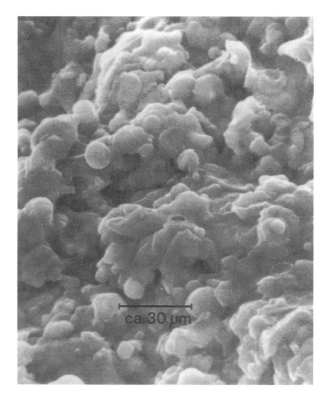

Fig. 4 Scanning electron micrograph showing the textured surface of a titanium plasma spray coating on an oral implant. Source: Ref 5

strong interfacial bonds with titanium implants, and this has been attributed to some chemical bonding between HA and the titanium substrate (Ref 8).

Hydroxyapatite coatings have been applied by the plasma spray process, which offers the attractive combination of economy and efficient deposition of HA (other coating methods have been used but with a far lesser degree of success). Plasma sprayed HA coatings can be applied to nonporous or porous substrates.

Bond coats based on bioinert ceramic materials such as titania and zirconia have been developed to increase the adhesion strength of HA coatings on Ti-6Al-4V alloy surfaces used for hip and dental implants (Ref 9). The bond coats improved adhesion strength, measured by a modified ASTM D 3167 peel test, by up to 100%. Figure 9 shows a cross section of a Ti-6Al-4V/titania bond coat/HA top coat system.

Functionally Graded Coatings Based on Calcium Phosphates. Functionally graded materials (FGMs) have a gradient compositional change from the surface to the interior of the material. With the unique microstructure of FGMs, materials for specific function and performance requirements can be designed (Ref 10). In the field of biomaterials, several approaches exist for the deposition of functionally graded coatings (FGCs) based on calcium phosphate compounds onto titanium alloy surfaces. Although still in the developmental stage, FGCs are being widely studied.

Figure 10 shows a calcium phosphate FGC graded in accordance to adhesive strength, bioactivity, and bioresorbability. Calcium phosphates have different phases. Hydroxyapatite has excellent chemical bonding ability with natural bone. Tricalcium phosphate (TCP), known in its two polymorphs of α-TCP and β-TCP, is a biosorbable ceramic that dissolves gradually in body fluid, and new bone will eventually replace it. The solubility of α-TCP is higher than that of β-TCP.

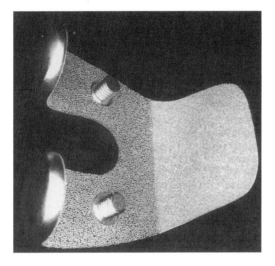

Fig. 5 Porous coated knee implant, as received. Insufficient bonding occurred at the tip of the patella flange.

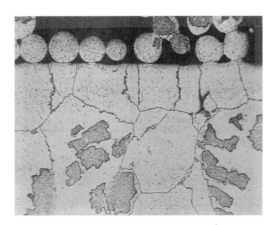

Fig. 6 Metallographic cross section through the region of insufficient bonding. Note that the substrate surface is free of the blocky carbides found in the interior of the casting. Decarburization was the cause of bond failure. Source: Ref 7

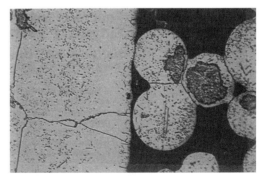

Fig. 7 Higher-magnification view of the low-bond-strength region shown in Fig. 6. Note the high degree of bead-to-bead bonding compared with bead-to-substrate bond. 158×. Source: Ref 7

Figure 11 shows a cross section of TCP/HA FGC. The top layer could provide calcium and phosphate materials for accelerated bone formation. The first layer coated on the titanium substrate is spheroidized HA (SHA) ranging from 20 to 45 μm (0.8 to 1.8 mils) (Fig. 12). The use

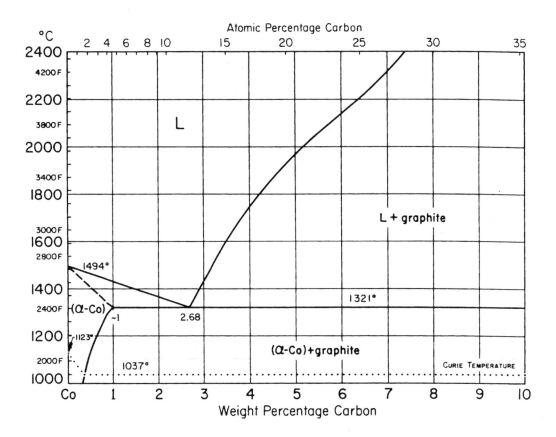

Fig. 8 The carbon-cobalt binary phase diagram. Source: ASM International

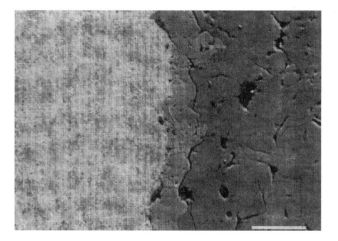

Fig. 9 Scanning electron micrograph of a cross section of a titania bond coat/HA top coat system. Left: substrate, light gray; center: titania bond coat, medium gray; HA, dark gray. Source: Ref 9

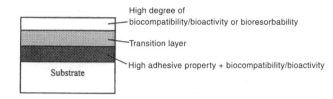

Fig. 10   Calcium phosphate functionally graded coating. Source: Ref 10

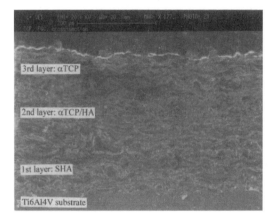

Fig. 11   Cross-sectional view of TCP/HA functionally graded coating. Source: Ref 10

of SHA powders can produce a very dense coating structure that may result in higher bond strength with Ti-6Al-4V substrates. The TCP/HA composite was deposited in the middle of HA and TCP coatings as a transition layer.

Ion Implantation

Ion implantation is an approach for modifying surface properties of materials similar to a coating process, but it does not involve the addition of a layer on the surface. Ion implantation uses highly energetic beam of ions (positively charged atoms) to modify the surface structure and chemistry of materials at low temperature. The process does not adversely affect component dimensions or bulk material properties.

Process Description. The ion implantation process is conducted in a vacuum chamber at very low pressure (10^{-4} to 10^{-5} torr, or 0.13 to 0.013 Pa). Large numbers of ions (typically 10^{16} to 10^{17} ions/cm^2) bombard and penetrate a surface interacting with the substrate atoms immediately beneath the surface. Typical depth of penetration is a fraction of a micrometer (or a few millionths of an inch). The interactions of the energetic ions with the material modify the surface, providing it with significantly different properties than the remainder (bulk) of the material. Specific property changes depend on the selected ion beam treatment parameters, for example, the particular ion species, energy, and total number of ions that impact the surface.

Ions are produced via a multistep process in a system such as that shown in Fig. 13. Ions are initially formed by stripping electrons from source atoms in a plasma. The ions are then extracted and pass through a mass-analyzing magnet, which selects only those ions of a desired species, isotope, and charge state. The beam of ions is then accelerated using a potential gradient column. Typical ion energies are 10 to 200 keV. A series of electrostatic and magnetic lens elements shapes the resulting ion beam and scans it over an area in an end station containing the parts to be treated.

Applications. Titanium and cobalt-chromium alloy orthopedic prosthesis for hips and knees are among the most successful commercial applications of ion-implanted components for wear resistance. In use, these components (Fig. 14) articulate against an ultrahigh-molecular-weight polyethylene mating surface (acetabular cup). Tests at several laboratories have indicated that wear reductions of 10× to 100× may be realized by implantation of nitrogen ions into the alloy (Ref 11). To date, tens of thousands of such components have been ion implanted prior to surgical implantation.

Ion-Beam-Assisted Deposition

Process Description. Ion-beam-assisted deposition (IBAD) is a thin-film deposition process wherein evaporated atoms produced by

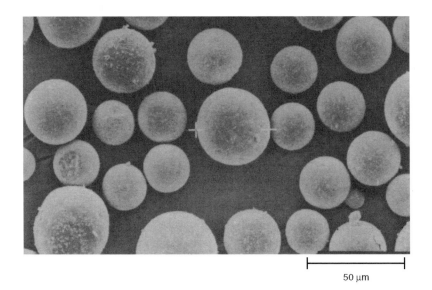

50 µm

Fig. 12   Spheroidized hydroxyapatite powder with a particle size range of ~20 to 45 µm. Source: Ref 10

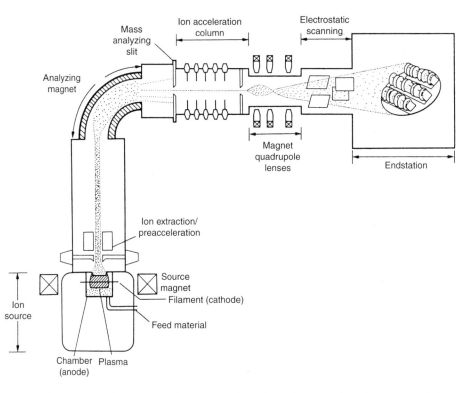

Fig. 13   Ion-implantation system for surface modification of metallic implants. The target in the end station is intended to represent an array of femoral components of artificial knee joints for implantation. Source: Spire Corporation

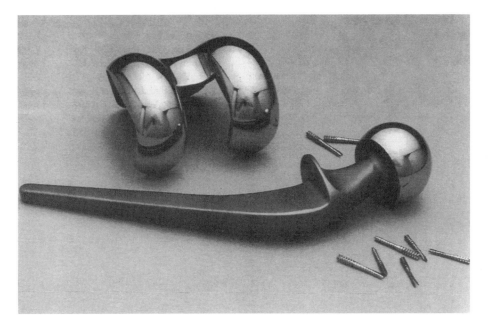

Fig. 14 Ti-6Al-4V alloy surgical prostheses that are ion implanted for enhanced wear resistance. Source: Ref 11

physical vapor deposition are simultaneously struck by an independently generated flux of ions (Ref 12). The evaporant (or coating) material is produced using a high-power electron beam. Components are placed in the vapor, and individual coating atoms or molecules condense and stick on the surface of the component to form the coating. Simultaneously, highly energetic ions (100 to 2000 eV) are produced and directed at the component surface. The component is situated at the intersection of the evaporant and ion beam (Fig. 15). The concurrent ion bombardment differentiates IBAD from other thin-film deposition techniques. It significantly improves adhesion and permits control over film properties such as morphology, density, stress level, crystallinity, and chemical composition. Ion bombardment intermixes the coating and substrate atoms and eliminates the columnar microstructure often observed with conventional PVD to create very dense, adherent thin-film structures.

Applications. The IBAD process is capable of depositing many different types of metallic and ceramic coatings. Examples of metallic coatings include silver, gold, platinum, and tita-

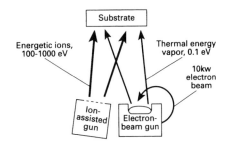

Fig. 15 Ion-beam-assisted deposition (IBAD) process. Source: Ref 12

nium. These films are typically used for increasing biocompatibility and providing conductivity or for increasing radiopacity. Silver coatings are also used to create antimicrobial surfaces on percutaneous and implantable medical devices. Representative ceramic coatings include aluminum oxide, silicon dioxide, titanium nitride, and aluminum nitride. These coatings are used for wear-resistant applications.

Vapor Deposition Processes

Vapor deposition processes can principally be divided into two types:

- *Physical vapor deposition* (PVD) processes, which require creation of material vapors (via evaporation, sputtering, or laser ablation) and their subsequent condensation onto a substrate to form the film
- *Chemical vapor deposition* (CVD) processes, which are generally defined as the deposition of a solid material from the vapor phase onto a (usually) heated substrate as a result of numerous chemical reactions

Physical vapor deposition and CVD processes can be classified as shown in Table 1. Details on these coating techniques can be found in various volumes of the *ASM Handbook* (see, for example, Ref 13).

Table 2 shows selected parameters of basic PVD and CVD processes. In general, CVD processes have the advantage over PVD processes of good throwing power, while PVD processes have higher deposition rates than those in CVD processes.

Physical Vapor Deposition. Since it was introduced to the medical device industry in the late 1980s, PVD has become widely used to deposit wear-resistant thin-film coatings on a variety of medical devices, including orthopedic implants, pacemakers, surgical instruments, orthodontic appliances, and dental instruments. The value of PVD technology rests in its ability to modify the surface properties of a device without changing the underlying material properties and biomechanical functionality. In addition to enhanced wear resistance, PVD coatings reduce friction, are compatible with sterilization processes, provide decorative colors, and improve corrosion resistance. The most commonly used coating is TiN, but ZrN, AlTiN, TiAlN, CrN, and amorphous carbon are being tested as alternative biomedical coatings. Properties of various PVD coatings are listed in Table 3.

Diamondlike carbon (DLC) films are hard (up to 80 GPa, or 12 psi $\times 10^6$) amorphous films produced by CVD, plasma-assisted CVD (PACVD), ion-beam processing, IBAD, and ion plating (Ref 14). Because the biocompatibility of DLC is excellent, these films are being considered as coatings for metallic implants to improve their compatibility with body tissues. Tissue can adhere well to carbon implants and sustain a durable interface. Also, in the presence of blood, a protein layer is formed that prevents the formation of blood clots at the carbon surface. Carbon-fiber implants can promote the rapid ingrowth of tissue and are used successfully for ligament repair. In bulk form, porous charcoal permits a similar ingrowth, but has low strength and may also present a site for infection.

Preliminary *in vitro* tests using mouse tissues as well as *in vivo* sheep tests have shown an encouraging degree of biocompatibility, but more laboratory tests are needed before it can be accepted in human trials. Carbon can also be impregnated with resin to improve the properties, but the ideal solution is probably to combine the strength of metals with the biocompatibility of carbon in the form of DLC-coated metal prosthetic implants such as hip and knee joints.

Diamond is extremely hydrophobic. Because of this, biological tissue does not adhere to diamond, so bacteria and viruses are thought to not readily cling to the surface. The combination of the hydrophobic nature of diamond, its nontoxicity, its corrosion-free properties, and its hardness combine to render it an ideal candidate for the coating and/or fabrication of artificial heart valves. Not only should valves fabricated with DLC not corrode, erode, or otherwise wear out, but the hydrophobic nature of the surface suggests that the major problem of conventional artificial heart valves—providing nucleation sites for blood clotting—may be overcome.

Another potential application for DLC is coatings for coronary stents. Studies have shown that DLC-coated stainless steel stents implanted in pigs resulted in decreased thrombogenicity and neointimal hyperplasia (Ref 15).

Diamond inserts are currently in widespread use as surgical scalpels (Ref 14). These scalpels are not only efficacious by virtue of their hydrophobic properties, but also because of their sharpness in comparison to surgical steel scalpels. The sharpness to which an edge may be polished is fundamentally dependent on the hardness of the material. With a radius of curvature some 30 times smaller than the steel equivalents, the diamond scalpels introduce much less tearing of the tissue. As a result, healing is much faster and scar-tissue formation is reduced. Although cutting can be faster when

Table 1 Classification of physical vapor deposition (PVD) and chemical vapor deposition (CVD) processes on the basis of material deposited on substrate

	Metals		Compounds	
Process	Basic	Hybrid	Basic	Hybrid
Physical vapor deposition				
Conventional	Evaporation deposition	Ion plating	. . .	. . .
	Sputter deposition	. . .	. . .	. . .
Plasma-assisted (PAPVD)	. . .	. . .	Activated reactive evaporation (ARE)	Reactive ion plating (RIP)
	. . .	. . .	Reactive sputtering (RS)	. . .
Chemical vapor deposition				
Conventional	Thermal	. . .	. . .	. . .
Plasma-assisted (PACVD)	. . .	. . .	rf excitation	. . .
	. . .	. . .	Microwave excitation	. . .
	. . .	. . .	Photon excitation	. . .

Source: Ref 13

Table 2 Selected parameters of basic PVD and CVD processes

	Physical vapor deposition		
Parameter	Evaporation	Sputtering	Chemical vapor deposition
Mechanism of production for depositing species	Thermal energy	Momentum transfer	Chemical reaction
Deposition rate	Can be very high (up to 7.5×10^5 Å/min)	Low except for pure metals (for example, copper, 10^4 Å/min)	Moderate (200–2500 Å/min)
Depositing species	Atoms and ions	Atoms and ions	Atoms
Throwing power	Poor line-of-sight coverage except by gas scattering	Good, but nonuniform thickness distribution	Good
Metal deposition	Yes	Yes	Yes
Alloy deposition	Yes	Yes	Yes
Refractory compound deposition	Yes	Yes	Yes
Energy of deposited species	Low (1.6×10^{-20} to 8.0×10^{-20} J, or 0.1 to 0.5 eV)	Can be high (1.6×10^{-19} to 1.6×10^{-17} J, or 1 to 100 eV)	Can be high with plasma-assisted CVD
Bombardment of substrate/deposit	Not normally	Yes	Possible
Growth interface perturbation	Not normally	Yes	Yes (by rubbing)
Substrate heating (by external means)	Yes, normally	Not generally	Yes

Source: Ref 13

Table 3 Properties of PVD biomedical coatings

	Coating					
Property	TiN	ZrN	AlTiN	TiAlN	CrN	Amorphous carbon
Hardness, HV(a)	2900 ± 200	2800 ± 200	4500 ± 500	2600 ± 400	2500 ± 400	8000
Adhesion, N(b)	70	70	70–80	60	70	80
Oxidation temperature, °C (°F)	500 (930)	600 (1110)	800 (1470)	800 (1470)	700 (1290)	500 (930)
Coefficient of friction(c)	0.65	0.61	0.42	1.70	0.55	0.10
Surface roughness(d) (R_a), µm	0.2	0.2	0.4	0.4	0.2	0.02
Ductility(e), %	1.19	1.01	1.2–1.5	1.2–1.5	. . .	. . .
Color	Gold	Gold	Black	Bronze	Silver	Black

(a) Vickers hardness test at 50 gf load. (b) Critical normal force in newtons required to detach the coating from the substrate. (c) Measured between 100Cr6 ball and coated substrate. (d) Measured by Dektak surface profilometer in micrometers. (e) Done by acoustic four-point bend test. Amount of deformation before cracking.
Source: IonBond

using a diamond scalpel, the much smaller radius of curvature on the diamond cutting edge provides less "springback" force to the surgeon's hand. The tough factor requires significant readjustment for the surgeon. With the advent of artificial diamond coatings, the cost and availability of diamond scalpels should be favorably affected.

Current applications for diamond surgical instruments include those for such microsurgical procedures as radial keratotomy, cataract extraction, and neurosurgery (Ref 14). Special diamond knives are used in coronary bypass surgery. Such a knife eliminates the need for changing to different knives and scissors during coronary surgery. Larger diamond knives are in use for extracting gristle in the hand in patients with Dupuytens syndrome.

Polymer Coatings

Many medical device coatings are polymer-based formulations. These coatings must meet a number of primary material characteristics for medical device use. These include (Ref 16):

- *Biocompatibility:* Coatings need to exhibit long-term compatibility and a nonreactive relationship with body fluids and tissues. The coating should not undergo any chemical interaction with the substrate to which it is being applied, nor should it produce any toxic by-products or extracts that could be harmful to a patient or to the function of the item being coated.
- *Coating inertness:* The coating must not contaminate the substrate with outgassing or with by-products from catalysts, cure agents, solvents, or plasticizers.
- *Hydrophobic characteristics:* Hydrophobic—or hydrophilic—characteristics may be important in certain medical applications, for example, a hydrophilic cardiovascular catheter (slippery when wet) for ease of insertion versus a wet hydrophobic guidewire that would be easy for the cardiologist to grip.
- *Cure temperature:* The cure temperature of a coating must be within the performance range of the substrate.
- *Cure forces:* The cure forces of a coating must not degrade or distort the underlying substrate.
- *Conformability:* The coating must offer conformability to highly variable surface geome-

tries. It must provide effective isolation of all surfaces, including hidden areas, crevices, and so forth, without bridging or pooling. The coating must be able to maintain conformability at all magnitudes of substrate and surface feature sizes, from macro to micro.
- *Finished thickness:* The finished thickness of a coating is important. The coating may need to meet extremely tight dimensional tolerances, and therefore be quite thin, while at the same time be able to provide uncompromised physical, chemical, or electrical protection for the substrate with coverage that is free of voids and pinholes.
- *Mechanical loading:* A coating often needs to function dependably without significantly altering the physical or mechanical properties of the substrate.
- *Resistance to flaking:* A coating needs to have considerable flaking resistance. It must be sufficiently robust and adherent to prevent flaking from substrates or from itself.
- *Sterilizability:* A coating must be capable of withstanding the effects of one or more sterilization processes.

Medical Coating Applications (Ref 16)

The U.S. Federal Drug Administration (FDA) specifies three contact-duration categories for medical devices: limited contact for a contact duration up to 24 h, prolonged contact for a duration of 24 h to 30 days, and permanent contact for any contact duration lasting longer than 30 days. Biomedical coating applications can be generalized into two primary categories: short-term, which are disposable or single-patient-use items and long-term, which are prosthetic hardware, reusable lab equipment, or various implants.

The primary coating requirement for short-term applications is surface isolation. This can be accomplished with a coating that creates a benign barrier between a substrate and body tissues. A short-term coating application may also require one or more secondary properties, however, such as lubricity or dielectric protection.

Long-term medical applications often demand the same coating performance, with the added necessity of functioning as intended for an extended period. There are other coating requirements, such as tissue growth promotion, that are unique to long-term applications.

Following are two lists of common medical products that may require conformal coating, along with the principal desired coating functions. The first list comprises short-term or temporary applications. These include:

- *Medical seals:* With medical seals, a coating may be used to eliminate tackiness, to supplement mechanical strength, and to provide dry-film lubricity and chemical isolation.
- *Pressure sensors and transducers:* Sensor coating entails the protection of delicate, sensitive elements without mechanically loading transducing surfaces or otherwise interfering with device function.
- *Guidewires:* The principal coating function for guidewires is to promote ease of insertion and to protect wires from potentially corrosive biofluids.
- *Catheters:* Coating increases lubricity and isolates surfaces from corrosive biofluids.
- *Mandrels:* An appropriate coating reduces the coefficient of friction, ensures a particulate-free surface, eliminates microscopic flaking, and extends the useful life of mandrels for the production of elastomer parts.
- *Brain probes:* Brain probes benefit from the increased lubricity of a coating and may require selective insulation to suit their conductive function.
- *Needles:* An effective coating should seal microporosity, minimize injection trauma with enhanced lubricity, and cover both inside and outside needle surfaces without measurably changing dimensions.

The following are examples of long-term or permanent coating applications:

- *Electronic circuits:* A coating should isolate the surface from moisture and corrosive biological effects and electrically insulate conductive elements.
- *Cardiac-assist devices:* Implanted cardiac-assist devices need to be isolated from corrosive biofluids and electrically insulated by a conformal coating.
- *Pipette and microplate trays and covers:* A coating should seal surfaces to eliminate microporosity; isolate surfaces from corrosive biofluids, moisture, and chemicals; and lubricate the cover attachment of the product.

Parylene Coatings (Ref 16)

Parylene is a thin, vacuum-deposited polymer that is widely used for demanding medical coating applications. It differs from conventional coatings in that it is deposited on objects at room temperature as a film and does not use solvents, catalysts, plasticizers, or other feature-enhancing additives. It is based on a high-purity raw material called diparaxylylene, which is a white, crystalline powder. A vacuum and thermal process converts the powder to a polymer film, which is formed on substrates at room temperature.

The unique properties of parylene include precise conformance to substrate topography, pinhole-free coverage in very thin layers, and the ability to penetrate and coat complex surfaces. Parylene film resists chemical attack from organic solvents, inorganic reagents, and acids; it adheres well to many surfaces, and offers dielectric strength above 5000 V dc at 25 μm (1 mil) of film thickness. It has a lubricious surface, with a coefficient of friction in the range of 0.25 to 0.33 (per ASTM D 1894), which approaches that of polytetrafluoroethylene (PTFE, or Teflon).

Parylene can be coated on such diverse substrates as glass, metal, paper, resin, plastics, ceramic, ferrite, and silicon, and even on powdered and granular substances. The coating achieves conformal coverage, moisture protection, dielectric protection, and freedom from pinholes in layers as thin as 500 Å.

A number of characteristics make parylene coatings particularly attractive for medical applications. Crystal-clear parylene film has very low thrombogenic properties and low potential for triggering an immune response. The film has also been shown to be highly resistant to the potentially damaging effects of corrosive body fluids, electrolytes, proteins, enzymes, and lipids. In addition, the film also forms an effective barrier against the passage of contaminants from a coated substrate to the body or the surrounding environment.

Because properly formulated parylene raw material is pure, no foreign substances are introduced that could degrade medical surfaces. Parylene is not a liquid at any stage in its application process, and thus it does not exhibit the surface-tension effects of pooling, bridging, or meniscus.

There are four versions of parylene currently available for medical surface-modification applications. The first two, parylene N and parylene C, are the most commonly used for medical products. Table 4 compares the properties of parylene N and C.

Parylene N provides particularly high dielectric strength and a dielectric constant that is independent of frequency. Because of its high molecular activity during deposition, parylene N has the highest penetrating power and is able to coat relatively deep recesses and blind holes. Its low dissipation factor and dielectric constant suit high-frequency substrates where the coating is in an electromagnetic field.

Parylene C has a chlorine atom added onto the parylene N benzene ring, and this gives it an excellent combination of electrical and physical properties, including a very low permeability to moisture and corrosive gases. Parylene C deposition is substantially faster than parylene N, and therefore its crevice-penetrating ability is reduced compared to the more active parylene N molecule.

Parylene D. With two chlorine atoms added to the benzene ring, parylene D has a higher degree of thermal stability than parylene C or parylene N, but its crevice penetration ability is the least pronounced of the three versions.

Parylene HT. Although standard parylene coatings can withstand temperatures up to about 150 °C (300 °F), fluorine-modified parylene coatings can be used at temperatures as high as 450 °C (840 °F). High-temperature parylene coatings are suitable for electrosurgical devices and other components that are subjected to high instantaneous temperatures.

Applications. Parylene coatings have found use in such diverse applications as temporary surgical hardware, prostheses components, catheters, stoppers, probes, needles, and cochlear implants. These coatings are also used on mandrels to manufacture catheters, on endoscopic surgical devices, and on implanted pacemakers and defibrillators.

Recent Developments in Polymer Coatings (Ref 17)

Traditionally, the goal of surface modification was to improve the physical or mechanical properties in a component or device—for example, by adding a nonstick coating to a catheter for easier insertion. Increasingly, however, surface modification also aims at inducing a specific desired bioresponse or inhibiting a potentially adverse reaction. This section briefly reviews some of the recently developed coatings for improving the function and durability of materials featured in a wide range of medical products. These coating formulations are highly proprietary, and some are still in the developmental stage. Nevertheless, they represent the future direction of research on polymer-based coatings for biomedical applications.

Blood-Compatible Coatings for Drug Delivery. Improved compatibility with blood is a desired feature for a variety of medical devices that must contact blood during clinical use. The materials used for manufacture of medical devices are not inherently compatible with blood and its components. The response of blood to a foreign material can be aggressive, resulting in surface-induced thrombus (clot) formation, which can impair or disable the function of the device and, most importantly, threaten the patient's health. Even with the use of systemic anticoagulants, the functioning of devices such as cardiopulmonary bypass circuits, hemodialyzers, ventricular-assist devices, and stents has been associated with thrombus formation, platelet and leucocyte activation, and other complications related to the deleterious effects of blood/material interactions.

Of the various biologically active substances used to improve the blood compatibility of synthetic surfaces, heparin is perhaps the most promising. Heparin is a pharmaceutical that has been used clinically for decades as an intravenous anticoagulant to treat inherent clotting disorders and to prevent blood clot formation during surgery and interventional procedures. Heparin-containing polymer coatings have been

Table 4 Property comparison of parylene coatings

Property	Parylene N	Parylene C
Crevice penetration	Best	Good
Molecular activity	Highest	Good
Coating uniformity	Best	Good
Hardness	Least	Moderate
Physical toughness	Least	Moderate
Moisture resistant	Moderate	Best
Cost-effectiveness	Moderate	Best
Dielectric strength	Best	Good
Dielectric constant	Low	Higher
Gas permeability	Good	Best
Chemical resistance	Good	Excellent
Elongation to break	Lower	Best
Thickness control	Good	Best
Masking complexity	Greatest	Moderate
Thermal stability	Moderate	Moderate
Coating speed	Lowest	Moderate
Dielectric strength	Good	Good
Dissipation factor	Low	Higher
Lubricity (CFE)	Best	Good

CFE, coefficient of friction. Source: Ref 16

developed for use on implants and indwelling catheters to render them blood compatible for sustained periods. The coating system consists of an inert, biocompatible hydrogel matrix that entraps heparin complexes on the surface of medical devices. The coating acts as a reservoir for the heparin complex, releasing the agent slowly over time upon exposure to blood, thereby increasing the duration of anticoagulant activity. In this manner, a high local heparin concentration at the device surface results in prolonged antithrombogenic protection while keeping the systemic concentrations low.

Nonheparin synthetic blood compatibility coatings are also being developed. These are polyvinylpyrrolidone- and polyacrylamide-based polymers. Nonheparin polymer coatings face fewer regulatory restrictions than do the heparin-containing coatings due to the side effects of heparin treatments.

Coatings for Added Lubricity. There are a number of coatings that have been developed for adding lubricity to device component surfaces. For example, cores that are made into balloon catheter hypotubes and various types of guidewires are coated with PTFE. These coatings reduce the friction coefficients of such devices by as much as 50%. Components can be spray coated or pulled through a PTFE coating bath.

Lubricious coatings based on nonreactive hydrophilic/hydrophobic polymer matrices have also been developed. When the coating is exposed to aqueous body fluids, moisture is absorbed and retained in the coating by the hydrophilic components. These fluids create a slippery surface, with a high fluid concentration at the surface. The hydrophobic components hold the matrix together and firmly anchor it the substrate. Lubricity can easily be tailored by varying the proportions of the hydrophilic and hydrophobic components in the matrix to make the device more or less slippery. Typical applications for these coatings include catheters, guidewires, shunts, and endoscopes. A wide variety of polymer and metallic substrates can be coated.

Coatings for ultrasonic imaging technology are designed to make medical devices used within the body more visible to ultrasound. Applied to products such as biopsy needles, the polymer coating incorporates micropores that trap air at the surface of the device. Rather than simply sending signals back to the transducer, the bubbles reflect the signals in all directions. This enables ultrasound imaging systems to show the position of a device in the body even when it is at an angle to the transducer. As a result, ultrasound can be used in place of MRI and fluoroscopy in many device-placement procedures.

Antimicrobial Coatings. Despite the efforts to combat it, device-associated infection remains a major problem in medical care. Infection at indwelling catheters, for example, can result from contaminated disinfectants, from the hands of medical personnel, or as a result of autoinfection from a patient's own microflora. Such infections are not easily treated, since proliferating bacteria on the surface of the catheter can secrete a polysaccharide biofilm or "slime" difficult for systemic antibiotics to penetrate. One way of addressing device-related infection is to incorporate antimicrobial agents directly onto the surface of the device. Silver compounds (silver chloride or silver oxide) are a popular choice for infection-resistant coatings, but many commercially available silver-coated catheters are of marginal effectiveness because the hydrophobic polymer matrix limits the silver ion concentration near the device surface. A process has been developed, however, that incorporates silver compounds in a nonreactive hydrogel polymer system that provides greater aqueous diffusion from the coating and thus a greater concentration of silver ions at and just above the device surface. The coatings can be formulated for short-intermediate-, or long-term effects; offer controllable lubricity and elution; can be applied inside lumens; and demonstrate superior adhesion, durability, and flexibility. Polymer substrates that can be treated with the technique include polyurethanes, polyolefins, polyesters, polyvinyl chlorides, polyamides, polyimides, and silicones.

Coating Adhesion-Resistant Devices. Some difficulty is encountered when lubricious coatings such as PTFE must adhere to catheters and other devices made from adhesion-resistant silicone. Hydrophilic coatings have been developed that give silicone devices both a dry and wet lubricity. To begin the coating process, the device is placed in a water bath that contains a monomer. This monomer forms polymer chains by reacting with the surface of the device. Chemical bonds hook the chains to the surface of the device. Treated catheters slide more easily into a patient's urinary tract than do untreated catheters with high coefficients of friction.

REFERENCES

1. "Biocompatible Coatings: The Impact of Surface Technology on Medical Markets," Technical Insights, John Wiley & Sons Inc., June 2000 (find summary at www.mindbranch.com)
2. "Medical Coatings," Technology Assessment Associates, March 2002 (find summary at www.tech-assessment.com)
3. R.M. Pilliar, Porous Biomaterials, *Concise Encyclopedia of Medical & Dental Materials,* D. Williams, Ed., Pergamon Press and The MIT Press, 1990, p 312–319
4. J.D. Bobyn et al., Biologic Fixation and Bone Modeling, with an Unconstrained Canine Total Knee Prosthesis, *Clin. Orthopaedics Related Res.,* No. 166, 1982, p 307
5. J.D. Brunski, Metals, *Biomaterials Science: An Introduction to Materials in Medicine,* B.D. Ratner, A.S. Hoffman, F.J. Schoen, and J.E. Lemons, Ed., Academic Press, 1996, p 37–50
6. T. Smith, The Effect of Plasma-Sprayed Coatings on the Fatigue of Titanium Alloy Implants, *JOM,* Feb 1994, p 54–56
7. M. Lisin and R.R. Peterson, Failure of the Bond between a Cobalt Alloy Prosthetic Casting and a Sintered Porous Coating, *Handbook of Case Histories in Failure Analysis,* Vol 1, K.A. Esaklul, Ed., ASM International, 1992, p 449–451
8. K.A. Khor, P. Cheang, and Y. Wang, Plasma Spraying of Combustion Flame Spheroidized Hydroxyapatite (HA) Powders, *J. Therm. Spray Technol.,* June 1998, p 254–260
9. R.B. Heimann, Design of Novel Plasma Sprayed Hydroxyapatite-Bond Coat Bioceramic Systems, *J. Therm. Spray Technol.,* Dec 1999, p 597–603
10. Y. Wang, K.A. Khor, and P. Cheang, Thermal Spraying of Functionally Graded Calcium Phosphate Coatings for Biomedical Implants, *J. Therm. Spray Technol.,* March 1998, p 50–57
11. J.K. Hirvonen and B.D. Sartwell, Ion Implantation, *Surface Engineering,* Vol 5, *ASM Handbook,* ASM International, 1994, p 604–610
12. G.K. Hubler and J.K. Hirvonen, Ion-Beam-Assisted Deposition, *Surface Engineering,* Vol 5, *ASM Handbook,* ASM International, 1994, p 593–601
13. R.F. Bunshah, PVD and CVD Coatings, *Friction, Lubrication, and Wear Technology,* Vol 18, *ASM Handbook,* ASM International, 1992, p 840–849
14. R. Jethanandani, The Development and Application of Diamond-Like Carbon Films, *JOM,* Feb 1997, p 63–65
15. I. De Scheerder, et al., Evaluation of the Biocompatibility of Two New Diamond-Like Stent Coatings (Dylyn) in a Porcine Coronary Stent Model, *Eur. Heart J.,* Aug 2000, p 389–394
16. L. Wolgemuth, Assessing the Performance and Suitability of Parylene Coating, *Med. Dev. Diagn. Ind.,* Aug 2000, p 42
17. W. Leventon, New Coatings and Processes Add Value to Medical Devices, *Med. Dev. Diagn. Ind.,* Aug 2001, p 48

CHAPTER 10

Biomaterials for Dental Applications

DENTAL MATERIALS for restorative dentistry include:

- *Amalgam alloys* for direct fillings
- *Noble metals and alloys* for direct fillings, crowns and bridges, and porcelain fused to metal restorations
- *Base metals and alloys* for partial-denture framework, porcelain-metal restorations, crowns and bridges, orthodontic wires and brackets, and implants
- *Ceramics* for implants, porcelain-metal restorations, crowns, inlays, and veneers, cements, and denture teeth
- *Composites* for replacing missing tooth structure and modifying tooth color and contour
- *Polymers* for denture bases, plastic teeth, cements, and other applications

These materials must withstand forces during either fabrication or mastication, retain their strength and toughness, and be resistant to corrosion, friction, and wear. Similar to implantable devices for nondental applications, they must also be biocompatible.

Biocompatibility is defined as the ability of a material to elicit an appropriate biological response in a given application in the body (Ref 1). Inherent in this definition is the concept that a single material will not be biologically acceptable in all applications. For example, a material that is acceptable as a full cast crown may not be acceptable as a dental implant. Also implicit in this definition is the expected biological performance of the material. In a bone implant, the material is expected to allow the bone to integrate with the implant. Thus, an appropriate biological response for the implant is osseointegration (close approximation of bone to the implant material). In a full cast crown, the material is expected to not cause inflammation of pulpal or periodontal tissues. Osseointegration, however, is not expected. Whether a material is biocompatible is therefore dependent on what physical function is asked of the material and what biological response is required from it.

This chapter reviews some of the important properties of biomaterial used in dentistry with emphasis on mechanical properties. The complex oral environment and the corrosion behavior of metallic restorative materials is discussed in chapter 11, "Tarnish and Corrosion of Dental Alloys." The tribological behavior of dental materials is reviewed in chapter 12, "Friction and Wear of Dental Materials." Additional information on the properties and applications of dental materials can be found in Ref 1.

Dental Amalgam Alloys

Dental amalgam has been in use since the 1800s, generally with limited known detrimental effects on humans. Dental amalgam is made by mixing mercury and a powdered alloy containing silver, tin, and copper, and sometimes zinc, palladium, indium, and selenium. The amalgam has a composition close to the Ag_3Sn γ-phase (amalgam microstructures are described in chapter 11, "Tarnish and Corrosion of Dental Alloys"). The amalgamation reaction produces a solidified alloy over a short time range, allowing the dentist to manipulate the pasty amalgam in the tooth cavity. Dental amalgam is used to restore chewing surfaces and is subject to heavy forces. The aim of the amalgam is to develop an acceptable compressive strength in the restoration within several hours without compromising the manipulative ability of the amalgam. The dimensional stability of the amalgam during setup is important for its clinical application.

Long-time phase changes can occur in amalgam, which may affect performance.

When a tooth cavity is restored by using an amalgam, there is no adhesion between the amalgam and the tooth material. This can cause marginal leakage of the restoration (filling). The dimensional stability of the amalgam during setup and its ability to reproduce the convolutions of the cavity walls, along with the technique of the dentist in mixing and applying the amalgam, affect leakage. Deterioration of fillings can occur by localized or crevice corrosion in crevices, pores, and cracks or at margins.

Dental amalgam is brittle, which can lead to failure in tension or creep. Dentists avoid this by feathering edges and minimizing chances for high tensile loads. Dental amalgam creeps under load; the mercury content of the amalgam affects creep resistance.

Amalgam chemistry has changed over the years. Production of improved spherical powder shapes enhanced setup of the amalgam restoration. In addition, copper was introduced to modify the phase reaction by eliminating the so-called γ_2 phase, which is the tin-mercury phase responsible for most long-term corrosion of fillings.

Compositions. The approximate compositions of commercial amalgam alloys are listed in Table 1 along with the shape of the particles. The alloys are broadly classed as low-copper (5% or less Cu) and high-copper alloys (13 to 30% Cu). Particles are irregularly shaped, microspheres of various sizes, or a combination of the two. The low-copper alloys are either irregular or spherical. Both morphologies contain silver and tin in a ratio approximating the Ag_3Sn intermetallic compound. High-copper alloys contain either all spherical particles of the same composition (unicompositional) or a mixture of irregular and spherical particles of different or the same composition (admixed).

More than 90% of the dental amalgams currently in use are high-copper alloys (Ref 1).

Properties. As stated earlier, important properties for dental amalgam include:

- Dimensional changes during setting of the amalgam
- Compressive strength
- Creep resistance
- Corrosion resistance

These properties are influenced by the composition, microstructure, and manipulation of the amalgam. Tables 2 and 3 list some of the physical and mechanical properties of dental amalgam alloys.

Biocompatibility Issues. Controversy has existed over the use of dental amalgams for the restoration of teeth ever since the technique was introduced. Mercury is a known toxic metal with a high vapor pressure and evaporates freely. Thus, there has always been a belief that amalgam restorations could cause mercury poisoning by chronically exposing the dental personnel and patient to mercury vapor. Strict limiting values on mercury exposure have been issued by such organizations as the World Health Organization (WHO) and the Occupational Safety and Health Administration (OSHA).

Although occupational exposure to mercury is a potential hazard for dental personnel, mercury can be handled in the dental office without exceeding limiting values. There is no evidence in the published literature that the minute amounts of mercury released from amalgam restorations into oral air, saliva, or tooth structure can cause mercury poisoning to patients, except for those who have allergies to mercury (Ref 1). Although allergic reactions to mercury in amalgam do occur, such allergies are rare and the allergic responses usually disappear in a few days, or, if not, on removal of the amalgam.

Table 1 Typical composition ranges for dental amalgam alloys

Alloy	Particle shape	Content, wt%					
		Ag	Sn	Cu	Zn	In	Pd
Low copper	Irregular or spherical	63–70	26–28	2–5	0–2	0	0
High copper							
Admixed regular	Irregular	40–70	26–30	2–30	0–2	0	0
	Spherical	40–65	0–30	20–40	0–1	0	0–1
Admixed unicomposition	Irregular	52–53	17–18	29–30	0	0	0.3
	Spherical	52–53	17–18	29–30	0	0	0.3
Unicompositional	Spherical	40–60	22–30	13–30	0	0–5	0–1

Source: Ref 1

Noble Metals and Base Metals Used in Dentistry

In addition to the amalgam alloys described in the previous section, dental alloys can be placed into two broad categories: noble metals and base metals.

Noble metals are elements with a good metallic surface that retain their surface in dry air. They react easily with sulfur to form sulfides, but their resistance to oxidation, tarnish, and corrosion during heating, casting, soldering, and use in the mouth is very good. The noble metals include:

- Gold
- Platinum
- Palladium
- Iridium
- Rhodium
- Osmium
- Ruthenium

Gold, in either pure or alloyed form, is the most commonly used noble metal used for dental restorations. Gold casting alloys are typically used for crowns and bridgework and ceramic-metal restorations. Pure gold is used in wrought form for fillings or as a cast material for bridges and crowns. Some palladium-base alloys are also used for similar applications. Although many in the metallurgical field also consider silver a noble metal, it is not considered a noble metal in dentistry because it corrodes considerably in the oral cavity.

Base (nonnoble) metals and their alloys for dental restorations include:

- Cast cobalt-chromium alloys used for partial dentures and porcelain-metal restorations

Table 2 Compressive strength and creep of dental amalgams

Product	Mercury in mix, %	1 h compressive strength, MPa (ksi) at 0.5 mm/min	7 day compressive strength, MPa (ksi)		Creep, %
			0.2 mm/min	0.05 mm/min	
Low-copper alloys					
Fine-cut, Caulk 20th Century Micro Cut Spherical	53.7	45 (6.5)	302 (44)	227 (33)	6.3
Caulk Spherical	46.2	141 (20)	366 (53)	289 (42)	1.5
Kerr Spheraloy	48.5	88 (13)	380 (55)	299 (43)	1.3
Shofu Spherical	48.0	132 (19)	364 (53)	305 (44)	0.50
High-copper alloys					
Admixed, Dispersalloy	50.0	118 (17)	387 (56)	340 (49)	0.45
Unicompositional					
Sybraloy	46.0	252 (37)	455 (66)	452 (66)	0.05
Tytin	43.0	292 (42)	516 (75)	443 (64)	0.09

Source: Ref 1

Table 3 Tensile strength and dimensional change of dental amalgams

Product	Tensile strength at 0.5 mm/min, MPa (ksi)		Dimensional change, μm/cm
	15 min	7 days	
Low-copper alloys			
Fine-cut, Caulk 20th Century Micro Cut Spherical	3.2 (0.46)	51 (7.40)	–19.7
Caulk Spherical	4.7 (0.68)	55 (7.98)	–10.6
Kerr Spheraloy	3.2 (0.46)	55 (7.98)	–14.8
Shofu Spherical	4.6 (0.67)	58 (8.41)	–9.6
High-copper alloys			
Admixed, Dispersalloy	3.0 (0.44)	43 (6.24)	–1.9
Unicompositional			
Sybraloy	8.5 (1.23)	49 (7.11)	–8.8
Tytin	8.1 (1.17)	56 (8.12)	–8.1

Source: Ref 1

- Cast nickel-chromium alloys used for partial dentures, crowns and bridges, and porcelain-metal restorations
- Cast titanium and titanium alloys used for crowns and bridges, partial dentures, and implants
- Wrought titanium and titanium alloys used for implants, crowns and bridges, and orthodontic wires
- Wrought stainless steels used for dental instruments, orthodontic wires and brackets, and preformed crowns
- Wrought Co-Cr-Ni alloys used for orthodontic wires
- Wrought nickel-titanium alloys used for orthodontic wires and endodontic files

Because of the significant increases in the price of noble metals during the past three decades, alloys with considerably less noble metal content have been developed. In addition, base metal alloys have replaced noble metals systems in many applications. The metals and alloys used as substitutes for gold alloys in dental applications must have the following fundamental characteristics (Ref 1):

- The chemical nature of the alloy should not produce harmful toxicologic or allergic effects in the patient.
- The chemical properties of the appliance should provide resistance to corrosion and physical changes when in the oral environment.
- The physical and mechanical properties—such as thermal conductivity, coefficient of thermal expansion, and strength—should all be satisfactory, meeting specified minimum values and that are variable for differing applications.

- The base metals and alloys for fabrication should be plentiful, relatively inexpensive, and readily available

Noble Metal Casting Alloys

Gold-base alloys used for cast restorations (e.g., crowns and bridges) are specified by American Dental Association (ADA) specification No. 5 (1997). Before the current revision of this specification, these alloys were classified as types I (highest gold content) through IV (lowest gold content) and by their hardening mechanism. Alloys under the old system contained a noble metal content of 75 to 83%. Details of the former ADA specification and the hardening mechanisms of noble metal castings can be found in chapter 11, "Tarnish and Corrosion of Dental Alloys."

The current ADA specification also classifies alloys by composition into three broad groups:

- *High-noble* alloys with a noble metal content of ≥60 wt% and a gold content of ≥40%
- *Noble* alloys with a noble metal content of ≥25%
- *Predominantly base metal* alloys with a noble metal content of <25%

Under the current specification, all of the older alloy types are considered high-noble alloys.

As shown in Table 4, the current ADA specification also uses a type I through type IV classification in addition to the composition groups described previously. However, rather than these alloy types being based on composition, the current classification scheme is based on the amount of stress the restoration is likely to

Table 4 Applications and properties of noble alloy castings per ADA specification No. 5

Alloy type	Description	Use	Yield strength (annealed), MPa (ksi)	Elongation (annealed), %
I	Soft	Restorations subjected to low stress: some inlays	<140 (<20)	18
II	Medium	Restorations subjected to moderate stress: inlays and onlays	140–200 (20–29)	18
III	Hard	Restorations subjected to high stress: crowns, thick-veneer crowns, short-span fixed partial dentures	201–340 (29–49)	12
IV	Extra-hard	Restorations subjected to very high stress: thin-veneer crowns, long-span fixed partial dentures, removable partial dentures	>340 (>49)	10

Source: Ref 1

receive with yield strength and elongation being emphasized (refer to Table 4).

Compositions. Although there are hundreds of high-noble and noble alloys that have been developed, they can be categorized into seven classes (Table 5). There are three classes of high-noble alloys:

- Gold-silver-platinum (>70% Au + Pt)
- Gold-copper-silver-palladium-I (>70% Au)
- Gold-copper-silver-palladium-II (50 to 65% Au)

Table 5 also shows that there are four classes of noble alloys:

- Gold-copper-silver-palladium-III (40% Au)
- Gold-silver-palladium-indium (20% Au)
- Palladium-copper-gallium (77% Pd and 2% Au)
- Silver-palladium (25% Pd and 0% Au)

Properties of importance for noble metal castings include:

- Color
- Melting range
- Density
- Yield strength
- Elongation
- Hardness

Table 6 summarizes the properties of the high-noble and noble alloys.

Crown and Bridge and Partial Denture Base Metal Alloys

There are three groups of base metal casting alloys that are used for crowns and bridges and partial denture frameworks: cobalt-chromium alloys, nickel-chromium alloys, and titanium

Table 5 Typical compositions of noble dental casting alloys

Alloy type	Content, wt%						
	Ag	Au	Cu	Pd	Pt	Zn	Other
High noble							
Au-Ag-Pt	11.5	78.1	. . .	. . .	9.9	. . .	Ir (trace)
Au-Cu-Ag-Pd-*I*	10.0	76.0	10.5	2.4	0.1	1.0	Ru (trace)
Au-Cu-Ag-Pd-*II*	25.0	56.0	11.8	5.0	0.4	1.7	Ir (trace)
Noble							
Au-Cu-Ag-Pd-*III*	47.0	40.0	7.5	4.0	. . .	1.5	Ir (trace)
Au-Ag-Pd-In	38.7	20.0	. . .	21.0	. . .	3.8	In 16.5
Pd-Cu-Ga	. . .	2.0	10.0	77.0	. . .	. . .	Ga 7.0
Ag-Pd	70.0	. . .	. . .	25.0	. . .	2.0	In 3.0

Source: Ref 1

Table 6 Physical and mechanical properties of noble dental casting alloys

Alloy	Solidus, °C (°F)	Liquidus, °C (°F)	Color	Density, g/cm^3	0.2% yield strength (soft/hard), MPa (ksi)	Elongation (soft/hard), %	Vickers hardness (soft/hard), kg/mm^2
High noble							
Au-Ag-Pt	1045 (1915)	1140 (2085)	Yellow	18.4	420/470 (61/68)	15/9	175/195
Au-Cu-Ag-Pd-*I*	910 (1670)	965 (1770)	Yellow	15.6	270/400 (39/58)	30/12	135/195
Au-Cu-Ag-Pd-*II*	870 (1600)	920 (1690)	Yellow	13.8	350/600 (51/87)	30/10	175/260
Noble							
Au-Cu-Ag-Pd-*III*	865 (1590)	925 (1695)	Yellow	12.4	325/520 (47/75)	27.5/10	125/215
Au-Ag-Pd-In	875 (1605)	1035 (1895)	Light yellow	11.4	300/370 (44/54)	12/8	135/190
Pd-Cu-Ga	1100 (2010)	1190 (2175)	White	10.6	1145 (166)	8	425
Ag-Pd	1020 (1870)	1100 (2010)	White	10.6	260/320 (38/46)	10/8	140/155

Source: Ref 1

and titanium alloys. Each is briefly discussed in this section. For information relating to the effects of alloying elements on the properties and microstructures of these alloy castings, the reader is referred to chapter 11, "Tarnish and Corrosion of Dental Alloys."

Cobalt-Chromium and Nickel-Chromium Casting Alloys

The cobalt, nickel, and chromium contents in cobalt-chromium and nickel-chromium castings account for about 82 to 92% of most alloys used for dental restorations. Chromium is responsible for the tarnish and corrosion resistance of these alloys. Cobalt, and to a lesser extent nickel, increases the elastic modulus, strength, and hardness. According to ADA specification No. 14 for base metal dental castings, these materials must meet the following minimum values:

- Yield strength, 500 MPa (72.5 ksi)
- Elastic modulus, 170 GPa (25×10^6 psi)
- Elongation, 1.5%

Cobalt-chromium alloys are used extensively for partial denture frameworks. One commercially available alloy (Vitallium) for such applications has the following composition:

Element	Content, wt%
Chromium	30.0
Cobalt	bal
Molybdenum	5.0
Iron	1.0
Carbon	0.5
Silicon	0.6
Manganese	0.5

Nickel-chromium alloys are used extensively for cast crowns and bridges, although some alloys are also used for partial dentures. However, cobalt-chromium alloys far exceed any other alloy for use in this application.

The nickel-chromium alloys can be divided into two groups: beryllium-containing alloys and alloys containing no beryllium. The addition of beryllium lowers the melting temperature of nickel-chromium alloys about 100 °C (212 °F). Most of the alloys contain 60 to 80% Ni, 10 to 27% Cr, and 2 to 14% Mo. Those alloys that contain beryllium contain about 1 to 2% Be. These alloys may also contain small amounts of aluminum, carbon, cobalt, copper, cerium, gallium, iron, manganese, niobium, silicon, tin, titanium, and zirconium. One commercially available alloy (Ticonium) for crown and bridge applications has the following composition:

Element	Content, wt%
Chromium	17.0
Nickel	bal
Molybdenum	5.0
Aluminum	5.0
Iron	0.5
Carbon	0.1
Beryllium	1.0
Silicon	0.5
Manganese	5.0

Properties. Important mechanical properties for cobalt-chromium and nickel-chromium castings include yield strength, tensile strength, elongation, elastic modulus, and hardness. Table 7 summarizes these properties for two commercially available alloys. For comparison, values for type IV gold casting alloys subjected to hardening heat treatments are also provided.

Density is another important consideration for the use of base metals for crown and bridge and partial denture applications. The average density of cast base metals is between 7 and 8 g/cm³, which is about half the density of most dental gold alloys. Density is important in bulky maxillary appliances, in which the force of gravity causes the relative weight of the casting to place additional forces on the supporting teeth.

Table 7 Mechanical properties of alloys used in partial dentures

	Yield strength (0.2% offset), MPa (ksi)	Tensile strength, MPa (ksi)	Elongation, %	Elastic modulus, GPa (10^6 psi)	Vickers hardness, kg/mm²
Cast base-metal alloys(a)					
Vitallium	644 (93)	870 (126)	1.5	218 (32)	380
Ticonium	710 (103)	807 (117)	2.4	186 (27)	340
Hardened partial-denture gold alloys	480–510 (70–74)	700–760 (102–110)	5–7	90–100 (13–15)	220–250

(a) See text for composition of base metal alloys. Source: Ref 1

Cast Titanium and Titanium Alloys

Although pure titanium has been cast into crowns, partial dentures, and complete denture bases, the use of cast titanium and titanium alloy has been limited. This is due to a number of difficulties associated with cast titanium for dental purposes including its high melting point and high reactivity, low casting efficiency, inadequate expansion of investment, casting porosity, and difficulty in finishing titanium and its alloys.

Currently there are a number of binary and ternary titanium alloys being examined for crowns and partial dentures. These include Ti-13Cu-4.5Ni, Ti-6Al-4V, Ti-15V, Ti-20Cu, Ti-30Pd, and alloys in the titanium-cobalt system.

Properties. The mechanical properties of cast commercially pure titanium are similar to those of types III and IV gold alloy, whereas cast Ti-6Al-4V and Ti-15V exhibit properties, except for modulus, similar to those of nickel-chromium and cobalt-chromium alloys. Because of their coarse and heterogeneous microstructure, the properties of cast titanium can be nonuniform.

Porcelain-Fused-to-Metal Alloys

All-ceramic anterior (front teeth) restorations can appear very natural. Unfortunately, the ceramics used in these restorations are brittle and subject to fracture. Conversely, all-metal restorations are strong and tough, but from an aesthetic viewpoint are acceptable only for posterior restorations. Fortunately the aesthetic qualities of ceramic materials can be combined with the strength and toughness of metals to produce restorations that have both a natural tooth-like appearance and very good mechanical properties. As a result they are more successful as posterior restorations than all-ceramic crowns. A cross section of a ceramic-metal anterior crown is shown in Fig. 1. The cast metal coping provides a substrate on which a ceramic coating is fused. The ceramics used for these restorations are porcelains, hence the common name, porcelain-fused-to-metal (PFM) restorations.

Fabrication of PFM Restorations

As shown in Fig. 1, PFM restorations consist of a cast preoxidized metallic coping on which at least two layers of ceramic are baked. The first layer applied is the opaque layer, consisting of a ceramic rich in opacifying oxides. Its role is to mask the darkness of the oxidized metal core to achieve adequate aesthetics. As the first layer, it also provides a ceramic-metal bond (see the discussion of "Bonding Mechanism" below). The next step is the buildup of mostly translucent dentin and enamel ceramics to obtain an aesthetic appearance similar to the natural tooth. Opaque, dentin, and enamel ceramics are available in various shades. After building up the porcelain powders, the ceramic-metal crown is sintered in a porcelain furnace.

Requirements for PFM Alloys

The specific requirements for PFM alloys are (Ref 2):

- A melting range starting at no less than 1100 °C (2010 °F)

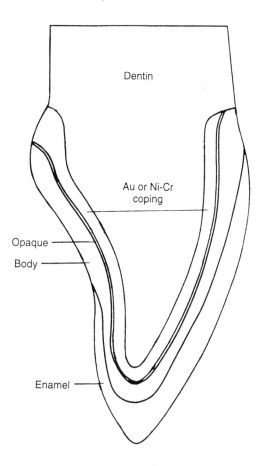

Fig. 1 Cross section of a ceramic-metal crown showing a gold alloy or base metal coping and three porcelain baked-on layers. Source: Ref 1

- A coefficient of thermal expansion closely matched to that of the low-fusing-point dental porcelains (960 to 980 °C, or 1760 to 1795 °F) developed for the PFM technique—the values for these coefficients should stay in the ranges 12.7 to $14.8 \times 10^{-6}/°C$ for the alloys and 10.8 to $14.6 \times 10^{-6}/°C$ for the porcelains
- Minimal creep or sag during firing of the porcelain
- Good wetting of the alloy by the porcelain

The wettability of the porcelain is achieved by the formation of a layer of oxides at the surface of the alloy through a preoxidation treatment. These superficial oxides are essential to the porcelain-metal bond.

Bonding Mechanism

A mechanism leading to the formation of a chemical bond between the porcelain and metal core is shown in Fig. 2. Owing to the preoxidation treatment, oxides of base metals are formed on the surface of the cast alloy. When the opaque porcelain is then fired on the oxidized metal coping, the indium, iron, and tin oxides diffuse into the vitreous phase of the porcelain. A continuous solid is formed, with chemical bonds between metals, metal oxides, and aluminosilicates of the feldspathic porcelain.

Types of PFM Alloys

Both noble and base metals and alloys are used for PFM restorations. Both types are briefly reviewed in this section. Much more detailed information on PFM systems, including the relationships among composition and microstructure, bonding characteristics, mechanical properties, and advantages and limitations of specific alloys, can be found in chapter 11, "Tarnish and Corrosion of Dental Alloys."

Noble Metal PFM Alloys. As shown in Table 8, there are five types of noble alloys for

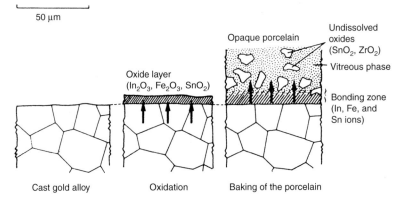

Fig. 2 Proposed mechanism of chemical bonding. The oxides of the base metals accumulated on the surface of the cast alloy during the oxidation treatment diffuse into the opaque porcelain during baking; a continuous solid is thus formed, with successive chemical bonds between metals, metal oxides, and aluminosilicates (feldspathic opaque porcelain). Source: Ref 2

Table 8   Composition ranges and colors of noble metal PFM alloys

Type	Content, wt%						Total noble metal content, %	Color
	Au	Pt	Pd	Ag	Cu	Other		
Au-Pt-Pd	84–86	4–10	5–7	0–2	. . .	Fe, In, Re, Sn 2–5	96–98	Yellow
Au-Pd	45–52	. . .	38–45	0	. . .	Ru, Re, In 8.5, Ga 1.5	89–90	White
Au-Pd-Ag	51–52	. . .	26–31	14–16	. . .	Ru, Re, In 1.5, Sn 3–7	78–83	White
Pd-Ag	. . .	. . .	53–88	30–37	. . .	Ru, In 1–5, Sn 4–8	49–62	White
Pd-Cu	0–2	. . .	74–79	. . .	10–15	In, Ga 9	76–81	White

Source: Ref 1

PFM restorations. In chronological order, they are:

- Gold-platinum-palladium (Au-Pt-Pd) alloys
- Gold-palladium-silver (Au-Pd-Ag) alloys
- Palladium-silver (Pd-Ag) alloys
- Gold-palladium (Au-Pd) alloys
- Palladium-copper (Pd-Cu) alloys

These alloys have noble metal contents ranging from about 50% to nearly 100%. The properties of noble metal PFM alloys are listed in Table 9.

Base Metal PFM Alloys. The range of compositions of base metal alloys for ceramic-metal restorations are given for nickel-chromium, cobalt-chromium, and titanium types in Table 10. Typical properties of these alloys are listed in Table 11. Considerable variations in compositions and properties are shown in these tables.

Comparison of PFM Alloy Characteristics. The noble alloys have good corrosion resistance, but only the Au-Pt-Pd alloys have a desirable yellow color. The other types are white

Table 9   Properties and casting temperatures for noble metal PFM alloys

Type	Ultimate tensile strength, MPa (ksi)	0.2% yield strength, MPa (ksi)	Elastic modulus, GPa (10^6 psi)	Elongation, %
Au-Pt-Pd	480–500 (70–73)	400–420 (58–61)	81–96 (11.7–13.9)	3–10
Au-Pd	700–730 (102–106)	550–575 (80–83)	100–117 (14.5–17.0)	8–16
Au-Pd-Ag	650–680 (94–99)	475–525 (69–76)	100–113 (14.5–16.4)	8–18
Pd-Ag	550–730 (80–106)	400–525 (58–76)	95–117 (13.8–17.0)	10–14
Pd-Cu	690–1300 (100–189)	550–1100 (80–160)	94–97 (13.6–14.1)	8–15

Type	Vickers hardness, kg/mm^2	Density, g/cm^3	Casting temperature, °C (°F)
Au-Pt-Pd	175–180	17.4–18.6	1150 (2100)
Au-Pd	210–230	13.5–13.7	1320–1330 (2410–2425)
Au-Pd-Ag	210–230	13.6–13.8	1320–1350 (2410–2460)
Pd-Ag	185–235	10.7–11.1	1310–1350 (2390–2460)
Pd-Cu	350–400	10.6–10.7	1170–1190 (2140–2175)

Source: Ref 1

Table 10   Composition ranges for base metal PFM alloys

Type	Ni	Cr	Co	Ti	Mo	Al	V	Fe	Be	Ga	Mn	Nb	W	B	Ru
											Content, wt%				
Ni-Cr	69–77	11–20	...	...	4–14	0–4	...	0–1	0–2	0–2	0–1	...	...	0–3	...
Co-Cr	...	15–25	55–58	...	0–4	0–2	...	0–1	...	0–7	...	0–3	0–5	0–1	0–6
Ti	...	...	...	90–100	...	0–6	0–4	0–0.3	...	...	...	...	...	...	...

Source: Ref 1

Table 11   Properties of base metal alloys for PFM restorations

Type	Ultimate tensile strength, MPa (ksi)	0.2% yield strength, MPa (ksi)	Elastic modulus, GPa (10^6 psi)	Elongation, %	Vickers hardness, kg/mm^2	Density, g/cm^3	Casting temperature, °C (°F)
Ni-Cr	400–1000 (58–145)	255–730 (37–106)	150–210 (22–30)	8–20	210–380	7.5–7.7	1300–1450 (2370–2640)
Co-Cr	520–820 (75–119)	460–640 (67–93)	145–220 (21–32)	6–15	330–465	7.5–7.6	1350–1450 (2460–2640)
Titanium	240–890 (35–129)	170–830 (25–120)	103–114 (15–17)	10–20	125–350	4.4–4.5	1760–1860 (3200–3380)

Source: Ref 1

(gray), which is more difficult to mask with the ceramic. The Au-Pd, Au-Pd-Ag, and Pd-Ag types have excellent mechanical properties coupled with high fusion temperatures and ease of casting and soldering. However, the palladium-silver type has caused some problems with discoloration of the ceramic. The palladium-copper types are characterized by the formation of dark oxides, which may cause problems with masking by the ceramic. The nickel-chromium and cobalt-chromium types are noted for high hardness and elastic modulus, although some nickel-chromium alloys have lower yield strengths (Table 11). They are also noted for high casting temperatures. In general, the titanium types have lower mechanical properties than the other base metal alloys, but notably lower density and higher casting temperatures. Good bonding of ceramic and alloy can be achieved with all alloys, but bonding with some base metal alloys is more technique sensitive.

Wrought Alloys for Orthodontic Wires

Orthodontic wires function to deliver force to misaligned teeth in order to change their configuration to approximate an ideal dental arch. This change is mediated by physiological remodeling of the supporting bones of the upper and lower jaws.

The capability of maintaining remodeling activity is a function of the ratio of yield strength to elastic modulus. The term "springback," meaning maximum elastic deflection, is used to define this property. Materials for orthodontic wires must have a low elastic modulus and high yield strength. Alloy ductility must be sufficient to allow the fabrication of complex low-radius bends. Since orthodontic appliances must function for long periods in the oral environment, the material must have good corrosion resistance.

There are four groups of alloys that currently meet the aforementioned requirements:

- Austenitic stainless steels
- Cobalt-base alloys
- Nickel-titanium shape memory alloys
- β-titanium alloy

These are all wrought alloys; that is, they are cast alloys that have been cold worked and formed by mechanical processes such as rolling, extrusion, and drawing. These processes estab-

lish the internal structure of the alloy as well as it mechanical properties.

It should be noted that wrought gold alloys were once widely used. However, their high cost and volatile market conditions have largely precluded the use of gold alloys. There is no longer an active ADA specification for wrought dental gold wire (formerly, ADA specification No. 7 covered these materials).

Stainless Steels. Austenitic stainless steels with a relatively low carbon content (<0.15% wt%) containing 18% Cr and 8% Ni are the most widely used alloys for orthodontic wires. Types 302 and 304 are widely used. In the annealed condition, these wires have a minimum yield strength of 205 MPa (30 ksi). Cold-worked 18-8 wires have yield strengths as high as 1380 MPa (200 ksi) and an elastic modulus of 190 GPa (28×10^6 psi). Stress-relief treatments improve the properties of austenitic stainless steels.

Cobalt-Base Alloys. Elgiloy, a Co-Cr-Ni alloy originally developed for the watch industry as a main spring, is widely used as an orthodontic alloy. The composition limits for Elgiloy are:

Element	Content, wt%
Cobalt	39.0–41.0
Chromium	19.0–21.0
Nickel	14.0–16.0
Molybdenum	6.0–8.0
Manganese	1.5–2.5
Carbon	0.15 max
Beryllium	0.10 max
Iron	Bal

Elgiloy has a yield strength of 690 MPa (100 ksi) in the non-cold-worked condition. Depending on the amount of cold reduction, yield strengths can range from 1240 MPa (180 ksi) to as high as 2240 MPa (325 ksi). The room-temperature elastic modulus is 190 GPa (28×10^6 psi). Because of its ductility, Elgiloy is also easily deformed and shaped.

Nickel-Titanium Alloys. A wrought nickel-titanium alloy known as Nitinol was introduced as a wire for orthodontic applications in 1972. The industrial alloy contains 55 wt% Ni and 45% Ti. The orthodontic alloy contains several percent of cobalt. A number of variations of nickel-titanium alloys have been developed in dentistry.

Nitinol is corrosion resistant and possesses a unique shape-memory property whereby plastically deformed wire can be returned to their original shape by an appropriate heat treatment. Nitinol has an elastic modulus of ~40 GPa (~6 × 10^6 psi) and a yield strength that ranges from 70 to 560 MPa (10 to 80 ksi) depending on the crystallographic orientation of the alloy (i.e., martensite or austenite).

β-Titanium Alloy. The first applications of β-titanium alloy (also known as Beta III in industry) were in the late 1970s. The composition of this alloy for dental use is 78Ti-11.5Mo-6Zr-4.5Sn. β-titanium has a yield strength of ~620 MPa (~90 ksi) and an elastic modulus that ranges from 70 GPa (10 × 10^6 psi) to as high as 110 GPa (16 × 10^6 psi) depending on the pro-

cessing conditions. This alloy exhibits good ductility, weldability, and corrosion resistance.

Alloys for Dental Implants

Implant Design. Dental implants are intended to support various dental appliances in the mouth. Dental implant designs can be separated into two categories called endosteal (endosseous), which enter the bone tissue, or subperiosteal systems, which contact the exterior bone surfaces. These are shown in Fig. 3 and 4. The endosteal implant designs, such as

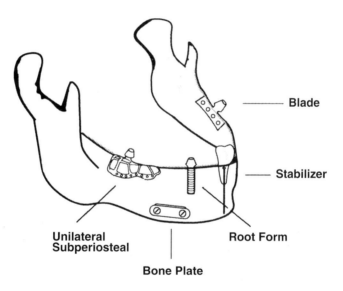

Fig. 3 Different dental implant designs. Source: Ref 3

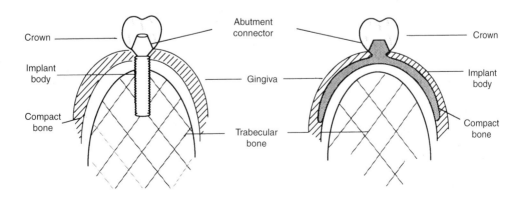

Fig. 4 Interfacial regions of dental implant systems. Idealized cross sections through mandibular bone. Source: Ref 3

root forms (cylinders, screws, wires, etc.), blades (plates) as shown in Fig. 5, and staples are placed into the bone as shown. In contrast, the subperiosteal devices are fitted to the bone surface as customized shapes while bone plates are placed onto the bone under the periosteum and fixed with endosteal screws.

Material Selection. Synthetic materials for dental implants include metals and alloys, ceramics, carbon and carbon-base materials, and various polymers. The nonmetallic materials are discussed later in this chapter. Metallic materials that have been used for implants include:

- Commercially pure titanium and Ti-6Al-4V
- Zirconium and tantalum (99% purity)
- Co-27Cr-5Mo
- 18Cr-14Ni austenitic stainless steel
- Gold
- Platinum-iridium alloys

Of these materials, commercially pure titanium is the most widely used implant alloy, particularly for endosteal designs (Co-Cr-Mo alloys are used for subperiosteal designs). Titanium dental implants have remarkably good integration with the bony structure of the jaw.

Coatings. Calcium phosphate ceramic, glass ceramics, porous layers added to metals, and other biomaterial surface modifications have been introduced and developed to enhance bone adaptation to endosteal and subperiosteal implant surfaces (see chapter 9, "Coatings," for further details). In terms of porous metal coatings, both powder and wire porous coatings sintered to metallic substrates have been used to enhance bonding between the device and the bone. Examples of Co-Cr-Mo and titanium wire-coated implants are shown in Fig. 6.

Soldering Alloys

It is often necessary to construct a dental appliance in two or more parts and then join them together by either a soldering or brazing technique (soldering is the preferred term used in dentistry for joining operations). Two types of solder alloys are used in dentistry. Gold-base solders have good tarnish and corrosion resistance and are used extensively in crown and bridge applications. Silver-base solders are commonly used in orthodontic appliances. Additional information on the applications, microstructures, and corrosion resistance of gold and silver solders can be found in chapter 11, "Tarnish and Corrosion of Dental Alloys."

Gold-base solders for dental use are primarily alloys of gold, silver, and copper, with small quantities of tin, zinc, and sometimes phospho-

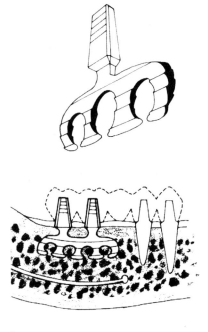

Fig. 5 Uncoated dental implants (blade design)

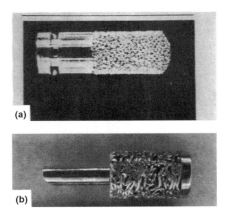

Fig. 6 Typical dental implants. (a) Cobalt-chromium-molybdenum powder coated dental implant. (b) Titanium wire-coated dental implant

rus included to modify the fusion temperature and flow qualities. The typical composition and resulting fusion temperature values of various gold-base solders are given in Table 12. Mechanical properties of three of the solders listed in Table 12 are given in Table 13.

Silver-base solders are used when a low-fusion point solder is needed for soldering onto stainless steel or other base metal alloys. Silver solders are basically Ag-Cu-Zn alloys to which small amounts of cadmium, tin, or phosphorus are added to modify the fusion temperature. The liquidus temperature for these solders range from 620 to 700 °C (1150 to 1290 °F), which is slightly below those of the gold alloys listed in Table 12.

Alloys for Dental Instruments

Important considerations for materials for dental instruments are their corrosion resistance, machinability, edge retention, and formability. Many dental instruments are fabricated from various types of stainless steels. Nickel-titanium alloys are being used increasingly for endodontic instruments.

Stainless Steels

Martensitic Grades. Most of the stainless steels used for dental instruments are of the harder and stronger martensitic types. Generally, these heat treatable stainless steels contain a higher carbon content than do the austenitic grades discussed earlier in this chapter, and most contain little or no nickel. Chromium content is in the range of 10.5 to 18%, and carbon content can exceed 1.2%. The chromium and carbon contents are balanced to ensure a martensitic structure. Examples of martensitic stainless steels used for dental applications include:

- Type 416 is a free-machining grade (increased phosphorus and sulfur for improved machinability) that has good nongalling and nonseizing characteristics.
- Type 420 contains a higher carbon content (0.15% C min) than does type 416 for extra strength and hardness.
- Type 431 contains higher chromium (16% Cr), and nickel is added for increased corrosion resistance.
- Type 440A contains 0.60 to 0.75% C and can achieve hardness levels as high as 56 HRC.

Table 12   Typical compositions and fusion temperatures for gold-base dental solders

Solder	Fineness(a)	Au	Ag	Cu	Sn	Zn	Fusion temperature, °C (°F)
		\multicolumn{5}{c}{Composition, wt%}	
1	0.809	80.9	8.1	6.8	2.0	2.1	868 (1594)
2	0.800	80.0	3–8	8–12	2–3	2–4	746–871 (1375–1600)
3	0.729	72.9	12.1	10.0	2.0	2.3	835 (1535)
4	0.650	65.0	16.3	13.1	1.7	3.9	799 (1470)
5	0.600	60.0	12–32	12–22	2–3	2–4	724–835 (1335–1535)
6	0.450	45.0	30–35	15–20	2–3	2–4	691–816 (1276–1501)

(a) Fineness is the gold content in weight percent related to a proportional number of units contained in 1000. Source: Ref 1

Table 13   Mechanical properties for three of the solder compositions listed in Table 12

Solder	Fineness(a)	Tensile strength (soft/hard), MPa (ksi)	Proportional limit (soft/hard), MPa (ksi)	Elongation (soft/hard), %	Brinell hardness (soft/hard), kg/mm^2
1	0.809	259 (38)	142 (21)	18	78
3	0.729	248/483 (36/70)	166/424 (24/61)	7/<1	103/180
4	0.650	303/634 (44/92)	207/532 (30/77)	9/<1	111/199

(a) Fineness is the gold content in weight percent related to a proportional number of units contained in 1000. Source: Ref 1

- Trimrite stainless steel was specifically designed to provide the attributes needed for cutting and scraping. It has better corrosion resistance than types 420 and 440A, improved resistance to tempering during edge sharpening, superior cold formability, and improved ductility and toughness to 50 HRC.

Age-hardenable martensitic stainless steels are also used for dental instruments. Two examples are Custom 450 and 455, which contain low carbon contents (0.05% C), 11 to 16% Cr, 5 to 9.5% Ni, and age-hardening additions such as niobium and copper. These steels have corrosion resistance similar to type 304 stainless steel, but they can develop higher strength, with good ductility and toughness, by means of a simple heat treatment, as opposed to cold working.

Austenitic grades fabricated into dental instruments include type 304 stainless steel and a proprietary grade referred to as Gall-Tough, which contains 15 to 18% Cr, 4 to 6% Ni, and 4 to 6% Mn. Compared to the conventional type 304, Gall-Tough possesses superior self-mated galling and metal-to-metal wear resistance.

Alloys for Endodontic Instruments

The term "endodontic" literally means "within the tooth." Examples of common endodontic instruments are handheld or motor-driven root canal files and reamers. Root canals are rarely straight. Therefore, endodontic files need to be able to follow a curved path. As such, bending and torsional properties of files are important.

Material Selection. Endodontic instruments have long been fabricated from 18-8 austenitic stainless steels. Files and reamers are made by machining a stainless steel wire into a pyramidal blank, and then twisting the blank to form a spiral edge.

In recent years, nickel-titanium alloys have been used increasingly for these applications. The alloys used in root canal instruments contains about 56% Ni and 44% Ti. In some instances, <2% of cobalt may be substituted for nickel. The superelasticity of nickel-titanium permits deformation of 8% strain in endodontic files with complete recovery. This value compares with <1% for stainless steels. Drawbacks associated with nickel-titanium endodontic instruments includes their susceptibility to fatigue failure and difficulties in their fabrication; that is, because of their superelasticity,

they must be made by machining rather than by twisting of tapered wire blanks.

Ceramics

The ceramic materials described in this section fall into two broad categories: implant materials and dental porcelains that have the general composition of vitrified feldspar along with additions of metallic oxide pigments that simulate natural tooth enamel shades. Dental porcelains can be classified according to their fusion temperature, application, fabrication technique, or crystalline phase (Table 14). The high-fusing ceramics have a fusing range from 1315 to 1370 °C (2400 to 2500 °F); the medium-fusing ceramics, from 1090 to 1260 °C (1995 to 2300 °F); and the low-fusing ceramics, from 870 to 1065 °C (1600 to 1950 °F).

Ceramics for Dental Implants (Ref 4)

Fully Dense Ceramics. Although considerable use has been made of titanium in endosseous implants, there has been an increasing amount of interest shown in nonmetallic systems, and especially the alumina ceramics. The material used is usually a high-purity fine-grained alumina (Al_2O_3).

The implants may be shaped as tapered cylinders, with a series of circumferential stops providing the taper. This design is aimed at achieving optimal load transfer to the implant. The coronal end of the implant contains a polished circular groove, into which the gingival tissue will be adapted; the anticipated contrac-

Table 14 Classification of dental ceramics for fixed restorations and denture teeth

Type	Fabrication	Crystalline phase/amount present(a)
All-ceramic	Machined	Alumina (Al_2O_3)/NR
		Feldspar ($KAlSi_3O_8$)/NR
		Mica ($KMg_{2.5}Si_4O_{10}F_2$)/50–70%
	Slip cast	Alumina (Al_2O_3)/>90%
		Spinel ($MgAl_2O_4$)/NR
	Heat pressed	Leucite ($KAlSi_2O_6$)/35–55%
		Lithium disilicate ($Li_2Si_2O_5$)/60%
	Sintered	Alumina (Al_2O_3)/40–50 wt%
		Leucite ($KAlSi_2O_6$)/45 vol%
Ceramic-metal	Sintered	Leucite ($KAlSi_2O_6$)/10–20%
Denture teeth	Manufactured	Feldspar

(a) Amount present is usually given as the volume percentage. NR, not reported.
Source: Ref 1

tion of the circumferential fibers provides a seal between the surface tissue (the epithelium) and the alumina. The external surfaces of the stepped cylinder are polished, but contain regularly spaced circular recesses of approximately 900 μm diameter, which are described as lucunae and allow some ingrowth of bone. A longitudinal groove also gives stability against rotation after bone ingrowth.

Other ceramic materials that have been used for dental implants include zirconia, carbons (99.9% C and C-15Si), and bioinert glasses (see the discussion of "Glass Implant Materials" in this chapter). Alumina, however, is used far more than these other materials.

Coatings. Hydroxyapatite, a relatively nonresorbable form of calcium phosphate, has been used with some success as a coating material for titanium implants and as a ridge augmentation material. Studies indicate that the hydroxyapatite increases the rate of bony ingrowth toward the implant. However, the long-term corrosion of these coatings and the stability of the bond of the coating to the substrate are still being studied.

Denture-Teeth Porcelains

Porcelain denture teeth are commercially manufactured, not fabricated by a dental technician. They are reacted and vitrified in metal molds to form the shape of the denture teeth. The compositions and properties of these dental porcelains set them apart from dental ceramics for fixed restorations.

Denture-teeth raw materials are based on feldspar with additions of around 15% quartz, 4% kaolin, and the pigment oxides. The kaolin improves the molding qualities of the mixture. This general composition in relation to other triaxial whiteware bodies is shown in Fig. 7. The product of the fusion is self-glazing and nonporous. Since the 1950s, denture teeth have been fired under vacuum to further reduce the porosity. Denture teeth are used in full dentures that replace all of the teeth of the upper or lower arch. Porcelain denture teeth show a natural translucency that simulates that of natural teeth; in fact, the main aesthetic problem of denture teeth is that they have the appearance of perfect teeth without the minor defects and nonalignment of natural teeth. This is a problem that some dentists attempt to solve by staining of the denture teeth and even simulating artificial restoration in some of the teeth. The main mechanical prob-

lems with porcelain denture teeth are their brittleness and the clicking sound they make during biting. Acrylic resin teeth have been gradually replacing porcelain denture teeth, as they are tougher and do not produce the clicking sound. Also, the acrylic denture teeth can be chemically bonded to an acrylic denture base, eliminating the gap between porcelain denture teeth and an acrylic denture base. Although acrylic denture teeth have aesthetics equal to that of porcelain teeth, they have lower long-term wear and stain resistance.

Ceramics for PFM Restorations

As discussed in the section "Fabrication of PFM Restorations," ceramic-metal restorations consist of a metallic coping on which at least two layers of ceramic are baked (see Fig. 1). The ceramics used for PFM restorations must fulfill the following five requirements (Ref 1):

- They must simulate the appearance of natural teeth.
- They must fuse at relatively low temperature.
- They must have thermal expansion coefficients compatible with the metals used for ceramic-metal bonding (most porcelains have coefficients of thermal expansion between 13.0 and 14.0 × 10^{-6}/°C and metals between 13.5 and 14.5 × 10^{-6}/°C).
- They must withstand the oral environment.
- They must not excessively abrade opposing teeth.

Ceramics for PFM restorations must be carefully formulated to meet these requirements. These ceramics are composed of crystalline

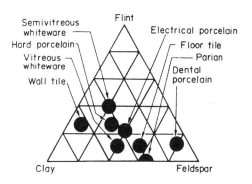

Fig. 7 Dental porcelain raw-material composition in relation to other triaxial materials. Source: Ref 5

phases in an amorphous and glassy (vitreous) matrix. They comprise primarily SiO_2, Al_2O_3, Na_2O, and K_2O (Table 15). Opacifiers (TiO_2, ZrO_2, SnO_2) and various heat-stable pigments are also added to the ceramic. Because of their composition, they can be considered a type of glass. To match the appearance of tooth structures, small amounts of fluorescing pigments such as rare earth oxides (CeO_2) are added. The nature of ceramics, with their glassy matrix and crystalline phases, produces a translucency much like that of teeth, whereas pigments and opacifiers control the color and translucency of the restoration. The ceramic is supplied as a fine powder.

In developing ceramics for ceramic-metal bonding, a major breakthrough was formulating products that had sufficiently high thermal expansion coefficients to match those of dental alloys. This higher expansion was made possible by the addition of potassium oxide and the formation of a high-expansion crystalline phase

called leucite ($KAlSi_2O_6$). This phase increased the thermal expansion of the porcelain so it could match that of dental alloys. Sodium and potassium oxides in the glassy matrix are responsible for lowering the fusing temperatures to the range of 930 to 980 °C (1705 to 1795 °F). The ceramics used to bond to metals have tensile strengths of 35 MPa (5 ksi), compressive strengths of 860 MPa (125 ksi), shear strengths of 120 MPa (17 ksi), and flexural strengths of 60 MPa (9 ksi).

All-Ceramic Restorations

All-ceramic crowns, inlays, onlays, and veneers are used when aesthetics is a priority. Materials for all-ceramic restorations use a wide variety of crystalline phases as reinforcing agents and contain up to 90 vol% of the crystalline phase. The nature, amount, and particle size of the crystalline phase directly influences the properties of the material. As summarized in Table 14, these materials are fabricated by sintering, heat pressing (also referred to as high-temperature injection molding), slip casting, and machining. The flexural strengths of various dental ceramics are compared in Table 16.

Glass-Ceramic Prosthetics Formed by a Casting Process

The lost-wax method of casting glass objects of art was developed in the 1930s by Frederick Carder of the Steuben Division of Corning Glass Works. The transition from weaker glass to stronger castable ceramics occurred in 1957 with the development of glass-ceramics by S.D. Stookey of Corning Glass Works. This group of materials employs a nucleating agent to initiate the controlled growth of crystals within the amorphous glass matrix. The properties of glass-ceramics are affected by the type of crystals formed and the amount of growth within the glass matrix. The microstructures produced are nonporous, and the grain size ranges from several hundred angstroms to a few microns.

Compared with the conventional porcelains used for all-ceramic dental restorations, castable ceramic systems offer great promise for dental applications because of their ease of fabrication, low processing shrinkage, high strength, translucency control, insensitivity to abrasion damage, thermal shock resistance, chemical durability, and polishability. McMillan (Ref 6) reported

Table 15   Composition ranges of dental porcelains for ceramic-metal restorations

Component	Opaque powder, %	Dentin (body) powder, %
SiO_2	50–59	57–62
Al_2O_3	9–15	11–16
Na_2O	5–7	4–9
K_2O	9–11	10–14
TiO_2	0–3	0–0.6
ZnO_2	0–5	0.1–1.5
SnO_2	5–15	0–0.5
Rb_2O	0–0.1	0–0.1
CeO_2	. . .	0–3
Pigments	. . .	Trace

Source: Ref 1

Table 16   Flexural strengths of various dental ceramics

Processing technique	Crystalline phase	Flexural strength, MPa (ksi)
Sintered ceramic-metal	Leucite	60–70 (9–10)
Sintered all-ceramic	Leucite	104 (15)
	Alumina	139 (20)
Heat pressed all-ceramic	Leucite	121 (17.5)
	Lithium disilicate	350 (51)
Slip-cast all-ceramic	Alumina	446 (65)
	Spinel-alumina	378 (55)
	Zirconia-alumina	604 (88)
Machinable all-ceramic	Fluormica	229 (33)
	Feldspar	122 (18)

Source: Ref 1

that of all glass-ceramics available, the greatest flexure strength has been achieved with Li_2O-SiO_2 materials nucleated with P_2O_5. Several other glass-ceramics have been introduced for dental applications that must be externally colored with shading porcelain to achieve acceptable aesthetics.

Compositions and Properties

The potential for using glass-ceramics for dental applications was first recognized by MacCulloch (Ref 7). Because of the excessive shrinkage, loss of contour, and porosity that occurred during processing of aluminous porcelain, he attempted to fabricate denture teeth from a Li_2O-ZnO-SiO_2 system.

The first demonstrated use of a castable glass-ceramic system for the fabrication of dental inlays, onlays, crowns, dentures, and veneers was reported by Hench et al. in 1971 (Ref 8). This system was based on a composition of 20 wt% Li_2O and 80% SiO_2. Although a nucleating agent was not used for this system, lithium ions are believed to induce phase separation in this system (Ref 9). Its diametral tensile strength is 124 MPa (18 ksi), which is approximately twice that of conventional feldspathic porcelain (61 MPa, or 8.85 ksi). The crystalline phase formed in this system was lithium disilicate (Li_2O·$2SiO_2$). Coloring elements and oxides were also added to a frit of the parent glass, and the mixture was melted, cast, and annealed. The resulting glass-ceramic produced a range of colors that could be varied further with control of the time of ceramming. One of the main problems with this system was the presence of microcracks around the crystals, which presumably formed because of a large volume change during crystallization.

Abe and Fukui (Ref 10) reported the use of a CaO-P_2O_5 glass-ceramic system for use in the production of dental crowns with the use of the lost-wax technique. Small concentrations of Al_2O_3 (1.5 wt%) were added to CaO to achieve an atomic percent ratio of 0.5 to 1.7. The frits were melted at 1300 °C (2370 °F) for 1 h and after reheating to 635 °C (1175 °F), the glass was transformed to the glass-ceramic. A molar ratio, CaO/P_2O_5, of 55/45 (1.22) was found to produce the most favorable results. The strength of this material is reported as 117 MPa (17 ksi) compared with 61 MPa (8.85 ksi) for feldspathic dental porcelain. Linear shrinkage resulting from conversion of glass to glass-ceramic

was less than 1%. The hardness (370 to 380 HV) and expansion coefficient (11.3×10^{-6}/°C) of this glass-ceramic are similar to those of tooth structure. Coloration is produced by an external layer of shading porcelain.

Improvements in the castability, chemical durability, and resistance to microcracks of the lithia-silica glass-ceramics were reported by Barrett (Ref 11) and Barrett, Clark, and Hench (Ref 12) for lithium-silicate glass-ceramics through the addition of CaO in amounts of 1.0 to 11.0 wt% and Al_2O_3 from 1.0 to 10.0 wt% to a glass frit containing 25 to 33 mole% Li_2O and 53 to 73.5 mole% SiO_2. It was claimed that these additions substantially improved both the castability of the glass and the chemical durability of the glass-ceramic. Mechanical properties were further improved by combining platinum metal and Nb_2O_5 as nucleating agents. Through the use of these nucleating agents, the crystallization process for these lithia-alumina-calcia-silica (LACS) glass-ceramics resulted in a fine-grained crystal phase uniformly dispersed within a vitreous matrix. Flexural strengths of 214 MPa (31 ksi), which are 31 to 42% higher than the corresponding values reported for Dicor glass-ceramic (discussed below), indicate that the LACS glass-ceramic may be more resistant to posterior failures when used for crowns and onlays. After exposure to a test bath of H_2O at 100 °C (212 °F) over a period of 6 h, these compositions released 17.2 to 22.0 ppm Li^+ for 0.01 wt% Pt and crystallization times of 0.5 h and 4.0 h, respectively, compared with 169 ppm Li^+ for the original Li_2O-SiO_2 glass-ceramic.

Additional improvements in properties of LACS glass-ceramics were claimed in the patent of Wu, Cannon, and Panzera (Ref 13). They used P_2O_5 as a nucleating agent, which was found to produce greater flexure strengths (275 to 360 MPa, or 40 to 52 ksi) and higher softening temperatures.

Kihara et al. (Ref 14) introduced a castable calcium phosphate glass-ceramic composed of 30.1 wt% CaO, 68.4 wt% P_2O_5, and 1.5 wt% Al_2O_3. The glass can be melted and cast into cristobalite investment preheated to 600 °C (1110 °F). Thermal processing at 645 °C (1195 °F) for 12 h is required for crystal growth, and this heat treatment yields a glass-ceramic with a hardness of 380 HV and a flexure strength (modulus of rupture) of 116 MPa (16.8 ksi). Thus, this material appears to be too weak for crown and bridge applications, especially in posterior sites.

Hobo and Iwata (Ref 15–17) and Hobo (Ref 18) have reported the development of a castable apatite ceramic, CeraPearl, which is composed of 45 wt% CaO, 15% P_2O_5, 5% MgO, and 34% SiO_2. This material is melted at 1460 °C (2660 °F), heated to 750 °C (1380 °F) for 15 min, and crystallized at 870 °C (1600 °F) for 1 h to form $Ca_{10}(PO_4)_6O$. This structure is unstable and reacts with H_2O to form hydroxyapatite, $Ca_{10}(PO_4)_6(OH)_2$. The tensile strength of Cera-Pearl (150 MPa, or 21.8 ksi) is more than twice the diametral tensile strength of feldspathic porcelain. It has an elastic modulus of 103 GPa (15×10^6 psi), a Knoop hardness of 350, a compressive strength of 590 MPa (85.5 ksi), and an expansion coefficient of 11.0 ppm/°C. Cera-Pearl crowns are colored externally by applying stains formulated from $K_2O\text{-}Al_2O_3\text{-}B_2O_3\text{-}SiO_2$ with traces of various metal oxides. The stains are fired at 790 °C (1455 °F). As is true for most other ceramics and glass-ceramics, crowns of hydroxyapatite can be mechanically and chemically treated to promote adhesion of the interior surface of the crown to glass ionomer cements.

The use of a machinable glass-ceramic that can be melted and cast into the form of dental inlays, onlays, and crowns was introduced by Adair (Ref 19) and Grossman (Ref 9). This glass-ceramic system is based on the growth of fluorine-containing, tetra-silicic mica crystals which was first reported in a patent by Grossman in 1973. Compositions enriched in K_2O and SiO_2 can be melted from 1350 to 1400 °C (2460 to 2550 °F) and subsequently be cerammed to yield a tetra-silicic fluormica glass-ceramic ($K_2O\text{-}MgF_2\text{-}MgO\text{-}SiO_2$). Addition of ZrO_2, in amounts up to 7 wt%, is believed to improve chemical durability and enhance translucency. Glass-ceramics are formed by a fine-scale phase separation that occurs at 625 °C (1160 °F), followed by crystallization of spherical mica grains approximately 400 μm in diameter (Ref 20). Heating to 940 °C (1725 °F) causes recrystallization into block-shaped crystals. The mica platelets grow by a dissolution and reprecipitation mechanism at 1075 °C (1970 °F). A holding time of 6 h is considered optimum for strength and other desirable properties. Like all other castable glass-ceramics, this product, which is marketed under the commercial name Dicor, must be stained on the external surface with shading porcelain to achieve acceptable aesthetics. If too thin a layer is applied, the entire colorant layer may be lost during routine dental prophylaxis because of the abrasiveness of the prophy paste. In addition, the daily use of acidulated fluoride gels may cause the dissolution of the shading porcelain. This situation would require costly remakes, loss of wages, and additional trauma to the patient. One of the uses of Dicor or other machinable glass-ceramics (see Table 14) is as a material to be used for the production of machined inlays, onlays, and crowns by means of computer-aided design and manufacturing (CAD-CAM) systems.

Glass Implant Materials

For many years it was considered that the normal interfacial tissue response to implant materials was the formation of a fibrous capsule. This viewpoint came into question in the early 1970s with the discovery that a certain compositional range of calcium phosphate silicate-based glasses did not produce a fibrous capsule when implanted in bone, but instead produced a strongly adherent bonded interface, where the strength of the interface was equal to or exceeded that of the bone with which it was bonded. These glasses contain SiO_2, Na_2O, CaO, and P_2O_5 in specific proportions. Three key compositional features distinguish these glasses from traditional soda-lime-silica glasses that do not bond to tissues containing: less than 60 mol% of SiO_2, high Na_2O and CaO content (up to 30 mol%), and a high Ca/P_2O_5 ratio. These features make the surface highly reactive when exposed to an aqueous medium and result in rapid formation of hydroxycarbonate apatite on the surface. The tradename Bioglass was coined to describe this compositional range of bioactive glasses. Subsequently the term "bioactive" has been used to describe implant materials that form a bond with living tissues. Other examples of bioactive-glass containing systems include:

- The $SiO_2\text{-}CaO\text{-}MgO\text{-}P_2O_5$ system, which contains apatite and wollastonite as crystalline phases and are referred to as AW glass-ceramics (Ref 21)
- The machinable glass-ceramics based on the $Na_2O/K_2O\text{-}MgO\text{-}Al_2O_5\text{-}SiO_2\text{-}F$ system containing phlogopite and apatite crystals (Ref 22)
- The $Na_2O\text{-}CaO\text{-}P_2O_5\text{-}B_2O_3\text{-}Al_2O_5\text{-}SiO_2$ system (Ref 23)

An example of a bioactive glass product is based on a Bioglass composition 45 wt% SiO_2, 24.5 wt% CaO, 24.5 wt% Na_2O, 6 wt% P_2O_5.

The product is called an ERMI (endosseous ridge maintenance implant). These implants, which are solid glass cones of various sizes, are designed to be placed into tooth sockets immediately after extraction of teeth. Their purpose is to maintain the bone level and contours, which under normal circumstances resorb after tooth extraction. The ERMIs are totally buried and not subjected to direct occlusal loading. They are indicated for patients scheduled to receive complete dentures after the loss of all their teeth as well as for individuals who have lost one or more teeth and will be restored with fixed bridge-work or removable partial dentures.

Composite Dental Materials

Resin-composites have been used to repair and rebuild teeth at an ever-expanding rate since their introduction to dentistry in the early 1960s based on the original patent by Bowen (Ref 24). These materials consist of an organic polymer matrix, an inorganic filler phase, and a coupling agent that serves as a filler-matrix binder. Typically, a composite resin is available as either a paste-paste system (which when mixed, undergoes a chemically activated polymerization) or as a single-paste system (in which polymerization is activated by either an ultraviolet or visible light source). Most dentists prefer the light-activated systems as they provide more working time. To ensure longevity, several important requirements should be met. To rebuild or replace tooth structure, a restoration must have sufficient resistance to material loss whether from stresses generated by loading, wear, or other factors. Ideally, the margin or interface between the tooth and the restorative material should be sealed to prevent microleakage and the resultant caries that will occur. The restoration should be aesthetically acceptable to the patient. From the perspective of the dentist, the material should be easy to manipulate and insensitive to technique. Finally, the material must be compatible with biological tissues. Because this article describes materials already in use, biocompatibility is not stressed. However, in the development of any new material, biocompatibility is a critical factor that must be addressed. For any dental material, assessment of biocompatibility falls under guidelines detailed in the American National Standard/American Dental Association Document No. 41 for Recommended Standard Practices for the Biological Evaluation of Dental Materials. This document has been approved by the Council on Dental Materials, Instruments and Equipment of the American Dental Association.

Dental composites have gained a wide acceptance in large part due to their superior aesthetic properties. Traditionally, the most extensively used material to restore teeth has been dental amalgam, a Ag-Sn-Cu-Hg alloy. Amalgam restorations have demonstrated excellent durability over long periods of time in millions of patients. However, the dark silver-colored appearance associated with amalgam restorations is objectionable to many patients. An additional complicating factor is a concern over potential health effects associated with the mercury in amalgam alloys. While the documented evidence to date does not support the removal of serviceable amalgam restorations for the purpose of removing a toxic substance from the body (Ref 25–28), nevertheless there is increased pressure to develop a dependable cost-equivalent alternative to amalgam. Dental composites currently are potential replacement materials.

Polymer Matrix

The polymer phase most commonly used in dental composites is an aromatic dimethacrylate monomer, bisphenol A-glycidyl methacrylate (BIS-GMA). A few systems employ diurethane dimethacrylates. In general, the properties of an unfilled resin are inadequate for a restorative material. Properties that affect clinical performance include polymerization shrinkage, thermal expansion, water sorption, modulus of elasticity, tensile strength, polymerization shrinkage, and wear resistance.

Inorganic Filler Phase

Filler particles are incorporated into the resin-matrix phase to improve properties and enhance the clinical longevity of restorative resins. The properties of the different filler materials, the particle size, shape, and filler fraction all affect the properties of the composite.

Typically, the filler phase particles are made of quartz, colloidal silica, or silicate glasses containing strontium or barium. The coupling agent that is coated onto the filler particles is a silane. A key factor in the performance of filled resins is the effective long-term bonding of these particles to the matrix via the coupling agent.

Quartz. From the mid 1960s to the late 1970s, quartz was the primary filler used in dental composites. Quartz is chemically inert, improves the hardness, and reduces the thermal expansion of an unfilled restorative resin. However, its hardness also contributes to difficulty in producing fine particles and in polishing to a smooth surface. Rough surfaces on restorations facilitate plaque accumulation that can lead to pulpal and periodontal problems. An additional problem associated with rough surfaces is an increased tendency to discolor via retention of food stains. Discoloration is a primary indication for replacement. Because of the lack of x-ray opacity of quartz, diagnoses of recurrent caries and identification of improper contours or voids in a restoration are compromised. An unexpected problem identified with quartz-filled materials was excessive wear noted in posterior restorations subjected to the forces of occlusion (Ref 29). The particles of the early materials were in the range of 30 to 50 μm, and they had irregular shapes produced by grinding. Because quartz is considerably harder than the resin matrix, stresses are concentrated at localized sites where the particles are embedded in the matrix. Cracking develops in the matrix and particle loss occurs. The abrasive particles thus contribute to the wear process.

Silicate Glasses and Colloidal Silica. To address these problems, two main types of filler materials have been developed: silicate glasses and colloidal silica. The silicate glasses typically contain (in mol%) 30 to 70% SiO_2, 0 to 30% B_2O_3, 0 to 15% Al_2O_3, 0 to 20% BaO, 0 to 23% ZnO, 0 to 30% SrO. Because these glasses are softer than quartz, powder production is facilitated. Particle sizes of 1 to 5 μm are used, and the number of filler particles per unit volume is significantly increased. Compared with the quartz-containing materials, there is a decrease in the stress around the particles. Furthermore, the softer glass particles absorb more of the stresses encountered during chewing and exhibit increased wear. The net effect is an improvement in clinical wear resistance. Polishing to a smoother finish is possible, enhancing appearance and reducing plaque accumulation. The radiopacity associated with the barium or strontium filler particles also enhances radiographic interpretation of caries around the restoration as well as inappropriate contours or bulk defects within the restoration (Ref 30).

The second major alternative to large quartz filler particles is colloidal amorphous silica particles. So-called pyrogenic silica is synthesized by burning silicon tetrachloride in a mixture of hydrogen and oxygen gas. Sol-gel processing can also be employed to manufacture these particles. The resultant filler particles are less than 0.05 μm in diameter and cannot be detected visually. These microfilled composites, as they are termed, can be polished to a smoother finish than composites containing the 1 to 5 μm glass particles. Thus, the tendency for plaque accumulation and food staining is reduced. In applications where aesthetics is of paramount importance, the microfilled materials currently are used almost exclusively.

Coupling Treatments

As mentioned previously, a key to the enhanced properties of composite resins is associated with effective coupling or bonding of the filler to the matrix. Silane treatment is most often done with gamma-methacryloxypropyltrimethoxy silane from an aqueous solution or by dry blending. In an aqueous solution, the silane coupling agent is hydrolyzed to form a triol with the fourth silicon bond linked to a reactive organic group. Upon drying, a condensation of the silanol groups occurs with bonding between silane molecules as well as hydrolyzed silicon atoms in the glass particles (Ref 30).

Properties

In general, many mechanical properties of microfilled composites are inferior to composites with the 1 to 5 μm size particles. For example, the thermal expansion, polymerization shrinkage, and water absorption are greater for the microfilled materials. Also, the modulus of elasticity, tensile strength, and hardness are lower for the microfilled materials. These differences can be accounted for when one considers the amount of filler incorporated into the polymer. Typical composites with 1 to 5 μm size particles have a 75 to 85 wt% filler content. The microfilled composites have a 35 to 50 wt% filler content. The extremely small silica particles have such a high surface area that when they are added to the unpolymerized resin matrix, the viscosity rapidly increases producing a consistency that is very difficult to manipulate. One technique that is utilized to increase the filler content involves loading of the resin with as much colloidal silica as possible despite the increased viscosity. The mixture is polymerized and then ground to produce filled polymerized composite particles in the 20 μm size range. The prepolymerized particles are then added to a resin matrix that also contains colloidal silica. The resulting mixture can be adequately manipulated; however, the filler content still is only in the 50 wt% range.

Regardless of the filler type, filler shape, or filler content, resin composites have not demonstrated the longevity of amalgams for posterior restorations (Ref 31). Failure models associated with posterior composites include wear, recurrent caries, pain, and bulk fracture. The failures have been attributed to limitations in properties and to the degree of difficulty in manipulating composite materials during their placement. Two critical factors in placing any restorative material are the achievement of intimate interfacial contact with the remaining tooth structure and the reestablishment of any contact that had existed with adjacent teeth. Both of these goals are much more difficult to achieve with composites compared to amalgams. Furthermore, the shrinkage associated with polymerization as well as expansion and contraction associated with thermal cycling can compromise the interfacial integrity and lead to caries around the restoration.

The failures associated with wear and/or bulk fractures may be due in large part to a breakdown in the bond between the filler particles and the matrix (Ref 32). It has been documented that water exposure can leach out filler elements and induce filler failures and filler-matrix debonding (Ref 33). With the increasing demand for a more durable, easier-to-manipulate composite resin, emphasis is being placed on improving the filler-matrix bond strength as well as its resistance to breakdown.

Dental Cements

Applications of dental cements include:

- Cementation of crowns, fixed partial dentures (bridges), or orthodontic bands
- Bases underneath other restorative materials
- Restorations themselves

Thus, the term cement is somewhat misleading. Furthermore, when actually used as cementing agent, mechanical retention rather than true adhesion is usually achieved. One of the few cements with documented chemical bonding to tooth structure is a glass-ionomer cement

that is described later in this chapter. Retention is determined by a number of factors such as the strength and stiffness of the cement, the surface roughness of the preparation, the degree of taper of the preparation, and the proper manipulation of the material. Properties important to the performance of any cement include:

- Adequate strength and stiffness
- Resistance to dissolution in the oral environment
- Biocompatibility with pulpal tissues
- Ability to set with a low (25 to 50 μm) film thickness
- Bonding mechanism to tooth structure and to restorative materials (ideally chemical but usually mechanical)
- Ability to release fluoride to prevent caries

Types of Cement Systems

Cement systems used for luting or cementing applications are differentiated by their matrix or a combination of their matrix and filler phase. Five of the more popular systems used include:

- Zinc phosphate
- Zinc oxide eugenol (phenolate)
- Polycarboxylate (with zinc powder component)
- Carboxylate (with glass ionomer particles)
- Polymethacrylate (with borosilicate or silicate glass powder)

Zinc Phosphate and Zinc Oxide Eugenol. The two cement systems with the longest history of use are the zinc phosphate and zinc oxide eugenol (ZOE) systems. Zinc oxide is the main powder constituent in both, and the liquid component is either phosphoric acid or eugenol (oil of cloves). Zinc phosphate typically is used for permanent cementation, and ZOE is used for temporary cementation. There are modified ZOE cements available for long-term cementation. These systems rely on retention and not adhesion. Both of these cement systems can also be used as a base. Bases are used in situations where a significant amount of tooth structure (dentin) has been removed and the pulp tissues are approximated (0.5 to 2 mm). Rather than placing a metallic restorative material (amalgam or a casting) with a relatively high thermal conductivity near the pulp, an insulating base is first placed to protect the pulp.

Polycarboxylate. A cement system that has zinc oxide as the main powder component and a solution of polyacrylic acid as the liquid component was developed in the late 1960s (Ref 34), it is called a polycarboxylate. With this cement, bonding to clean enamel (Ref 35) and dentin can occur via chelation of carboxyl groups to calcium ions. It should be noted that bonding to dentin as compared to enamel is often limited by debris or contamination. Bond strength to dentin can be improved by treatment of the dentin with a remineralizing solution (Ref 36). The contribution of retention provided by the adhesion is still unknown, but carboxylate cements are used both as luting agents and as bases.

Glass Ionomer Cement. A modified class of carboxylate cement was developed by replacing the zinc oxide powder component with silicate glass particles (Ref 37–39). These are referred to as glass ionomer cements. Typical compositional ranges (in wt%) of the glass particles are: 20 to 36% SiO_2, 15 to 40% Al_2O_3, 0 to 40% CaO, 0 to 35% CaF_2, 0 to 5% Na_3AlF_6, 0 to 6% AlF_3, 0 to 10% AlP. When the glass particles are mixed with an aqueous solution of polyacrylic acid, a series of reaction steps occur. Hydrogen ions are removed from the carboxyl groups of the acid solution. Simultaneously the glass particles undergo a solution reaction in which Al^{3+}, Ca^{2+}, Na^+, F^-, and PO_4^{3-} ions are released into solution to form a silica-rich gel on the particle surfaces. Polyacrylate salts of calcium and aluminum undergo precipitation and gelation. The calcium salts form first, followed by the aluminum salts. The set cement consists of a matrix phase of aluminum and calcium polyacrylates interspersed with glass particles with a silica gel surface layer. As was noted earlier, the fluoride content can be quite high. Fluoride ions perform two important functions. For any dental cement, the mixed powder and liquid should remain in a smooth consistency for the entire working time and then go through a rapid set. Initially, the fluoride complexes with the calcium and aluminum ions as they are removed from the glass, temporarily preventing these ions from bonding to the polycarboxylate chains; later, a rather sharp setting reaction occurs. Once the cement has set, there is still a significant amount of residual fluoride that can be released to exhibit a potential cariostatic effect.

The glass ionomer cements demonstrate adhesion or bonding to enamel, dentin, and metals via the same mechanism as the zinc polycarboxylate cements. They are used as cementing or luting agents and as bases. In addition, due to the translucency imparted by the glass particles, glass ionomer cement is used as a restorative material. Most commonly, they are placed in what are termed class V lesions, which typically occur on the facial surface of teeth near or below the gum line. Their appearance and release of fluoride are primary indicators for this specific application. Glass ionomer cements used for cementation typically contain particle sizes of less than 25 μm, while the materials used for restorative applications contain particle sizes of 40 μm.

Because the complete setting reaction extends over several hours and the cement is subject to breakdown on exposure to water prior to complete setting, it is recommended that any exposed material be coated with a varnish that will provide temporary protection.

Polymethacrylates. The fifth cement system based on polymethacrylates is the most recent to be developed and does not have the history of use of the previous four. One class based on the dimethacrylates (BIS-GMA) contains borosilicate or silicate glass powder as a filler (Ref 40). These materials are used to cement cast restorations that have been etched to produce an increased irregular surface to a similarly etched enamel surface. Thus, mechanical interlocking is the bonding mechanism. A problem with these cements is the potential for microleakage at the margin or tooth interface created by the polymerization shrinkage during setting.

Polymers

In terms of quantity, the primary use of polymers in dentistry has been in the construction of prosthetic appliances such as denture bases and artificial teeth. Materials used for these applications are the focus of this section. However, polymers have also been used for other highly important applications, some of which have already been discussed in this chapter (see the sections on "Composite Dental Materials" and "Dental Cements"). In addition, polymeric materials have been used for:

- Orthodontic space maintainers and elastics
- Crown and bridge facings
- Obturators for cleft palates
- Inlay patterns
- Implants
- Impressions
- Dies
- Temporary crowns

- Endodontic fillings
- Athletic mouth protectors

Information on these applications can be found in Ref 1.

Denture Base Materials

Polymethyl methacrylate (PMMA) polymers were introduced as denture base materials in 1937. Previously, materials such as vulcanite, nitrocellulose, phenol formaldehyde, vinyl plastics, and porcelain were used for denture bases. The acrylic resins were so well received by the dental profession that by 1946, 98% of all denture bases were constructed from methyl methacrylate polymers or copolymers. Other polymers developed since that time include vinyl acrylic, polystyrene, epoxy, nylon, vinyl styrene, polycarbonate, polysulfone-unsaturated polyester, polyurethane, polyvinylacetate-ethylene, hydrophilic polyacrylate, silicones, light-activated urethane dimethacrylate, rubber-reinforced acrylics, and butadiene-reinforced acrylic.

Material Requirements

The following list indicates the requirements for a clinically acceptable denture base material (Ref 1):

- Strength and durability
- Satisfactory thermal properties
- Processing accuracy and dimensional stability
- Chemical stability (unprocessed as well as processed material)
- Insolubility in and low sorption of oral fluids
- Absence of taste and odor
- Biocompatible
- Natural appearance
- Color stability
- Adhesion to plastics, metals, and porcelain
- Ease of fabrication and repair
- Moderate cost

Although there are many commercially available materials that meet these requirements, the vast majority of dentures currently made are fabricated from heat-cured PMMA, polyvinyl acrylics, and rubber-reinforced PMMA. These denture-base materials are commonly supplied in a powder-liquid form (Table 17).

Properties. Strength properties of heat-cured PMMA and polyvinyl acrylics are shown in Table 18. These materials are typically low in

strength, soft and fairly flexible, brittle on impact, and fairly resistant to fatigue failure. In addition to the strength characteristics listed in Table 18, acrylic denture-base materials must meet a number of physical property requirements (water sorption, low density, tasteless

Table 17 Components of dental PMMA systems

Component	Remarks
Powder	
PMMA	In the form of beads, produced from monomer by emulsion polymerization
Benzoyl peroxide	An initiator of polymerization—some may remain from initial preparation of PMMA beads
Pigment	Sometimes added during production of polymer, or may be milled into the polymer beads; the cadmium compounds that are used are believed to present no systemic toxicological problems
Fibers	Colored fibers (acrylic or rayon) may be added for aesthetic effect
Liquid	
Monomer	Methyl methacrylate
Ethylene glycol dimethacrylate	This or other similar difunctional monomer may be added to give a degree of cross linking in the polymer.
Hydroquinone or its mono-methyl ether	Prevents polymerization on storage: concentration must be kept low to avoid undue interference with the rate of polymerization
Dibutyl phthalate	Such a plasticizer is sometimes added (it may also be added to polymer during ball milling stage).
Tertiary amine	Only used in autopolymerizing resins

Source: Ref 38

Table 18 Strength properties of acrylic denture base materials

Property	Polymethyl methacrylates	Polyvinyl acrylics
Tensile strength, MPa (ksi)	48.3–62.1 (7–9)	51.7 (7.5)
Compressive strength, MPa (ksi)	75.9 (11)	70.0–75.9 (10–11)
Elongation, %	1–2	7–10
Elastic modulus, GPa (10^6 psi)	3.8 (0.5)	2.8 (0.4)
Proportional limit, MPa (ksi)	26.2 (3.8)	29.0 (4.2)
Impact strength, Izod, kgf · m	0.011	0.023
Transverse deflection, mm (in.)		
At 3500 g	2.0 (0.08)	1.9 (0.076)
At 5000 g	4.0 (0.16)	3.9 (0.156)
Fatigue strength (cycles at 17.2 MPa, or 2.5 ksi)	1.5×10^6	1×10^6
Recovery after indentation, %		
Dry	89	86
Wet	88	84
Knoop hardness, kg/mm^2		
Dry	17	16
Wet	15	15

Source: Ref 1

Table 19 Physical properties and processing characteristics of acrylic denture base materials

Property	Polymethyl methacrylates	Polyvinyl acrylics
Density, g/cm^3	1.16–1.18	1.21–1.36
Polymerization shrinkage, vol%	6(a)	6(a)
Dimensional stability	Good	Good
Water sorption, mg/cm^2; ADA Test	0.69	0.26
Water solubility, mg/cm^2	0.02	0.01
Resistance to weak acids	Good	Excellent
Resistance to weak bases	Good	Excellent
Effect of organic solvents	Soluble in ketones, esters, and aromatic and chlorinated hydrocarbons	Soluble in ketones and esters and swells in aromatic hydrocarbons
Processing ease	Good	Good
Adhesion to metal and porcelain	Poor	Poor
Adhesion to acrylics	Good	Good
Colorability	Good	Good
Color stability	Yellows very slightly	Yellows slightly
Taste or odor	None	None
Tissue compatibility	Good	Good
Shelf life	Powder and liquid, good; gel, fair	Gel, fair

(a) Monomer shrinkage in mixes with polymer/monomer ratios of approximately 3 to 1. Source: Ref 1

Table 20 Comparison of properties of plastic and porcelain teeth

Plastic teeth	Porcelain teeth
High resilience	Very brittle
Tough	Friable
Soft—low abrasion resistance	Hard—high abrasion resistance
Insoluble in mouth fluids—some dimensional change	Inert in mouth fluids—no dimensional change
Low heat-distortion temperature, cold flow under pressure	High heat-distortion temperature; no permanent deformation under forces of mastication
Bond to denture base plastic	Poor bond-to-denture base plastic (a); mechanical retention provided in tooth design
Natural appearance	Natural appearance
Natural feel—silent	Possible clicking sound in use
Easy to grind and polish	Grinding removes surface glaze
Crazing and blanching—if non-cross-linked	Occasional cracking

(a) Does not apply if silane-treated. Source: Ref 1

and odorless, insoluble or no loss of constituents, etc.), processing requirements, and cost and aesthetic considerations. These requirements are summarized in Table 19. More detailed information can be found in Ref 1.

Denture Teeth

Plastic teeth are prepared from acrylic and modified acrylic materials similar to denture plastics. Different pigments are used to produce the various tooth shades, and usually a cross-linking agent is used to improve strength and prevent crazing (ultrafine cracking).

Plastic versus Porcelain Denture Teeth (Ref 1). The main difference between porcelain and plastic teeth is that plastic teeth are softer but tougher than porcelain teeth. Other differences are the low elastic modulus, low resistance to cold flow, low abrasion resistance, and high impact strength of plastic teeth. Both plastic and porcelain teeth are insoluble in oral fluids. Porcelain teeth are resistant to organic solvents such as ketones and aromatic hydrocarbons, which will react with non-cross-linked plastic teeth. Plastic teeth composed of polymethyl methacrylate show small dimensional changes when placed in water. As expected, vinyl acrylic teeth do not show as much dimensional change as the totally acrylic teeth. Porcelain teeth show no dimensional change when stored in water and exhibit no permanent deformation from forces exerted on them in the mouth. Table 20 compares the properties of plastic and porcelain denture teeth.

ACKNOWLEDGMENT

Portions of this chapter were adapted from A.E. Clark and K.J. Anusavice, Dental Applications, *Ceramics and Glasses,* Vol 4, *Engineered Materials Handbook,* ASM International, 1991, p 1091–1099.

REFERENCES

1. R.G. Craig and J.M. Powers, Ed., *Restorative Dental Materials,* 11th ed., Mosby Inc (an affiliate of Elsevier Science), 2002

2. J.-M. Meyer, Porcelain-Metal Bonding in Dentistry, *Concise Encyclopedia of Medical & Dental Materials,* D. Williams, Ed., Pergamon Press and MIT Press, 1990, p 307–312

3. J.E. Lemons, Dental Implants, *Biomaterials Science: An Introduction to Materials in Medicine,* B.D. Ratner, A.S. Hoffman, F.J. Schoen, and J.E. Lemons, Ed., Academic Press, 1996, p 308–319

4. D.F. Williams, Dental Implants, *Concise Encyclopedia of Medical & Dental Materials,* D. Williams, Ed., Pergamon Press and MIT Press, 1990, p 134–140

5. W.J. O'Brien, Dental Porcelain, *Concise Encyclopedia of Medical & Dental Materials,* D. Williams, Ed., Pergamon Press and MIT Press, 1990, p 149–152

6. P.W. McMillan, The Properties of Glass-Ceramics, *Glass-Ceramics,* 2nd ed., 1979

7. W.T. MacCulloch, Advances in Dental Ceramics, *Br. Dent. J.,* Vol 124, 1968, p 361–365

8. L.L. Hench, R.E. Going, F.A. Peyton, B.H. Bell, N. Ingersoll, and G. Kluft, Glass-Ceramic Dental Restorations, *IADR Prog. Abstr.,* Vol 51 (No. 322), 1971

9. D.G. Grossman, Cast Glass Ceramics, *The Dental Clinics of North America,* W.J. O'Brien, Ed., W.B. Saunders, 1985, p 725–739

10. Y. Abe and H. Fukui, Studies of Calcium Phosphate Glass-Ceramics Development of Dental Materials (Part I), Shika Rikogaku Zasshi, *J. Jpn. Soc. Dent. Appl. Mater.,* Vol 15, 1975, p 196–202

11. J.M. Barrett, "Chemical and Physical Properties of Multicomponent Glasses and Glass-Ceramics," M.S. thesis, University of Florida, 1978

12. J.M. Barrett, D.E. Clark, and L.L. Hench, "Glass-Ceramic Dental Restorations," U.S. patent 4,189,325, Feb 1980

13. J.M. Wu, W.R. Cannon, and C. Panzera, "Castable Glass-Ceramic Composition Useful as a Dental Restorative," U.S. patent 4,515,634, May 1985

14. S. Kihara, A. Watanabe, and Y. Abe, Calcium Phosphate Glass-Ceramic Crown Prepared by Lost-Wax Technique, *Commun. Am. Ceram. Soc.,* Vol 67, 1984, p C100–C101

15. S. Hobo and T. Iwata, Castable Apatite Ceramics as a New Biocompatible Restorative Material. I. Theoretical Considerations, *Quint. Int.,* Vol 16 (No. 2), 1985, p 135–141

16. S. Hobo and T. Iwata, Castable Apatite Ceramics as a New Biocompatible Restorative Material. II. Fabrication of the Restorative, *Quint. Int.,* Vol 16 (No. 3), 1985, p 207–216

17. S. Hobo and T. Iwata, A New Laminate Veneer Technique Using a Castable Apatite Ceramic Material. I. Theoretical Considerations, *Quint. Int.,* Vol 16 (No. 7), 1985, p 451–458

18. S. Hobo, Castable Hydroxyapatite Ceramic Restorations, *Dental Ceramics, Proc. Fourth International Symposium on Ceramics,* J.D. Preston, Ed., Quintessence Publishing, 1988, p 135–152

19. P.J. Adair, "Glass-Ceramic Dental Products," U.S. patent 4,431,420, Feb 1984

20. D.G. Grossman, The Science of Castable Glass Ceramics, *Dental Ceramics, Proc. Fourth International Symposium on Ceramics,* J.D. Preston, Ed., Quintessence Publishing, 1988, p 117–133

21. T. Kukubo, S. Ito, S. Saka, and T. Yamamuro, Formation of a High-Strength Bioactive Glass-Ceramic in the System $MgO-CaO-SiO_2-P_2O_5$, *J. Mater. Sci.,* Vol 21, 1986, p 536–540

22. W. Vogel, W. Holand, W. Naumann, and J. Gummel, Development of Machinable Bioactive Glass Ceramics for Medical Uses, *J. Non-Cryst. Solids,* Vol 80, 1986, p 34–51

23. O.H. Andersson, K.H. Karlsso, K. Kangasniemi, and A. Yli-Urpe, Models for Physical Properties and Bioactivity of Phosphate Opal Glasses, *Glastech. Ber.,* Vol 61, 1988, p 400–405

24. R.L. Bowen, "Dental Filling Material Comprising Vinyl Silane Treated Fused Silica and a Binder Consisting of the Reaction Product of Bisphenol and Glycidyl Acrylate," U.S. patent 3,066,112, Nov 1962

25. T. Axell, K. Nilner, and B. Nilsson, Clinical Evaluation of Patients Referred with Symptoms Related to Oral Galvanism, *Swedish Dent. J.,* Vol 7, 1983, p 169–178

26. B. Johansson, E. Steniman, and M. Bergman, Clinical Study of Patients Referred for Investigation Regarding So-Called Oral Galvanism, *Scand. J. Dent. Res.,* Vol 92, 1984, p 469–475

27. M. Alqwist, C. Bentsson, B. Furnunes, L. Hollender, and L. Lapidus, Number of Amalgam Tooth Fillings in Relation to Subjectively Expressed Symptoms in a Study of Swedish Women, *Commun. Dent. Oral Epidemiol.,* Vol 16, 1988, p 227–231

28. T. Kallus, Incidence of Adverse Reactions from Dental Materials, *J. Dent. Res.,* Vol 64 (Abst. No. 21), 1985, p 758

29. K.F. Leinfelder, Current Developments in Posterior Composite Resins, *Adv. Dent. Res.,* Vol 2, 1988, p 115–121

30. K.J. Söderholm, Filler Systems and Resin Interface, *Posterior Composite Resin Dental Restorative Materials,* G. Vanherle and D.C. Smith, Ed., International Symposium, The Netherlands, Peter Szulc Publishing, 1985, p 139–160

31. J.P. Moffa, Comparative Performance of Amalgam and Composite Resin Restorations and Criteria for Their Use, *Quality Evaluation of Dental Restorations, Criteria for Placement and Replacement,* K.J. Anusavice, Ed., Quintessence Publishing, 1989, p 125–138

32. K.J. Söderholm and M.J. Roberts, Influence of Water Exposure on the Tensile Strength of Composites, *J. Dent. Res.,* Vol 69, 1990, p 1812–1816

33. K.J. Söderholm, M. Zigan, M. Regan, W. Fischlchewiger, and M. Bergman, Hydrolytic Degradation of Dental Composites, *J. Dent. Res.,* Vol 63, 1984, p 1248–1254

34. D.C. Smith, A Review of the Zinc Polycarboxylate Cements, *J. Can. Dent. Assoc.,* Vol 37, 1971, p 22–29

35. A.D. Wilson and H.J. Prosser, A Survey of Organic Polyelectrolyte Cements, *Br. Dent. J.,* Vol 157, 1984, p 449–484

36. D.R. Beech, R. Soloman, and R. Bermer, Bond Strength of Polycarboxylate Cements to Treated Dentin, *Dent. Mater.,* Vol 1, 1985, p 154–157

37. S. Crisp and A.D. Wilson, Reactions in Glass Ionomer Cements—I Decomposition of the Powder, *J. Dent. Res.,* Vol 53, 1974, p 1408–1413

38. S. Crisp and A.D. Wilson, Reactions in Glass Ionomer Cements—II An Infrared Spectroscopic Study, *J. Dent. Res.,* Vol 53, 1974, p 1414–1419

39. S. Crisp and A.D. Wilson, Reactions in Glass Ionomer Cements—III The Precipitation Reaction, *J. Dent. Res.,* Vol 53, 1974, p 1429–1424

40. R. Simonsen, V.P. Thompson, and G. Barrack, *Etched Cast Restorations: Clinical and Laboratory Techniques,* Quintessence Publishing, 1983

41. E.C. Combe, Acrylic Dental Polymers, *Concise Encyclopedia of Medical & Dental Materials,* D. Williams, Ed., Pergamon Press and MIT Press, 1990, p 8–14

CHAPTER 11

Tarnish and Corrosion of Dental Alloys

DENTAL ALLOYS placed in the ever-changing oral environment are subject to two main forms of attack: sulfide tarnishing and chloride corrosion. Chloride corrosion causes deterioration of less noble metals; the attack is usually in the form of pitting and sometimes penetrates deep into the structure. The effect can range from degradation of appearance to loss of mechanical strength. Corrosion can also release metallic ions into the digestive tract or directly into the tissues.

Electrochemical processes in the oral cavity can be accelerated if different metals come into contact, forming a galvanic cell. The galvanic currents have been reported to cause pain and pathological changes.

This chapter reviews how dental alloys react with the complex oral environment, the electrochemical properties of dental alloy restorations, and the effects of alloy composition and microstructure on corrosion characteristics. Tribological characteristics of dental alloys are described in Chapter 12, "Friction and Wear of Dental Materials."

Overview of Dental Devices and Alloys

Dental alloy devices serve to restore or align lost or misaligned teeth so that normal biting function and aesthetics can prevail. Depending on the application, the particular design can take a number of different forms. The dental specialties of restorative, crown and bridge, prosthodontia, orthodontia, endodontia, implant, pedodontia, periodontia, and geriatric find applications. Alloys are used for direct fillings, crowns, inlays, onlays, bridges, fixed and re-movable partial dentures, full denture bases, implanted support structures, and wires and brackets for the controlled movement of teeth. In addition to applications calling for cast or wrought alloys, other uses of alloys include soldered assemblies, porcelain fused to metal, and resin bonded to metal restorations. Figures 1 to 6 show a number of typical restorations and appliances fabricated from dental alloys.

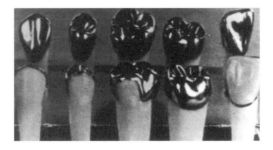

Fig. 1 Various types of crowns. Source: Ref 1

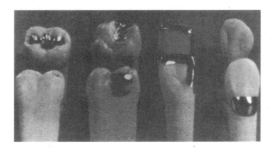

Fig. 2 Various types of inlays. Source: Ref 1

Dental Alloy Categories

The compositions of alloys utilized to fulfill the diverse applications germane to dentistry include the following elements: Au, Pd, Pt, Ag, Cu, Co, Cr, Ni, Fe, Mo, W, Ti, Zn, In, Ir, Rh, Sn, Ga, Ru, Si, Mn, Be, B, Al, V, C, Ta, Zr, and others. Alloys utilizing the aforementioned elements fall into seven distinct categories. These are briefly reviewed in this section. More detailed information on these dental alloys, including their compositions and microstructures, can be found in the section "Characterization and Classification of Dental Alloys" in this chapter.

Direct filling alloys usually consist of dental amalgams formed by the reaction of liquid mercury with alloy powders containing silver, tin, copper, and zinc. Pure gold in the form of cohesive foil, mat, or powder is used in limited applications. Gold cavity restorations are preferred by some patients concerned about the health aspects of mercury in silver-tin amalgams.

Crown and Bridge Alloys. Alloys for all-alloy cast crown and bridge restorations are usually gold-, silver-, or nickel-base compositions, although iron-base and other alloys have also been used. The gold-base alloys contain silver and copper as principal alloying elements, with smaller additions of palladium, platinum, zinc, indium, and other noble metals as grain refiners.

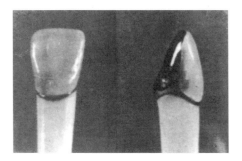

Fig. 3 Porcelain veneer fused to alloy. Source: Ref 1

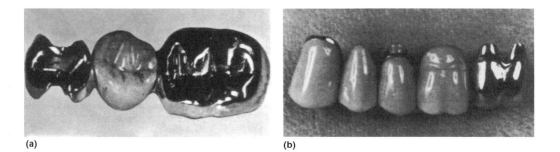

(a)   (b)

Fig. 4 Fixed bridges. (a) Three-unit bridge consisting of inlay (left member), onlay (right member), and porcelain fused to alloy pontic (center member). Source: Ref 2. (b) Five-unit bridge consisting of four porcelain fused to alloy members and one crown. Source: Ref 1

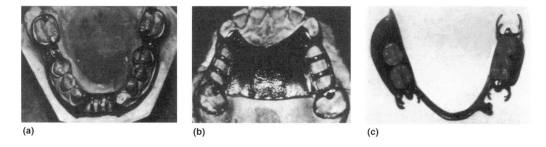

(a)   (b)   (c)

Fig. 5 Removable partial dentures, lower (a) and upper (b) cobalt-chromium frameworks, and a completed unit in (c). Source: Ref 3

The silver-base alloys contain palladium as a major alloying element, with additions of copper, gold, zinc, indium, and grain refiners. The nickel-base alloys are alloyed with chromium, iron, molybdenum, and others.

Porcelain Fused to Metal (PFM) Alloys. Alloys for porcelain fused to alloy restorations are gold-, palladium-, nickel-, or cobalt-base compositions. The gold-base alloys are divided into Au-Pt-Pd and Au-Pd-Ag, and Au-Pd types. The palladium-base alloys are palladium-silver alloys or palladium-gallium alloys with additions from either copper or cobalt. The nickel- and cobalt-base alloys are alloyed primarily with chromium and with minor additions of molybdenum and other elements. In contrast to alloys for crown and bridge use, alloys fused to porcelain contain low concentrations of oxidizable elements, such as tin, indium, iron, gallium for the noble-metal-containing alloys, and aluminum, vanadium, and others for the base metal alloys. During the heating cycle, these elements form oxides on the surface of the alloy and combine with the porcelain at the firing temperatures to promote chemical bonding.

Partial Denture Alloys. Alloys for removable partial dentures are primarily nickel- and cobalt-base compositions and are similar to alloys used for porcelain fused to alloy applications. However, carbon is present in amounts up to 0.3 to 0.4% with the partial denture alloys. Carbon is not added to alloys to be used for porcelain bonding.

Wrought Wire Alloys. Wrought orthodontic wires are composed of stainless steel, Co-Cr-Ni, Ni-Ti, and β-titanium alloys.

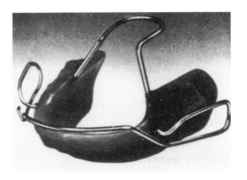

Fig. 6 Removable orthodontic appliance. Source: Ref 4

Soldering alloys, which consist of silver- and gold-base alloys, are used for the joining of components.

Implant Alloys. Alloys that have found applications for support structures implanted in the lower or upper jaws are composed primarily of titanium and titanium alloys, although cobalt-chromium, nickel-chromium, and stainless steels have also been used.

Properties

The diversity in available alloys exists so that alloys with specific properties can be used when needed. For example, the mechanical property requirements of alloys used for crown and bridge applications are different from the requirements of alloys used for porcelain fused to alloy restorations. Even though crown and bridge alloys must possess sufficient hardness and rigidity when used in stress-bearing restorations, excessively high strength is a disadvantage for grinding, polishing, and burnishing. Also, excessive wear of the occluding teeth is also likely to occur. Alloys used with porcelain fused to metal restorations are used as substrates for the overlaying porcelain. In this case, the high strength and rigidity of the alloys more closely matches the properties of the porcelain. Also, a higher sag resistance of the alloy at temperatures used for firing the porcelain means less distortion and less retained residual stresses.

Similarly, alloys used for partial denture and implant applications must possess increased mechanical properties for resistances to failures. However, clasps contained within removable partial denture devices are often fabricated from a more ductile alloy, such as a gold-base alloy, than from cobalt-chromium or nickel-chromium alloys. This ensures that the clasps possess sufficient ductility for adjustments without breakage from brittle fractures.

Other properties required in specific systems include the matching of the thermal expansion coefficients between porcelain and substrate alloy, negligible setting contractions with the direct filling amalgams, and specific modulus to yield strength ratios with orthodontic wires. Due to the use of lower gold content alloys because of the gold price market, alloy color is often a consideration. Lighter and pale-yellow gold alloys, as well as white gold alloys, are currently more prevalent. Tarnish and corrosion of all dental alloy systems have been and will remain of prime importance. Table 1 presents some typical mechanical properties for a number of different alloy systems used in dentistry.

Tarnish and Corrosion Resistance

Dental alloy devices must possess acceptable corrosion resistance because of safety and efficacy. Aesthetics is also a consideration and is discussed in "Efficacy" in this section.

Safety

Dental alloys are required to have acceptable corrosion resistance so that biocompatibility is maintained during the time the metallic components are used (Ref 5–7). No harmful ions or corrosion products can be generated such that toxicological conditions result. The effects of the dental alloys on the oral environment have the capabilities for producing local, remote, or systematic changes that may be short-term, long-term, or repetitive (sensitization) in nature (Ref 8). Dental-alloy oral-environment interactions have the potential for generating such conditions as metallic taste, discoloration of teeth, galvanic pain, oral lesions, cariogenesis, allergic hypersensitive dermatitis and stomatitis, endodontic failures, dental implant rejection, tumorgenisis, and carcinogenisis. Figure 7 shows a schematic of useful dental anatomy. Figure 8 shows three typical examples of restored teeth.

Metallic Taste. The symptom of metallic taste has been reported and related to the presence of metallic materials in the mouth (Ref 9). In addition, the release of ions and the formation of products through corrosion, wear, and abrasion can occur simultaneously, which can accelerate the process. Therefore, patients with metallic restorations and with an inclination toward bruxism (the unconscious gritting or grinding of the teeth) are likely to be more susceptible to metallic taste. Although this condition is not as prevalent as it once was when metallic materials with lower corrosion resistances were more often used, metallic taste is still known to occur on occasion.

Discoloration of teeth has occurred mainly with amalgam fillings (Ref 10) and with base alloy screwposts (Ref 11). With amalgams, tin and zinc concentrations have been identified in the dentinal tubules of the discolored areas, while with the screwposts, copper and zinc were

detected in both the dentin and enamel and the surrounding soft connective tissue. Discoloration is not, however, a definite indicator of the presence of metallic ions.

Galvanic pain results from contacting dissimilar-alloy restorations either continuously or intermittently (Ref 9, 12). An electrochemical circuit occurring between the two dissimilar-alloy restorations is short circuited by the contact. An instantaneous current flows through the external circuit, which is the oral tissues. The placement of dissimilar-alloy restorations in direct contact is ill advised.

Oral lesions resulting from the metallic prosthesis contacting tissue can be due to physical factors alone (Ref 9). An irritation in the opposing tissues of the oral mucosa can be generated because of the shape and location in the mouth of the prosthesis, as well as its metallurgical properties such as surface finish, grain size, and microstructural features. Tarnish and corrosion can change the nature of the alloy surface and be more of an irritant to the opposing tissues. Microgalvanic currents due to chemical differences of microstructural constituents and due to crevices, such as those created by the partial coverage of the alloy surface by the opposing tissues, must also be considered as possible causative factors in traumatizing and damaging tissue. However, no data have related *in vivo* galvanic currents from dental restorations to tissue damage. The released metallic ions from corrosion reactions can interact with the oral tissues to generate redness, swelling, and infection. Oral lesions can then occur. These reactions are discussed in the section "Allergic Hypersensitive Reactions" in this chapter.

Cariogenesis corresponds to the ability for released metallic ions and formed corrosion products to affect the resistance of either dentin or enamel to decay (caries). The mechanisms involved with caries formation (Ref 13, 14), which include the fermentation of carbohydrate by microorganisms and with the production of acid, are likely to become altered when metallic ions and products from corrosion reactions are included. This may be indicated by the reports that show tin and zinc concentrations originating from amalgam corrosion in softened, demineralized dentin and enamel (Ref 15–17).

Allergic Hypersensitive Reactions. With allergic hypersensitive contact reactions, some people can become sensitized to particular foreign substances, such as ions or products from the corrosion of dental alloys (Ref 9, 18). The metallic ions or products combine with proteins in the skin or mucosa to form complete antigens. Upon first exposure to the foreign substance by the oral mucosa, sensitization of the host may occur in times of up to several weeks and with no adverse reactions. Thereafter, any new exposures to the foreign substance will lead to biological reactions, such as swelling, red-

Table 1 Properties of some typical dental alloys

	Proportional limit		Yield strength, 0.1% offset		Modulus of elasticity		Strain, %	Ultimate tensile strength(b)		Brinell hardness, kg/mm²
	MPa	ksi	MPa	ksi	GPa	10⁶ psi		MPa	ksi	
Amalgam										
New True Dentalloy	...	...	...	...	21.3	3.1	...	54 (318)	7.9 (46.1)	...
Dispersalloy	...	...	...	...	33.8	4.9	...	48 (423)	6.9 (61.3)	...
Conventional gold alloys										
Type I, Ney Oro A	69	10	...	...	...	...	29.5	221	32	45
Type II, Ney Oro A-1	190	27.5	...	...	...	...	32	379	55	95
Type III, Ney Oro B-2										
Soft	221	32.0	...	...	...	...	35	421	61	110
Hard	262	38.0	...	...	...	...	34	448	65	120
Type IV, Ney Oro G-3										
Soft	286	41.5	...	...	99.3	14.4	24	469	68	140
Hard	572	83.0	...	...	...	...	6.5	758	110	220
Low-gold alloys										
40 Au-Ag-Cu (Forticast)										
Soft	...	...	379	55.0	...	...	18	562	81.5	177
Hard	...	...	738	107	...	...	2	889	129	252
10 Au-Ag-Pd (Paliney)										
Soft	438	63.5	...	...	...	...	17	558	81.0	150
Hard	583	84.5	...	...	...	...	7	731	106	205
Ag-Pd (Albacast)										
Soft	...	...	262	38.0	...	...	10	434	63	130
Hard	...	...	324	47.0	...	...	8	469	68	140
Porcelain fused to metal gold alloy										
Ceramco O	...	...	...	...	86.2	12.5	5	...	...	131
Nickel-chromium alloys										
Crown and bridge alloys	...	...	359	52	179.3	26.0	1.1	421	61	330 HV
Partial denture alloys	...	...	710	103	...	...	2.4	807	117	...
Porcelain fused to metal alloys	...	...	...	...	202.7	29.4	16	917	133	270 HV
Cobalt-chromium alloy										
Cast Vitallium	...	...	644	93.4	217.9	31.6	1.5	869	126	...
Wires										
Austenitic stainless steels	...	...	1372	199(a)	200.6	29.1	...	...	...	...
Elgiloy	...	...	1110	161(a)	171.0	24.8	...	...	...	...
β-titanium	...	...	586	85(a)	71.7	10.4	...	...	...	...
Nitinol	...	...	193	28(a)	42.1	6.1	...	...	...	...
Tooth structure										
Enamel	353	51.2	...	...	...	...	...	10 (384)	1.5 (55.7)	343 HV
Dentin	167	24.2	...	...	...	...	...	52 (297)	7.5 (43.1)	68 HV

(a) 0.05% offset. (b) Values in parentheses are ultimate compressive strengths.

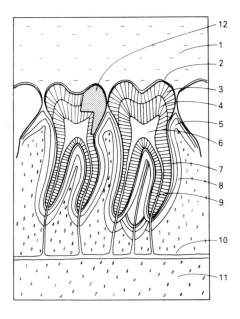

Fig. 7 Useful dental anatomy. 1, saliva; 2, integument; 3, enamel; 4, dentin; 5, gingiva; 6, pulp; 7, cementum; 8, periodontal ligament; 9, root canal; 10, artery; 11, alveolar bone; 12, restoration—amalgam filling

ness, burning sensation, vesiculation, ulceration, and necrosis. Abstinence from the foreign substance leads to healing. Identification and avoidance are the means for controlling these allergic hypersensitive reactions. Exposure of the oral mucosa to the foreign substance can lead not only to allergic stomatitis reactions (of the oral mucosa), but also to allergic dermatitis reactions (of the skin) at sites well away from the contact site with the oral mucosa. Because the oral mucosa is more resistant to allergic reactions than the skin, the reverse process usually does not occur.

Of the currently used metals contained in dental alloys, nickel, cobalt, chromium, mercury, beryllium, and cadmium need to be considered as inducing possible allergic or cytotoxic reactions. Nickel is the primary alloying element in nickel-chromium casting alloys (up to 80%), in nickel-titanium wires (up to 50%) and in lower concentrations in some cobalt-chromium alloys, and in austenitic stainless steels. Nickel from dental alloys is known to react with the oral tissues in some individuals to

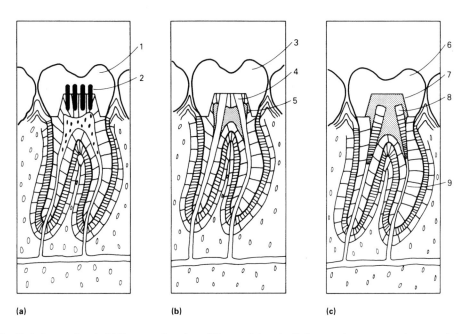

(a) (b) (c)

Fig. 8 Typical restored teeth. (a) Pin restored amalgam filling on vital tooth. (b) Cast metal crown restoration on endodontically treated tooth with silver cones and cement to seal root canals. (c) Cast metal crown restoration on endodontically treated tooth with cement core buildup and screwposts. 1, amalgam filling; 2, stainless steel pins; 3, metal crown; 4, silver cones; 5, cement; 6, metal crown; 7, cement core; 8, screw posts; 9, sealing material

produce allergic sensitization reactions (Ref 19). About 9% of women and 1% of men are estimated to be allergic to nickel. It is recommended that individuals be screened for possible nickel allergies prior to dental treatments. If an allergy arises from a dental restoration, it is recommended that the individual be tested for allergies to nickel and have the nickel-containing prosthesis replaced with a nickel-free alloy, if so indicated by the testing results.

Cobalt, also a component of some dental alloys, has been known to react with the oral mucosa and cause allergic reactions (Ref 19). However, the occurrences of such allergies are less than 1% of the population and mainly affect women. Testing for cobalt allergies should be performed if reactions to cobalt from cobalt-containing materials are suspected. Contact allergic reactions to chromium from dental alloys are also reported (Ref 19), but the occurrences of such reactions are rare.

Mercury is contained in amalgam fillings, which contain microstructural phases composed of silver-mercury and tin-mercury. Mercury ions may be released from microstructural phases through corrosion. However, the concentrations are low and not relatable to toxicological ramifications. Mercury vapors released from amalgam surfaces may also occur. Again, because of the low concentrations emitted, amalgam mercury vapors are not related to toxicity. Allergic reactions to mercury contained in dental amalgams have been reported (Ref 19). If mercury allergic reactions are suspected from the amalgam, it is recommended that testing for mercury allergies be conducted. Mercury vapors pose more of a health risk to dental personnel who routinely handle pure mercury than to individuals having amalgam restorations. Precautions should be followed in handling of pure mercury for amalgams.

Beryllium is contained in some nickel-chromium casting alloys in concentrations up to about 2 wt%. No biological reactions have been related to the beryllium contained in these alloys (Ref 19). More of a health hazard is posed to the dental personnel doing the actual melting and finishing of the alloy than to individuals having a prosthesis made from a beryllium-containing alloy. Precautions for working with beryllium must be followed.

Cadmium is contained in some dental gold and silver solders of up to 15% (Ref 20). No biological reactions have been related to the cadmium contained in these materials. Precautions should be taken in fusing solders containing cadmium.

Endodontic Failures. Root canals obturated with silver cones have occasionally been associated with corrosion (Ref 21). Development of a fluid-tight seal at the apex of the root canal is the primary objective of endodontic therapy. Corrosion of the silver points is known to lead to failure by allowing the penetration of fluids along the silver cone/root canal interface. Figure 8(b) shows a schematic of a tooth with cones.

Dental Implant Rejection. Dental implants, which are used for permanently attaching bridges, and so on, extend through or up to the maxillary or mandibular bones and must function in both hard and soft tissues as well as within a wide range of applied stresses (Ref 22, 23). Depending on the chemical inertness of the materials used for these devices, the thickness of the tissue connecting implant to bone varies. Released ions can infiltrate thick membranes surrounding loosely held implants, which can lead to an early rejection of the implant through immune response.

Tumorgenisis and Carcinogenisis. Even though dental alloy devices have not been implicated with tumorgenisis and carcinogenisis, their possible formation must never be ruled out and should always be considered as potential biological reactions, especially with new, untried alloys (Ref 23).

Efficacy

The oral environment must not induce changes in physical, mechanical, chemical, optical, and other properties of the dental alloy such that inferior functioning and/or aesthetics result. The effect of the oral environment on the alloy has the potential for altering dimensions, weight, stress versus strain behavior, bonding strengths with other alloys and with nonmetals, appearances, and creating or enhancing crevices. In combination with mechanical forces, the oral environment is capable of generating premature failure through stress corrosion and corrosion fatigue and of generating increased surface deterioration by fretting, abrasion, and wear.

Dimensions, Weight, Mechanical Properties, and Crevices. At least in theory, corrosion of precision castings and attachments, which rely on accurate and close tolerance for proper fit and functioning, can alter their dimensions, thus changing the fit and functionality of the restorations. Similarly, corrosion of margins on crowns and other cast restorations can lead to decreased dimensions and to enhanced crevice conditions. Increased seepage of oral secretions into the crevices created between restoration and tooth, microorganism invasion, generation of acidic conditions, and the operation of differential aeration cells can occur. Under these conditions, the bonding of the restoration to the dentinal walls through the underlying cement is likely to become weakened. In combination with the biting stresses, microcrack formation along the interface is likely to occur; this will cause the penetration of the crevice even further beneath the restoration. Eventually, the loosening of the entire restoration may occur.

With amalgam restorations, however, a slight amount of corrosion on these surfaces adjacent to the cavity walls may actually be beneficial, because corrosion product buildup increases dimensions and adaptability. The crevice between the amalgam and the cavity is reduced in width, which leads to a decreased seepage of fluids. On the other hand, corrosion of the amalgam deteriorates its subsurface structure; this is likely to lead to an increased occurrence of marginal fracture, a known problem with amalgams, through corrosion fatigue mechanisms with stresses generated from biting (Ref 24).

The loss of sufficient substance from any dental alloy through corrosion can lead to a reduction in mechanical strength, thus enhancing failure or reducing rigidity so that unacceptable strains occur. For silver-soldered wires, corrosion of the solder leads to a weakening of the entire joint (Ref 25). Loosening of crowns and bridges because of corrosion-induced fractures of posts and pins is also known to occur (Ref 26). Restorations featuring posts and pins are shown in Fig. 8(a) and (c). Still other possibilities include the reduction through corrosion in the bond strengths of metal brackets bonded to teeth, as well as the degradation of porcelain fused to metal restorations because of corrosion.

Appearance. Because of the various optical properties of corrosion products, the appearances of tarnished and corroded surfaces can become unacceptable. A degradation in surface appearance without a loss in the properties of the appliance can be taken to be either accept-

able or unacceptable, depending on individual preferences. If, however, the tarnished surface promotes additional consequences, such as the attachment of plaque and bacteria or a greater irritation to opposing tissue, then tarnishing must be deemed unacceptable.

Interstitial versus Oral Fluid Environments and Artificial Solutions

In order to select and/or develop dental alloys, an understanding of the environment to which these materials will be exposed is imperative. This section defines and compares interstitial fluid and oral fluid environments. In addition, artificial solutions developed for testing and evaluation of dental materials are also discussed.

Interstitial Fluid

Applications of metallic materials to oral rehabilitation are confronted with a number of environmental conditions that differentiate most dental uses from other biomedical uses (Ref 27). The one major exception is dental implants, because interstitial fluids (the fluids in direct contact with tissue cells) are encountered by both dental and other types of surgical implants. As discussed later in this chapter, other exceptions occur, because restorations in teeth have their interior surfaces in direct contact with the dentinal and bone fluids, which are more similar to interstitial fluids in composition than to saliva.

Other types of extracellular fluids, such as lymph and blood plasma, contain similar inorganic contents and are also likely to come into contact with dental implants, particularly with plasma during and shortly after surgery. Table 2 presents a composition of blood plasma. The inorganic content is similar to the inorganic content of interstitial and other types of extracellular fluids, while the protein concentration for plasma is higher than for other biofluids. For plasma, the major proteins are albumin, globulins, and fibrinogen. For all extracellular fluids, the inorganic contents are characterized by high sodium (Na) and chloride (Cl^-) and moderate bicarbonate (HCO_3^-) contents. Considerable variations in pH, pO_2, and pCO_2 can occur in the vicinity of an implant. In crevices formed between plates and screws, some extreme values ranging from 5 to 7 in pH, and <8 to 110 and <10 to 300 mm Hg, respectively, have been determined (Ref 28). Similar corrosive conditions are expected regardless of the extracellular fluid, provided the effects of the protein and cellular contents are minimal.

Tissue cells and other types of cellular matter can also directly contact implant material, with the possibility of intracellular fluid permeating through the cell membrane and effecting corrosion of the alloy. Separation by shearing of biological cells from alloy surfaces almost always generates cohesive failures through the cell instead of adhesive failures along the alloy/cell interface (Ref 29). In these situations, intracellular fluids can gain direct access to the surface of the alloy. In contrast to extracellular fluids, intracellular fluids contain high potassium and organic anion contents. The sodium is replaced by potassium and Cl^- by orthophosphate (HPO_4^{2-}). The effectiveness of intracellular fluids in corroding implant surfaces will be governed by the ability of the larger organic anions to pass through cell membranes, which are usually very restricted. Extracellular fluids are

therefore the fluids interacting with the implant in most cases, although the possible effects from intracellular fluids must not be dismissed.

Oral Fluids

Whole mixed saliva is produced by the paratid, submandibular, and sublingual glands, together with the minor accessory glands of the cheeks, lips, tongue, and hard and soft palates from the oral mucosa. Gingival or crevicular fluid is also produced, as well as fluid transport between the hard tissues of the teeth and saliva. The composition of the secretion from each gland is different and varies with flow rate and with the intensity and duration of the stimulus. Saliva composition varies from individual to individual and in the same individual under different circumstances, such as time of day and emotional state.

Although about 1 L of saliva is produced per day in response to stimulation accompanying chewing and eating; for the greater part of the day, the flow rate is at very low levels (0.03 to 0.05 mL/min). During sleep, there is virtually no flow from the major glands. At low flow rates, the concentrations of sodium, Cl^-, and HCO_3^- are reduced notably; the concentration of calcium is elevated slightly; and the concentrations of magnesium, phosphate (PO_4^{3-}), and urea are elevated decidedly when compared with stimulated flow rates (Ref 30). It is therefore impossible to define specific compositions and concentrations that are universally applicable. However, compilations of data encompassing large statistical populations have been made by a number of researchers. One typical analysis for the composition of human saliva that utilized the results from many investigators is shown in Table 3.

The inorganic ions readily detectable in saliva are Na^+, K^+, Ca^{2+}, Mg^{2+}, Cl^-, PO_4^{3-} HCO_3^- thiocyanate (SCN^-), and sulfate (SO_4^-). Minute traces of F^-, I^-, Br^-, Fe^{2+}, Sn^{2+}, and nitrite (NO_2^-) are also found, and on occasion, Zn^{2+}, Pb^{2+}, Cu^{2+}, and Cr^{3+} are found in trace quantities. Figure 9 shows the Cl^- and HCO_3^- variations in concentration as saliva is stimulated to flow at a rate of 1.5 mL/min. The O_2 and N_2 contents of saliva are 0.18 to 0.25 and 0.9 vol%, respectively. The carbon dioxide (CO_2) content varies greatly with flow rate, being about 20 vol% when unstimulated and up to about 150 vol% when vigorously stimulated. The buffer-

Table 2 Mean blood plasma composition

Compound	mg/100 mL
Inorganic	
Na^+	327
K^+	13
Ca^{2+}	10
Mg^{2+}	2
Cl^-	372
HCO_3^-	165
PO_4^-	20
SO_4^-	10
Nonprotein organic	
Urea	25
Uric acid	4
Carbohydrates	260
Organic acids	19
Lipids	530
Fatty acids	325
Amino acids	50
Major proteins	
Albumin	3650
Globulins	3250
Fibrinogen	300

Source: Ref 27

ing capacity is chiefly due to CO_2/HCO_3 system, with that of the PO_4^{3-} system only having a small, limited part. The redox potential of saliva indicates that it possesses reducing properties, which are likely due to bacteria reductions, car-

Table 3 Mean saliva composition

Compound	mg/100 mL
Inorganic	
Na^+	30
K^+	78
Ca^{2+}	6
Mg^{2+}	1
Cl^-	53
HCO_3^-	31
PO_4^{3-}	48
SCN^-	15
Nonprotein organic	
Urea	4
Uric acid	5
Amino acids	4
Citrate and lactate	5
Ammonia	0.6
Sugars	4
Carbohydrates	73
Lipids	2
Protein	
Glycoproteins	45
Amylase	42
Lysozyme	14
Albumin	2
Gamma-globulin	5

Source: Ref 30, 31

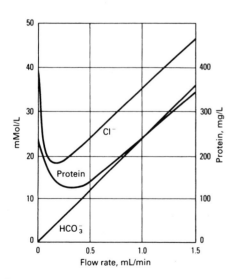

Fig. 9 Variations in the concentrations of Cl^-, HCO_3^- and protein in human saliva as a function of the flow rate of saliva. Source: Ref 30

bohydrate split-offs from glycoproteins, and nitrites. The normal pH of unstimulated saliva is in the 6 to 7 range and increases with flow rate.

The clearance of saliva involves its movement toward the back of the mouth and its eventual introduction into the stomach. Saliva is continually being secreted and replenished, especially during active times. A volume of about 1 L/day is considered average for saliva production. Chemical analysis of human mouth air showed hydrogen sulfide (H_2S), methyl mercaptan, and dimethyl sulfide to be some of the most important constituents (Ref 30).

Organic. Human saliva is composed of nonprotein organic and protein contents, as shown in Table 3. The largest contributions from the nonprotein ingredients are from the carbohydrates, while smaller amounts are from urea, organic acids, amino acids, ammonia, sugars, lipids, blood group substances, water-soluble vitamins, and others. Some of the lipids include the fatty acids, glycerides, and cholesterol. At least 18 amino acids have been identified, with glycine being the main constituent. Many of these species are produced directly by the salivary glands, while others, such as some carbohydrates and amino acids, are the result of the dissociations of glycoproteins and proteins by bacterial enzymes. Still others are derived from blood plasma. The protein content of human saliva is primarily of salivary gland origin, with a very small amount derived from blood plasma. The protein content may vary from less than 1 to more than 6 g/L. Detailed information on protein and glycoproteins that have been identified to be in saliva can be found in Ref 32 to 34.

Chemicals in Food, Drink, and Atmospheric Air. All of the ingredients found in food and drink are capable of becoming incorporated into saliva. However, most of the foods are ingested before the breakdown into basic chemicals occurs. Some foods and beverages, though, contain chemicals that are reactive by themselves without any reductions and may become dissolved in saliva and affect the tarnish and corrosion of metallic materials. Some of these include various organic acids, such as lactic, tartaric, oleic, ascorbic, fumaric, maleic, and succinic, as well as sulfates, chlorides, nitrates, sulfides, acetates, bichromates, formaldehyde, sulfoxylates, urea, and the nutrients themselves of lipids, carbohydrates, proteins, vitamins, and minerals (Ref 35).

The components found in atmospheric air and pollutants, coupled with the human respiratory function, have the potential of exposing the oral environment to additional aggressive chemical species. Some of the species known to be in atmospheric air and pollutants are O_2, CO_2, NO_2, carbon monoxide (CO), sulfur dioxide (SO_2), Cl_2, hydrogen chloride (HCl), hydrogen sulfide (H_2S), ammonia (NH_3), formaldehyde, formic acid, acetic acid, Cl^- salts, ammonium salts of sulfate and nitrate, and dust (Ref 36).

Because the volume of lung ventilation is of the order of 8.5 L/min, the amount of potentially hazardous and corrosive material possibly coming into contact with the oral environment is significant. In approximately 2 h, 1 m^3 of air for a mouth breather will have been used during respiration with the potential uptake of the normal urban SO_2 amount of 0.11 to 2.3 mg. Sulfur dioxide can be involved in many interactions, accelerating the tarnish and corrosion of metals. Hydrogen sulfide is another reactive gas. Ammonium salts are known for lowering of the surface tension of water and salt solutions. Dust particles may vary from organic to inorganic components of the earth's surface to industrial pollutants. The proteins in saliva combine with most of the aggressive external stimuli coming into contact with saliva. Therefore, most of these hazardous species are rendered inactive before they can cause tarnish and corrosion. However, the pathway from the atmosphere to the surfaces of dental alloys are certainly potential sources for introducing corrosive species.

A comparison between interstitial and oral fluids shows differences in both inorganic and organic contents. One important difference is the approximately sevenfold higher Cl^- concentration in interstitial fluid. Even though interstitial fluids do undergo variations in pH and pO_2, especially at the site of the implant, saliva is more susceptible to variations in composition. This comes about because the composition of saliva depends to a large degree on flow rate, which in turn depends on a number of physical and emotional factors. Saliva is also subjected to exposures from chemicals contained in the air, food, drink, pharmaceuticals, as well as temperature variations of 0 to 60 °C (32 to 140 °F) and microbiological involvement with the production of acid and plaque.

The operation of crevice conditions and mechanical-environment interactions are common to both saliva and interstitial fluid. Differential aeration cells and the generation of acidic conditions accompany crevices, while the biting stresses or the stresses generated in surgical implants, such as from walking, can develop creep, fatigue, wear, and abrasion process. Stress-corrosion cracking (SCC) and corrosion fatigue are additional potential mechanisms.

Artificial Solutions. Numerous solutions simulating human saliva have been formulated and used for testing the tarnish and corrosion susceptibility of dental alloys (Ref 37–42). Modifications to these solutions have also been made and used (Ref 43–48). Some of the solutions contain only inorganics (Ref 40–42, 46–48), while others include the addition of an organic component consisting mostly of mucin (Ref 37–39, 43–45). Some solutions also purge a $CO_2/O_2/N_2$ gas mixture through the solution to simulate pH control and buffering capacity controlled by the CO_2/HCO_3^- redox reaction. All compositions contain mostly chlorides (sodium, potassium, and calcium) and various forms (mono-, di-, or tri-basic, pyro) of phosphates in smaller amounts. Additional ingredients include bicarbonate, thiocyanate, sulfide, carbonate, organic acids, citrate, hydroxide, and urea.

Table 4 presents the composition for an artificial saliva that corresponds very well to human saliva with regard to the anodic polarization of dental alloys. Ringer's physiological saline solution used to simulate interstitial fluid is also included in Table 4. Both solutions are entirely inorganic. The Cl^- concentration of Ringer's is about seven times higher than that of the saliva. The anionic content of Ringer's is entirely chloride, but that of saliva also contains phosphate and sulfide. Urea is also a part of the saliva. Sodium, potassium, and calcium constitute the cationic content of both solutions.

Table 4 Composition of artificial solutions

| Compound | Composition, mg/100 mL | |
	Artificial saliva	Ringer's solution
NaCl	40	82–90
KCl	40	2.5–3.5
$CaCl_2 \cdot 2H_2O$	79.5	3.0–3.6
$NaH_2PO_4 \cdot H_2O$	69	...
$Na_2S \cdot 9H_2O$	0.5	...
Urea	100	...

Source: Ref 41, 49

A number of additional artificial physiological solutions, some of which are named Hanks, Tyrod, Locke, and Krebs, appear in the literature and have been used to simulate the interstitial fluids. Basically, these solutions contain small additions of modifying ingredients, such as magnesium chloride, glucose, lactate, amino acids, and organic anions. The Ringer's solution presented in this article, after the National Formulary Designation, does not contain sodium bicarbonate ($NaHCO_3^-$). Some solutions, however, referred to in the literature as Ringer's, do contain bicarbonate.

Effect of Saliva Composition on Alloy Tarnish and Corrosion

Chloride/Orthophosphate/Bicarbonate/Thiocyanate.
The interactions of the various salts contained in saliva are complex. The effects from the combined saliva solutions are not simply the additive effects from the isolated individual salts. This synergistic behavior is discussed for the corrosion of an amalgam in the $Cl^-/HPO_4^{2-}/HCO_3^-/SCN^-$ system in Ref 42. Chloride alone produces a powdery, finely crystalline corrosion product in heaps around the sites of attack, such as porosities and pits. The addition of HPO_4^{2-} which by itself produced very little effect, caused the corrosion products to become organized in conical structures, the bases being over the sites of corrosion. The addition of HCO_3^- to the $Cl^--HPO_4^{2-}$ system generated increased microstructural corrosion. On the contrary, addition of SCN^- to the Cl^-/HPO_4^{2-} system suppressed the microstructural corrosion. By adding all four salts together, an even more corrosion-resistant system was obtained. Corrosion was much reduced and more localized.

Artificial Salivas. The effect on alloy corrosion from different artificial saliva solutions has been studied (Ref 41). The polarization behavior of a number of dental alloys, including gold-base alloys, nickel-chromium, and cobalt-chromium, in artificial salivas without HCO_3^- and SCN^- but with protein provided the best correlation with the behavior observed with human saliva in both aerated and deaerated conditions. The artificial salivas containing HCO_3^- and SCN^- but no proteins constantly shortened the passivation range of the alloys. The specific contributions from Cl^- and SCN^- shortened the passivation range of the gold-base alloy, but phosphate increased the passivation range of all alloys.

Lowering the pH shifted the amalgam polarization curve to increased currents and potentials, while buffering capacity, which was increased by protein content, influenced corrosion behavior under localized corrosion conditions (Ref 50). In sulfide solution, the polarization curves of amalgams indicated increased corrosion (Ref 39, 51). Dissolved O_2 generated both inhibition and acceleration, as reflected by the formation of anodic films and the consumption of electrons by cathodic depolarization. The particular alloy-environment combination determines whether corrosion is inhibited or accelerated.

Chloride and Organic Content. Anodic polarization of amalgams in human saliva compared to Ringer's solution was shown to be shifted by up to several orders of magnitude to lower currents at constant potentials, depending on the amalgam system (Ref 52). These differences were related to the Cl^- concentration of the solutions. The effect of Cl^- on amalgam polarization is well documented (Ref 47, 53, 54). Pretreatment of gold-base alloys in human saliva prior to galvanic coupling with amalgams in a protein-free artificial saliva reduced the corrosion on some of the amalgams studied (Ref 55). Pretreatment of the amalgams had little effect.

Significant reductions in the weight gains of amalgams stored in artificial saliva with mucin as compared to mucin-free saliva have been reported (Ref 39). Anodic polarization of amalgams in artificial saliva or diluted Ringer's solution with and without additions of mucin or albumin was, however, shown to be very similar (Ref 39, 53). Proteins in artificial saliva on silver-palladium and nickel-chromium alloy polarizations were also reported to have little effect (Ref 50). For a copper-aluminum crown and bridge alloy, anodic polarization differences were detected in an artificial saliva with and without additions of a human salivary dialysate (Ref 56). The total accumulated anodic charge passed from corrosion potentials to +0.3 V versus saturated calomel electrode (SCE) was significantly reduced in protein-containing saliva. Similarly, the polarization resistance of the alloy was more than doubled by progressively adding up to 1.6 mg dialysate/mL to saliva initially free of proteins.

Microorganisms. The tarnishing of dental alloys by three microorganisms likely to be found in the mouth has been reported (Ref 57). Some specificity between the degree of tarnish and the type of microorganism was obtained. A likely tarnishing mechanism was due to the organic acids generated by the fermentation of carbohydrate by the bacteria. The section "Oral Corrosion Processes" in this chapter discusses in greater detail the effect of microorganisms on accelerating corrosion.

Oral Corrosion Pathways and Electrochemical Properties

The electrochemical properties of dental alloy restorations vary widely. Electrochemical potentials, current pathways, and resistances depend on whether there is no contact, intermittent contact, or continuous contact between alloy restorations. This section examines the effects of restoration contact on electrochemical parameters and reviews concentration cells developed by dental alloy-environment electrochemical reactions.

Noncontacting Alloy Restorations

Isolated. The total liquid environment of a restoration includes, in addition to saliva, fluids contained within the interior of dentin and enamel, which are more like extracellular fluids in composition than saliva. Figure 10 shows a schematic of a likely current path for a single metallic restoration. The current path encompasses a route that includes the restoration, enamel, dentin, membranes such as the periodontal ligament, soft tissues, and saliva (see Fig. 7). The conduction of current through hard tissues, including enamel, dentin, and bone, occurs through the extracellular fluids, which are compositionally similar in all hard and soft tissues. However, the current through these different hard tissues will take pathways of least resistances. For example, the resistance of dentin in a direction parallel to the tubules is about 18 times lower than in a perpendicular direction due to the calcification of the tubule walls. Structural details, including imperfections, orientations, and so on, control the actual resistances for particular hard tissue structures.

The restoration (R) develops electrochemical potentials with the extracellular fluids, E_{RE}, and with saliva, E_{RS}, while a liquid junction potential occurs between extracellular fluids and saliva, E_{ES}. Contact resistances occur between restoration and extracellular fluids, R_{RE}, and between restoration and saliva, R_{RS}. Resistances of the extracellular fluids, R_E, extracellular

fluid-saliva junction, R_{ES}, and of saliva, R_S, also occur. Figure 11 shows an electrical schematic for this system. Summing electromotive forces (emf) in one direction and equating to zero yields for the current I:

$$I = \frac{E_{RE} + E_{ES} - E_{RS}}{R_{RE} + R_{RS} + R_E + R_S + R_{ES}} \qquad \text{(Eq 1)}$$

Taken together, E_{ES} and R_S have negligible effect on current. The extracellular resistance

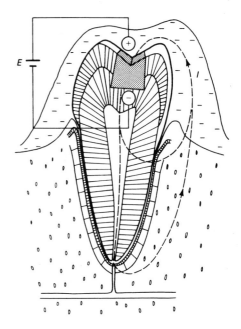

Fig. 10 Single metallic restoration showing two possible current (*I*) pathways between external surface exposed to saliva and interior surface exposed to dentinal fluids. Because the dentinal fluids contain a higher Cl⁻ concentration than saliva, it is assumed the electrode potential of interior surface exposed to dentinal fluids is more active and is therefore given a negative sign (–). The potential difference between the two surfaces is represented by *E*.

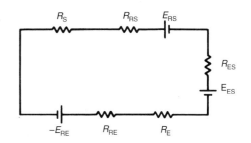

Fig. 11 Electrical schematic representing the equivalent circuit pathway shown in Fig. 10. Terminology is defined in text.

R_E is usually in the range between 10^4 and 10^6 Ω because of variations in particular hard tissue structures and possible variations in membrane/hard tissue interfacial characteristics. The potentials E_{RE} and E_{RS} are characteristic of the metal-electrolyte combinations, and the resistances R_{RE} and R_{RS} are dependent on the polarization characteristics for the particular combinations.

Polarization is related to the corrosion products that form. For soluble or loosely adhered products, the contact resistances will not be changed significantly. However, for tenaciously adhering products with semiconducting or insulating electrical characteristics, the contact resistances will be largely affected. These resistances are the primary parameters affecting the magnitude of the generated current. This reasoning is directly in line with the mixed-potential theory for electrochemical corrosion (Ref 58). The corrosion current, I_{corr}, without ohmic resistance control is:

$$I_{corr} = \frac{\beta_a \beta_c}{(\beta_a + \beta_c) R_p} \qquad \text{(Eq 2)}$$

where β_a and β_c are the Tafel slopes from the anodic and cathodic polarization curves, and R_p is the polarization resistance or the linear slope of the $\Delta E / \Delta I$ curve within ±10 mV of the corrosion potential

Nonisolated. For two restorations not in contact (Fig. 12), the extracellular fluid-saliva resistance, R_{ES}, determines the extent to which the current will be short circuited through the saliva/extracellular fluid interface. If R_{ES} is high, there is maximum interaction between the separated restorations (the currents are small, of the order of 1 to 10×10^{-9} A/cm^2 between an amalgam and a gold alloy restorations). As R_{RS} decreases, the current through the interface between saliva and extracellular fluids increases. The interaction between the separated restorations will then be minimized. Each restoration, though, will still generate its own current path loop (Ref 59).

Intraoral Electrochemical Properties. In a study comprising 115 people, the corrosion potentials from 243 restorations ranged between –0.55 and +0.4 V versus SCE. Amalgam restorations were the most active, followed by cobalt-chromium alloys and gold-base alloys. Variations in potential on different surfaces of the same restoration occurred routinely. This

was likely due to the effects from abrasion on the occlusal surfaces and from the accumulation of plaque and debris on nonocclusal surfaces (Ref 60).

For noncontacting amalgam and gold alloy restorations (78 fillings in 66 people), the average currents flowing through the restorations due to saliva-bone fluid liquid junction cells were calculated from measured intraoral potential and resistance data to be 0.48 and 0.26 μA, respectively (Ref 12).

Utilizing constant current pulses (1 to 10 μA) and measuring the corresponding potential changes, the intraoral polarization resistances for noncontacting amalgam restorations ranged between 50 and 300×10^3 Ω (Ref 61). With the use of linear polarization theory, corrosion currents are calculated to be 0.2 to 1.0 μA.

Restorations Making Intermittent or Continuous Contact

Intermittent Contact. A situation can occur in the mouth in which two alloy restorations, one in the upper arch and the other in the lower arch, come into contact intermittently by biting (Fig. 13). When the two restorations are in direct contact, a galvanic cell is generated with an associated galvanic current short cir-

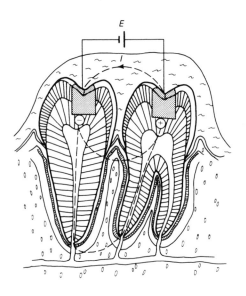

Fig. 12 Two nonisolated, noncontacting restorations. The alloy restoration on the left, which is an amalgam, is more active than the restoration on right, which is a gold-base alloy

cuited between the two restorations. The external current path can take a number of directions, with the least resistance path controlling. Figure 13 shows two possible pathways, one entirely through extracellular fluids and the other partly through extracellular fluids and partly through saliva.

The current-time transients have been measured and are presented in Fig. 14. Upon first making contact, currents of the order of 10 μA and more occur and decrease rapidly within a matter of minutes. If, however, the restorations are open circuited for a time interval and then again closed, the current level will again increase, but not to the same magnitude as from the previous closure. The amount of recovery will increase as the time lapse between closure

increases. This phenomenon is explained by the formation of protective surface films on the electrodes due to the passage of current. Upon making contact on succeeding occasions, the film offers additional resistance to the flow of current, even though the two restorations appear to be in direct intimate contact. The films dissipate with time, thus increasing the level of the initial current upon recontacting restorations.

A similar situation can occur because of an alloy restoration contacting, for example, eating utensils or dental instruments during dental treatment. Again a short-circuited galvanic current is generated. The external circuit will be partly through saliva and partly through extracellular fluids.

Continuous Contact. The fourth situation in which metallic restorations in the mouth are capable of generating galvanic currents involves two dissimilar metallic restorations in continuous contact, as shown in Fig. 15. Most attention has been given to the combination of amalgam-gold alloy couples (Ref 44). Other situations occur, for example, between two amalgam restorations (Ref 63)—one a conventional amalgam and the other a high-copper amalgam—and between two gold alloys with differences in noble metal content. Other situations have already been discussed. These include a stainless steel reinforced amalgam (Fig. 8a), an endodontically restored tooth with silver cones making contact with a gold crown (Fig. 8b), and an endontically restored tooth with steel screwposts making contact with a gold crown (Fig. 8c). Soldered appliances are also examples of dissimilar metals making continuous contact. Any multiphase microstructures are situations

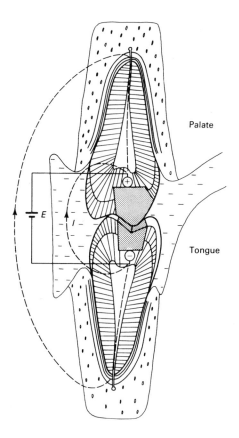

Fig. 13 Two restorations making intermittent contact due to biting. The restoration in the lower arch, which is an amalgam, is more active than the restoration in the upper arch, which is a gold-base alloy. Two possible current pathways are shown. An additional pathway very likely to occur would be directly through saliva between the two restorations.

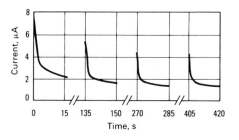

Fig. 14 Current-time responses between gold alloy and amalgam of the same cross-sectional areas. Short circuiting occurred for 15 s, followed by a 2 min delay before recontacting. Source: Ref 62

for galvanic corrosion to occur. Multiphase microstructures occur extensively with dental alloys.

For the amalgam-gold alloy couple making direct contact, the amalgam is the anode and suffers corrosive attack; the gold alloy is the cathode. As with galvanic couples making intermittent contact, large galvanic currents occur upon first contact and decrease rapidly with time. For silver-tin amalgams, the tin from the tin-mercury phase suffers corrosive attack. The freed mercury combines with the gold of the gold alloy to form a gold amalgam that is capable of producing surface discolorations on the gold alloy. In addition to becoming corroded, the amalgam is capable of being degraded in strength by the corrosion generated by the galvanic currents (Ref 63).

Currents calculated from polarization resistance and potential differences of various contacting dissimilar metallic restorations indicate most couples to pass 1 to 5 μA upon first contact (Ref 60). However, amalgam-gold alloy couples indicate a greater percentage of currents in the ranges of 6 to 10 and 11 to 15 μA. All couples initially show a sharp decrease in current with time, followed by a gradual leveling off as zero current is approached. However, disruption

of surface protective films is reason for considering possible increases in current at later times.

Concentration Cells

Interior-Exterior Surfaces. Because the interior surfaces of restorations adjacent to the cavity walls are exposed to extracellular fluids and higher concentrations of Cl^- than the exterior surfaces exposed to saliva, the interior instead of the exterior surfaces are more susceptible to anodic attack from Cl^-. However, if the electrons generated by the anodic oxidations are not consumed by reductions, the oxidation reactions will cease. Because the extracellular fluids have low concentrations of dissolved oxygen, corrosion of the interior surfaces would likely cease if it were not for the accessibility of electrons to the exterior surfaces exposed to saliva having a supply of dissolved oxygen from contact with the atmosphere.

Corrosion that is perpetuated by electrochemical reactions occurring on adjacent or opposite surfaces of the same restoration constitutes an important pathway for the tarnishing and corrosion of dental alloys. This pathway is germane to amalgams as well as all types of restorations, including crowns and inlays that are cemented into the cavity preparation. In the mouth, cements are likely to become electrical conductors because the absorption of oral fluids permits the passage of ions.

Marginal Crevices. A second pathway can occur because of the seepage of salivary fluids into crevices or marginal openings formed between the restoration (especially with amalgams) and the cavity walls. The pathway is distinguished from the first in that the conditions developed in the crevice are due to diffusion and charge balances resulting from the salivary fluids instead of the extracellular fluids. Because of a lack of diffusion of the large O_2 molecule into the crevice, low O_2 concentrations result within the crevice. With time, the acidity within the crevice increases because of the accumulation of H^+ ions from the oral environment and from corrosive reactions occurring within the crevice. Chloride and other anion concentrations will also tend to increase within the crevice over time because of charge equalization. Therefore, this pathway results in conditions that are similar to the interior-exterior pathway.

Alloy Surface Characteristics. Porosities, differences in surface finish, pits, weak micro-

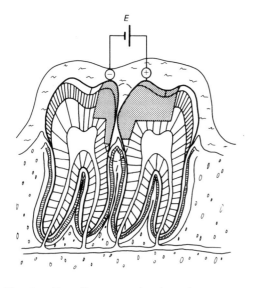

Fig. 15 Two adjacent restorations in continuous contact. Two possible current pathways are shown.

structural phases, and the deposition of organic matter can initiate corrosion by concentration cell effects. For example, gold-base alloys are known to become tarnished more easily when containing porosities and inhomogeneities (Ref 64). Rougher surface finishes of restorations generate increased corrosive conditions (Ref 65). Similarly, the pitting of base metal dental alloys of the stainless steel and nickel-chromium varieties occurs by concentration cell corrosion. Basically, the advancing pit front is free of O_2, but the surfaces of the alloy outside the pit have an ample supply of O_2 from the air. Because the anode-to-cathode surface area is very small, the corrosion occurring at the bottom of the pit is concentrated to a very small area, thus increasing intensity of the attack. Removal of only a small amount of metal has a large effect on advancing the pit front.

Amalgam γ_2 Phase. Deterioration of the weak, corrosion-prone tin-mercury phase (γ_2) in silver-tin amalgams has also been proposed to occur by concentration cell corrosion (Ref 59). In this model, partial removal of the γ_2 phase initially occurs by abrasion resulting from biting and chewing. After removal of the γ_2 phase has progressed to a sufficient depth, an occluded cell is formed between the bottom of the depression and the unabraded surface. Mass transport is restricted from and into the cell. The condition will approach conditions occurring in other types of concentration cells. In the present example, however, Sn^{2+} will be slowly released from the passivated γ_2 regions. The concentration of Sn^{2+} will slowly increase within the occluded cell and will be neutralized by an equivalent amount of Cl^- by migration from the bulk electrolyte.

Consumption of O_2 within the occluded cell will take place by its utilization in the consumption of electrons by cathodic depolarization. Replenishment of O_2 will be restricted, and the concentration of O_2 within the cell will become reduced. When the solubility product of stannous oxide (SnO) is exceeded, SnO precipitates and the H^+ concentration increases. At this point, activation of the γ_2 phase occurs. Dissolution of tin occurs freely. The Cl^- concentration within the cell continuously increases to maintain electrical neutrality. Galvanic coupling of the occluded cell to the external surface generates a galvanic cell by which the cathodic reduction of O_2 occurs. Corrosion of γ_2 tin within the cell continues. Under conditions of high acidity and high concentration of Cl^-, the formation of insoluble tin chloride hydroxide ($Sn(OH)Cl \cdot H_2O$) becomes thermodynamically possible.

Oral Corrosion Processes

Whether corrosion occurs between microstructural phases of a single restoration, between components having different environmental concentrations, or between individual restorations of different compositions and making intermittent or continuous contact, the corrosion processes involved consist of oxidation and reduction. The dissolution of ions is involved with the anodic reaction, and the consumption of electrons is involved with the cathodic reaction. The slowest step in the complete chain of events controls the overall corrosion rate. Corrosion of alloys in the mouth can be viewed as being the result of corrosive and inhibiting factors (Ref 66). Some corrosive factors consist of Cl^- (in most instances), H^+, S^- (at times), O_2, microorganisms, and the clearance rate of corrosion products from the mouth, while some inhibiting factors consist of proteins and glycoproteins (in most instances), CO_2/HCO_3^- buffering system, PO_4^-/PO_4^{3-} buffering system, and salivary flow rate.

Corrosive Factors

Chloride. The effect of Cl^- on the deterioration of passivated surface films on stainless steel, nickel-chromium, and cobalt-chromium alloys is well known. The susceptibility to pitting attack is increased. Increased Cl^- content also increases the attack of corrosion-prone phases in amalgam, other base metal alloys, and the low noble metal content alloys. Because the Cl^- concentration in saliva is about seven times lower than that in the extracellular fluids, the corrosiveness of Cl^- in saliva is usually less. Figure 16 illustrates the effect of Cl^- concentration on the polarization of amalgam by comparing the cyclic voltammetry in deaerated artificial saliva to that in Ringer's. Increases in Cl^- concentrations are also likely to occur in crevices, such as the interfaces between cavity walls and adjacent surfaces of restoration. The Cl^- concentration within crevices is expected to increase to preserve electrical neutrality from the increase in Sn^+ concentration resulting from the γ_2 tin and γ_1 corrosion (Ref 59).

Chloride is capable of generating numerous compounds as products of corrosion. Chloride combines with zinc, tin, copper, silver, and others contained in dental alloys. Some of the products formed include zinc chloride ($ZnCl$), stannous chloride ($SnCl_2$), stannic chloride ($SnCl_4$), SnCl compounds such as hydrated $SnOHCl \cdot H_2O$ and $Sn_4(OH)_6Cl_2$, copper chloride ($CuCl$), cupric chloride ($CuCl_2$), complex hydrated cupric chloride ($CuCl_2 \cdot 3Cu(OH)_2$), and silver chloride ($AgCl$). The solubilities are high for all compounds, except $CuCl$, $AgCl$, and the basic tin and copper chlorides. Many additional compounds are to be considered for a complete listing of all potential corrosion products that form from dental alloys. Certainly, the chlorides of indium, gallium, beryllium, iron, nickel, chromium, cobalt, and molybdenum should be included.

Hydrogen Ion. The pH in the mouth can vary from about 4.5 and lower to about 8. In addition to the normal variations in pH of saliva due to human factors (see the section "Oral Fluids" in this chapter), increased acidity can also result from a number of additional factors, such as the operation of crevice corrosion conditions, the production of plaque, and the effects of food, drink, and atmospheric conditions. The operation of crevice conditions in amalgams can increase acidity to well below a pH of 4. For amalgams, this acidity is mostly the result of the oxidation of γ_2 and γ_1 tin in aqueous solution. Under these conditions, the freed H^+ will become the cathodic depolarizers. With this

increased acidity, dissolution of the tooth structure is also likely to occur. Calcium and phosphorus are likely to be dissolved from enamel and dentin. Plaque is produced by the fermentation of carbohydrate by microorganisms (Ref 13, 14). Most of the fermentable carbohydrate responsible for acid production comes from the diet in the form of sugars or starchy foodstuffs.

Figure 17 shows a Stephan pH test curve of plaque. Stephan showed that the pH for all plaques decrease in value following a sugar challenge (Ref 13). This means that the production of acid by fermentable carbohydrate is greater than the rate at which acid can be removed. As time proceeds, the pH again rises. For caries-free and caries-active individuals, the qualitative shapes of Stephan pH curves are similar; however, the relative position of the curve for caries-active individuals is shifted to lower pH values. Values in pH of 4.5 and lower occur. Depending on the source of the sugar challenge, the pH minimum on the Stephan pH curves have been shown to remain for a number of hours. Even though no data are available to show the effect of plaque pH value on the tarnishing and corrosion of dental alloys, it follows from first principles that the reduction in pH will adversely affect tarnishing and corrosion resistance. Metallic restorations can become se-

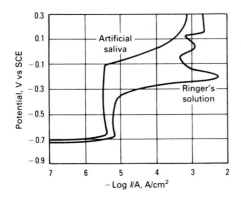

Fig. 16 Anodic polarization at 0.03 V/min of low-copper amalgam (Microalloy) in artificial saliva and Ringer's solution. Source: Ref 67

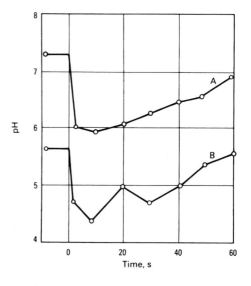

Fig. 17 pH versus time responses (Stephan curves) of plaque from caries-active (B) and caries-free (A) groups following a sugar challenge. Source: Ref 13

verely deposited with plaque and organic matter, as shown in Fig. 18.

Sulfide compounds, such as silver sulfide (Ag_2S), cuprous sulfide (Cu_2S), and cupric sulfide (CuS), have very low solubility product constants and often constitute the tarnished films on dental alloys. Mercury and tin sulfides may also be considered when amalgams are considered. The formation of thin insoluble films occurs with very small amounts of formed corrosion products, especially on the higher noble metal content alloys. In spite of even microgram quantities of tarnishing products at times, surface discolorations can still occur and elicit unsatisfactory personal responses. Tarnishing products under these conditions almost always maintain biocompatibility with the alloy system. With the lower noble metal content alloys, however, increased quantities of corrosion products can form, and tarnishing and corrosion can become more involved.

The corrosion potentials for many dental alloys in sulfide-containing solutions are often lower than the standard reduction potentials for the formation of the metal sulfides—an indication that the metal sulfides are thermodynamically stable. In some instances, particularly with amalgams, dissolution rates increase with S^- concentrations. This is probably due to the increased solubility for some of the sulfides (for example, Sn_2S_3 with amalgams) to form complexes with other species. Dietary factors are the main source for increasing S^- levels in saliva. Some foods, such as eggs and fish, as well as some drinking waters, are high in sulfur. Smokers have higher SCN^- saliva concentrations than nonsmokers (Ref 69). Sulfate-reducing bacteria may also generate S^- in the mouth. Hydrogen sulfide that is produced in the crevicular fluid and periodontal pockets can be easily dissolved in oral fluids. Atmospheric pollutants often contain high levels of So_2 and H_2S and may influence the concentrations of S^- in the oral fluids.

Dissolved oxygen participates in corrosion reactions by either depolarizing cathodic reactions or by reoxidizing disruptive passivated surface films on base metal alloys. The first case increases or perpetuates corrosion, while the second case reduces or inhibits corrosion. Oxygen depolarization occurs by the customary electrochemical redox reactions. Electrons from the anodic process are consumed by the depolarization process. For a typical restoration, the exterior surfaces are exposed to higher O_2 concentrations. Differential aeration conditions can become operative, with the outer surfaces cathodic to the anodic interior surfaces. In other situations, differential aeration cells are set up between the bottoms of pits and the surrounding surfaces. Other types of pores and porosities are also likely to generate concentration cells. In near-neutral solution that corresponds to saliva, the reaction $O_2 + 2H_2O + 4\ e^- \rightarrow 4OH^-$ occurs most prevalently. If a driving force exists for metal oxidation, dissolution will be perpetuated on surfaces exposed to the lower O_2 concentration.

Oxygen is involved with numerous corrosion products formed on dental alloys. The tin from the γ_1 and γ_2 phases from silver-tin amalgams generates tin oxide products. These products passivate the amalgam at potentials less negative than about –0.7 V versus SCE, as indicated by the passive regions on the anodic polarization curves shown in Fig. 16. At more noble potentials, basic tin chlorides of the type $SnO \cdot HCl \cdot H_2O$ are formed, as indicated by the large current increases on the polarization curves. For copper-containing amalgams, basic copper chlorides of the type $CuCl_2 \cdot 3Cu\ (OH)_2$ form. Some additional products containing oxygen that are likely to occur with the corrosion of dental alloys include SnO_2, $Sn_4(OH)_6Cl_2$, Cu_2O, CuO, ZnO, $Zn(OH)_2$, and the oxides of chromium, nickel, cobalt, molybdenum, iron, titanium, and so on.

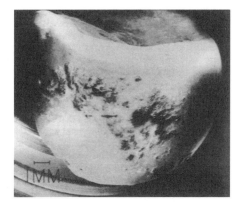

Fig. 18 Copper-aluminum alloy restoration after intraoral usage showing the severity of plaque buildup that can occur. Source: Ref 68

Oxygen is usually excluded from solutions during polarization testing with alloys. Dissolved O_2 interferes with the anodic processes. The generated anodic polarization curves obtained in O_2-containing solutions are usually cut off within the negative potential regions. For this reason, deaerated solutions are usually used to obtain entire anodic polarization curves. Passive breakdown potentials were observed to vary depending on whether aerated, dearated, or air-exposed solutions were used (Ref 70). Within the O_2 concentration range likely to occur for surgical implants, the anodic polarization of type 316L stainless steel in Ringer's solution was independent of oxygen concentration (Ref 71).

Microorganisms. Two types of organisms—sulfate-reducing (*Bacteriodes corrodens*) and acid-producing (*Streptococcus mutans*) bacteria—have been discussed with the corrosion of dental alloys in the mouth (Ref 66). With regard to sulfate-reducing bacteria, depolarization of cathodic sites is thought to occur by removing H^+ from the metal surface. The hydrogen is utilized by the bacteria for the reduction of sulfate to sulfide, such as by the reaction $SO_4^- + 8H^+ \rightarrow S_2^- + 4H_2O$. In the case of acid-producing bacteria, the adsorbed microorganisms on the surface establish differential aeration conditions. As the dissolution of the metal occurs underneath the deposited microorganisms, the released acidic metabolic products, which include organic acids such as lactic, pyruvic, acetic, proprionic, and butyric, increase corrosion of the already-formed anodic sites. Because anodic areas are relatively small compared to the larger cathodic areas, corrosion can be severe.

The fermentation of carbohydrates by microorganisms generates plaque. The effects of plaque on the tarnishing and corrosion of dental alloys are probably more significant than the effect on alloy corrosion of only the microorganisms themselves. The effects of plaque on corrosion are considered in the section "Hydrogen Ion" in this chapter.

Clearance Rate. The clearance of corrosion products from the mouth by the movement of saliva toward the back of the mouth and eventually by swallowing and replenishment affects the concentration of products in equilibrium with the metallic restorations. Therefore, a driving force for the continuation of the corrosion processes is maintained. Products of corrosion, like chemical species introduced through the diet, are cleared from the mouth by binding the exterior surfaces of the oral mucosa to the salivary glycoproteins and mucopolysaccharides lining. Detailed information on the binding ability of corroded metallic ions to proteins in human saliva can be found in Ref 32, 33, and 72.

Alloy Factors. Although the effects of alloy selection on tarnish and corrosion behavior are considered in more detail in the section "Tarnish and Corrosion under Simulated or Accelerated Conditions" in this chapter, some of the important factors are mentioned here. Alloy composition and microstructure are probably the two most important factors. The corrosion resistance of dental alloys is the result of nobility in composition or the protectiveness of oxide films formed on base metal alloys. Multiphase microstructures are capable of exhibiting increased tarnish and corrosion because of galvanic coupling of the individual components. The heat treatment state of cast alloys has an important influence on corrosion resistance (Ref 73). Surface state or finish also influence corrosion. Rougher surfaces are more prone to corrosion because of increased tendencies for galvanic coupling. Cast restorations with burnished margins are more susceptible to corrosion because of differences in surface cold-worked states. Rougher surfaces are prone to attachment of microorganisms and plaque, which usually increase corrosion (Ref 74).

Inhibiting Factors

Organics in the form of microorganisms and plaque usually have an accelerating effect on the tarnishing and corrosion of dental alloys (see the sections "Effect of Saliva Composition on Alloy Tarnish and Corrosion" and "Oral Corrosion Processes" in this chapter). Organics in the form of amino acids, proteins, and glycoproteins have received mixed reports. For the amino acids, the building blocks of proteins, the passivation of copper was shown to be improved in Ringer's solution with added cysteine, while nickel became more corrosion prone (Ref 75). Alanine had little effect. For Ti-6Al-4V, the amino acids proline, glycine, tyrosine, and others that constitute many salivary proteins were again shown to have very little effect. For the plasma proteins, which simulate the organic content in blood and which simulate dental and surgical implant applications more closely, additional evidence can be found implicating the effect of proteins on corrosion behavior.

For example, the corrosion rates of cobalt and copper powders increased significantly when exposed to saline solutions with albumin and fibrinogen (Ref 76); however, for chromium and nickel powders only slight increases occurred, and for molybdenum decreases occurred. Corrosion of stainless steel by applied external currents was shown to be increased when conducted in saline with added calf's serum (Ref 77). When conducted under fretting corrosion conditions, however, the degradation of stainless steel was shown to increase in saline without the added serum (Ref 78). For a copper-zinc alloy, the cyclic voltammetry was reported to be altered by addition of plasma proteins and at plasma concentrations to a phosphated physiological saline solution (Ref 79). Albumin and γ-globulin generated increased passivation currents, while fibrinogen generated decreased critical current densities. The anodic polarizations prior to the onset of critical current densities were also shifted to more active behavior in the protein solutions. Finally, the pitting potential for aluminum increased slightly in human plasma, and current-time transients were shifted to lower values in plasma (Ref 80).

Carbon Dioxide/Bicarbonate Buffering System. The major buffering system in saliva is the CO_2/HCO_3^- system, which has been found to inhibit corrosion processes on dental alloys. Inhibition results from the deposition of such elements as copper, zinc, and calcium as carbonate films. Carbon dioxide, above all other gases, is contained most abundantly in saliva. Up to about 150 vol% (~3000 ppm) is contained in vigorously stimulated saliva. The equilibrium concentration of HCO_3^- in saliva is identified by the redox reaction:

$$CO_2(g) + H_2O \rightarrow H^+ + HCO_3^- \qquad \text{(Eq 3)}$$

and with its equilibrium constant pK equal to (Ref 46):

$$pK = 7.9 = -\log \frac{[(H^+)(HCO_3^-)]}{p_{CO_2}} \qquad \text{(Eq 4)}$$

At pH = 7, rearranging terms yields:

$$\frac{p_{CO_2}}{HCO_3^-} = 7.9 \qquad \text{(Eq 5)}$$

Equation 5 states that the partial pressure, p, of CO_2 in units of atmospheres is 7.9 times larger than the HCO_3^- concentration in mol/L. Therefore, for p_{CO_2} of the order of 0.07 atm, HCO_3^- concentrations of the order of 0.009 mol/L are formed. This shows that relatively large concentrations of HCO_3^- can be made available in saliva to form carbonates with cations released from corrosion reactions on dental alloys and with other cations found in the mouth, such as calcium.

Many of the different carbonates likely to form are insoluble in aqueous solution. The calcium carbonates are known for making waters hard. Compounds of this type being deposited as thin-film tarnish and corrosion products on dental alloys are very likely to interfere with the corrosion activity. Deposition over cathodic sites effectively increases corrosion resistance by increasing resistance to depolarization reactions. Because the films of carbonates are also likely to increase the contact resistances between electrodes and saliva, galvanic-corrosion processes are likely to change from purely corrosion control to at least partial ohmic control. Under these conditions, local anodes and cathodes may change in order to maintain lower-resistance paths for both ionic and electronic conduction. The *in vivo* tarnishing of several silver-palladium alloys was shown to be due to the galvanic coupling between microstructural phases located very close to each other on the alloy surface (Ref 81). This was in contrast to laboratory tests in high-conductivity solutions indicating larger distances between microelectrodes.

Phosphate Buffering System. A secondary buffering system in saliva, the PO_4^-/PO_4^{3-} system, has also inhibited the corrosion of dental alloys. The progressive inhibition of chloride (10 millimolar NaCl) amalgam corrosion activity was shown to occur with increasing added phosphate concentrations (Ref 66). A 15 millimolar phosphate addition retarded the anodic polarization almost entirely, while concentrations of 10, 7, 5, and 1 millimolar generated anodic current peaks of about 2.5, 3.0, 3.5, and 6.0 $\mu A/mm^2$, respectively. The 10 millimolar NaCl solution without phosphate generated a continuous increase in current to much larger values. No passivation occurred within the potential range used.

For tin in neutral phosphate solutions, a passive film forms by precipitation or by a nucleation and growth processes (Ref 82). Tin phosphate, basic tin phosphate complexes, and tin hydroxides are formed.

Salivary Flow Rate. Increasing the salivary flow rate increases the concentration of most species in saliva. This tends to inhibit corrosion. The organic content, the CO_2/HCO_3^- content, and the PO_4^-/PO_3^- content, pH, and the Ca^{2+} content all increase with flow rate. Only the increases in Cl^- concentration promote corrosion. Figure 9 shows the effect of flow rate on the concentration of a number of species.

Overview. Saliva acts as an ocean of anions, cations, nonelectrolytes, amino acids, proteins, carbohydrates, and lipids flowing in waves against and into dental surfaces with a diurnal tide and varying degrees of intensity (Ref 83). Whether or not tarnish and/or corrosion of dental metallic materials will occur cannot be categorically stated. It has been discussed that the degree to which dental alloy corrosion occurs in the mouth is dependent on the oral environmental conditions for each person. In addition to effects from the dental alloy itself, competition between corrosive and inhibitory factors of the oral environment will dictate whether or not corrosion will occur and to what

extent. In addition to the factors listed above, still others have been isolated and should be included for a more complete assessment of the overall corrosiveness or protectiveness of the oral environment (Ref 66).

Nature of the Intraoral Surface

The composition and characterization of biofilms, corrosion products, and other debris that deposit on dental material surfaces are discussed in this section. The nature of these deposits depends on the substrate material (enamel, alloy, porcelain, and so on).

Acquired Pellicles

Characteristics. Most surfaces that come into contact with saliva, including enamel and metallic, polymeric, and ceramic dental materials, interact almost instantaneously with the proteins and glycoproteins to form a bacteria-free biofilm of the order of several nanometers in thickness (Ref 84–86). This most intimate layer of organic matter adsorbed to the substrate material is called the acquired pellicle. A Fourier transform infrared spectroscopy (FTIR) spectra of the surface of a low-gold dental crown and bridge alloy after *in vivo* exposure is shown in Fig. 19. Detection for protein, carbo-

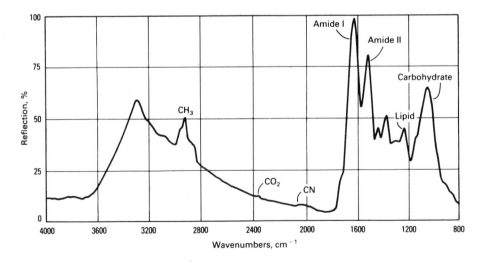

Fig. 19 Fourier transform infrared spectroscopy spectra from surface of a crown and bridge alloy (Midas) after several weeks of intraoral usage. Amide I and II are protein. Additional smaller peaks at 1375 and 1425 cm⁻¹ are also protein.

hydrate, and lipid is indicated. Thicknesses of the films increase only slightly with longer exposure times. The pellicles, in contrast to enamel and most dental alloys, are acid insoluble, although an acid-soluble fraction also occurs. The films are diffusion barriers against acids, thus reducing the acid solubility of enamel and metallic materials and inhibiting or at least reducing the adherence of organisms.

Composition. Chemical analysis of pellicles formed on enamel after 2 h indicated abundant amounts of glycine, glutamic acid, and serine (Ref 87). Carbohydrate contents of similar pellicles formed on enamel were found to contain about 70% glucose, with a number of other sugars and small molecules. Acidic proline-rich phosphoproteins have also been identified from *in vivo* enamel pellicles (Ref 88). The proline-rich proteins constitute as much as about 37% of the total proteins in new pellicles within the first hour. However, there is a gradual degradation beginning after about 24 h that is reflected by the fact that the proline-rich protein content in aged pellicles is less than 0.1%.

Substrate Effects on Pellicle Composition. Chemical analysis of the pellicles formed on several plastics and glass showed that the amino acid content varied and was different from that formed on enamel (Ref 89). It was concluded that the chemical composition of the substrate has an important influence on the type of proteins that become adsorbed. For the pellicle formed on dentures, it was concluded that a specific mechanism was controlling the deposition of protein and that specific proteins seemed to be precursors in forming the film (Ref 90). Isoelectric focusing of the extracted proteins adsorbed from a human saliva preparation onto a number of different powder substrate compositions, including palladium, silver, copper, silver-copper, tin, Ag-Sn-Cu alloy, bismuth, polymethyl methacrylate, porcelain, hydroxyapatite, and enamel, indicated that the same three to four proteins appeared to be involved with the adsorption process on all substrates regardless of composition (Ref 33). Therefore, from this study, substrate composition appeared not to affect the type of proteins becoming adsorbed.

Binding Mechanisms. The binding of salivary macromolecules to surfaces has been proposed to consist of electrostatic interactions between the charged groups in the molecule and the surface charges on the substrate (Ref 91). For enamel, only the hydroxyapatite, and not

the organic matrix, contributes a surface charge for binding. Because the negatively charged phosphate group comprises about 90% of the surface area of hydroxyapatite, the phosphate group rather than the calcium ions will be the primary binding sites. The hydration layer contains soluble calcium and phosphate ions as well as soluble cations and anions. Because the salivary molecules adsorbed to enamel are mainly acidic, binding to the negatively charged phosphate group appears to occur through a divalent cation, such as calcium. Phosphorylated and sulfated acidic proteins show a high affinity for hydroxyapatite. A direct replacement of the protein phosphate group and the phosphate in hydroxyapatite is also likely (Ref 92).

Direct binding to the calcium surface ions in enamel will also occur, but will be limited because of the relatively small surface area fraction occupied by the calcium ions. Adsorption of salivary proteins to metals may again occur through a divalent cation. The negative charges in the acidic proteins are likely to be bound to the negative anodic surface sites on the metal surface by the bridging cation. Additional information on protein binding and analyses of variations in protein binding to a metal surface through differential scanning calorimetry can be found in Ref 93.

Plaque, Corrosion Products, and Other Debris

Integument. In addition to the thin acquired biofilms, aged pellicles contain microorganisms, plaque, mineralized products, corrosion products, and other debris. Plaque, which is a by-product of the reaction between microorganisms and carbohydrates, may form in abundance in some environments. Plaque does not form directly onto teeth or other materials. It is deposited or adsorbed onto the acquired pellicle. The combined surface coating, including the adsorbed pellicle and plaque, which includes organic matter and any released ions or corrosion products generated by the substrate, is often referred to as the integument.

Substrate Effects on Integument Characteristics. A study was made of the effect of the restorative material type on plaque composition (Ref 94). The carbohydrate/nitrogen ratios (CHO/N) were similar for amalgam, gold inlay, gold foil, and resin. Plaque analyzed from freshly placed restorations had CHO/N = 1; this value increased to 1.3 and 1.2 at 3 and 6 months, respectively, and decreased to 0.5 at 1 year and for old restorations. It was proposed that the variation in plaque carbohydrate content with the age of the restoration was due to corrosion or to the absorption of impurities into surface porosities and pits. These mechanisms are supported by the data generated with silicate restorations. This was the only material to show significant differences in CHO/N. The CHO/N was 1.0 at 1 year. This suggests that the carbohydrate is metabolized less efficiently by the silicate. It is known that silicate restorations leach fluoride with time. Therefore, the fluoride acts as an enzyme inhibitor.

The thicknesses of the integuments formed in the mouth vary and may depend on the substrate material. For example, sputtering times in Auger electron spectroscopy depth profiling required only 0.3 min to reach the amalgam substrate, while 2.4 min was required to reach the gold alloy substrate (Ref 86). Carbon, nitrogen, and oxygen were distributed in much the same manner as films formed on different substrates. The main difference between the integuments formed on the amalgam and on the gold alloy was the presence of tin ions with the amalgam and the presence of copper ions with the gold alloy. The release of substrate ions is likely to interact with the attachment of microorganisms and therefore with the metabolism of plaque.

Substrate Corrosion. Corrosion reactions involve diffusion of ions—whether cations from oxidations or dissolved O_2 and H^+ for reductions—through the formed integument. The surface coating has the ability to act as a diffusion barrier to the movement of ions. Released ions are likely to become complexed, or bound, to the proteins and glycoproteins constituting the integument and free native proteins in the bulk saliva, provided diffusion is not restricted by the integument. Insoluble corrosion products of the oxides, chlorides, sulfides, carbonates, phosphates, and so on, have the capability of being deposited at the alloy/film interface or becoming an integral part of the integument. Soluble products, in addition, may be released into the bulk saliva.

For one dental restorative alloy, it was shown that the polarization resistance of the alloy increased with protein concentration, while at the same time, the concentration of soluble species in solution also increased (Ref 56). This situation was explained by the increased effect of proteins in solubilizing corrosion products.

Energy-dispersive spectroscopy (EDS) spectra of the corroded surfaces showed reduced peak intensities for chlorine and sulfur on surfaces exposed to the proteins. Therefore, even though the severity of corrosion is less in protein-containing solutions, increased levels of soluble products are still generated.

In Vivo Tarnished Film Compositions. Auger thin-film analysis of the surfaces of dental alloys with varying compositions and after functioning in the mouth indicated that the tarnished films were due to chemical reactions between alloy and inorganic species and to the adsorption and deposition of organic matter (Ref 35). Carbon was the dominant nonalloying element by about six times, followed by oxygen, calcium, nitrogen, chlorine, sulfur, magnesium, silicon, phosphorous, aluminum, sodium, and tin. Of the elements from the alloy itself, copper was dominant. In a microprobe analysis of *in vivo* discolorations on gold alloys, both silver sulfides and copper sulfides were detected, depending on the composition of the alloy. Sulfur was found isolated and carbon was present in greatest quantities (Ref 95).

Intraoral (in Vivo) versus Simulated (in Vitro) Exposures

Need for Laboratory Testing. The tarnish and corrosion behavior of dental alloys under actual oral environmental conditions is required. However, except for selected clinical trials, the initial testing of new and improved alloys for tarnish and corrosion resistance is usually carried out under laboratory conditions in either simulated or accelerated tests. This is so because of:

- The possible human exposure to harmful species
- The variability in the oral environmental conditions from person to person and even with the same person from location to location and with time
- As a result of the variability in the oral environment, the inability to follow the effects on tarnish and corrosion from changes in parameters in alloys and in solution

Most laboratory tests utilize an artificial saliva or a physiological saline solution, such as Ringer's solution (Table 4), diluted Ringer's solution, various concentrations of NaCl, and various concentrations of Na_2S. The main deficiencies with these solutions is that the nonelectrolytes, including the proteins, glyco-proteins, and microorganisms, are not included. This fails to produce the pellicle and integuments on laboratory samples that otherwise would have formed on all intraoral surfaces.

In spite of these shortcomings, for the most part, the inorganic salt solutions have become indicators for the aggressiveness of the oral environment. However, the inability to correlate *in vivo* to *in vitro* behaviors in some instances is likely because of the failure to account for the shortcomings (Ref 81).

The use of solutions with higher-than-normal concentrations accelerates the tarnish and corrosion processes. For example, 3200 immersions of 15 s/min duration in a 5% Na_2S solution with a Tuccillo and Nielsen tarnishing apparatus (Ref 96) is estimated to simulate 12 months of actual in-service use (Ref 97). Ringer's and 1% NaCl solutions, which contain about seven times the Cl^- concentration of human saliva, are used in anodic polarization tests to amplify peaks in current behavior (Ref 53, 54). Corrosion of conventional amalgams in Ringer's or 1% NaCl generates products that are morphologically similar to those from retrieved amalgams after intraoral use (Ref 98, 99).

A comparison of the tarnishing of three gold alloys, both *in vivo* and *in vitro,* indicated that the cyclic immersions in a 5% Na_2S-air environment predicted with considerable reliability the relative susceptibility for the alloys to tarnish (Ref 100). The tarnishing of 81 Au-Ag-Cu-Pd alloys also indicated accelerated laboratory exposures in Na_2S solution simulated *in vivo* use (Ref 101). The *in vivo* and *in vitro* (Na_2S solutions) tarnishing of gold alloys in Na_2S solutions has shown the same microstructural constituents to be attacked (Ref 102, 103). Silver- and copper-rich lamellae were the constituents exhibiting sulfide deposits. Utilizing linear polarization, good agreement with calculated current densities was obtained between measurements whether performed *in vivo* (baboons) or *in vitro* with an artificial saliva for times up to 45 days (Ref 104). Differences that occurred between *in vivo* and *in vitro* (0.1% NaCl) tarnish measurements as determined by colorimetry were attributed to the effects of abrasion and buildup of plaque that occurs on *in vivo* surfaces (Ref 105). Figure 18 shows the potential plaque buildup that can occur on a nonocclusal surface of a restoration.

Artificial Solutions in Corrosion and Tarnish Testing. As already indicated, the interior surfaces of restorations are exposed to the interstitial fluids and the exterior surfaces to the salivary fluids. A physiological saline solution, such as Ringer's, which contains a Cl^- concentration of about seven times larger than artificial saliva, is therefore more appropriate for simulating *in vivo* interior surfaces in laboratory testing methodologies. The O_2 content should be reduced to simulate *in vivo* levels in dentin. The use of Ringer's and even higher Cl^- concentrations is appropriate for the testing of corrosion that may occur within marginal crevices of restorations, because crevices can become chloride-rich and acidified. However, applying these results to the corrosion occurring on exterior surfaces of restorations may not be appropriate, even when considering that the increased Cl^- corrosion with Ringer's solution would be an even more stringent test and that the results would correspond to maximum corrosion conditions.

An artificial saliva is more appropriate for testing the corrosion of the exterior surfaces of restorations. The artificial saliva should take into account most of the species contained in saliva and not just a selected few that have been known to affect alloy corrosion. The artificial saliva should include the capabilities for generating organic films on the surfaces, even though their effects in isolated tests may prove unimportant. In order to simulate oral environmental conditions for the tarnishing of the exterior surfaces of restorations, an artificial saliva incorporating sulfide is appropriate. Even though the normal sulfide concentrations contained in saliva are within low ranges, accumulations of sulfide can occur along and within crevices to justify the use of higher than normal concentrations. However, the sulfur peak intensities detected with secondary ion mass spectroscopy (SIMS) on alloy surfaces exposed to low levels of sulfide solutions were similar to those from solutions containing higher sulfide concentrations. However, the alloy surface color changes responded more to higher sulfide concentrations.

Classification and Characterization of Dental Alloys

As indicated in the introduction to this chapter, a wide range of dental alloys exists. This section reviews the following types of alloys available for dental applications:

- Direct filling alloys
- Crown and bridge alloys
- Partial denture alloys
- Porcelain fused to metal alloys
- Wrought wire alloys
- Soldering alloys
- Implant alloys

The effects of composition and microstructure on the corrosion of each alloy group is discussed. Additional information on tarnishing and corrosion behavior of these alloys is discussed in the section "Tarnishing and Corrosion under Simulated or Accelerated Conditions," which immediately follows in this chapter.

Direct Filling Alloys

Amalgams. Two types of amalgams are used: low copper and high copper. The alloy particles of the low-copper type are all of the single-particle variety, whereas the high-copper type can also be of the dispersed (admixed) particle variety.

Amalgams are produced by combining mercury with alloy particles by a process referred to as trituration. About 42 to 50% Hg is initially triturated with the high-copper types, while increased quantities of mercury are used with the low-copper types. High-speed mechanical amalgamators achieve mixing in a matter of seconds. The plastic amalgam mass after trituration is inserted into the cavity by a process of condensation. This is accomplished by pressing small amalgam increments together until the entire filling is formed. For amalgams using excess mercury during trituration, the excess mercury is condensed to the top of the setting amalgam mass and scraped away. Dental amalgam alloys can become certified by complying with the requirements of American National Standards Institute (ANSI)/American Dental Association (ADA) Specification No. 1, which covers alloys for dental amalgams (Ref 106, 107). Table 5 presents compositions for a number of different amalgam alloys.

Low-Copper Amalgams. The alloy particles with the low-copper type are basically Ag_3Sn, the γ phase of the Ag-Sn binary system, even though smaller amounts of the β phase, a phase richer in silver, may be present. Copper can be added in amounts up to about 5 wt% and zinc up to 1 to 2%. About 2 to 4% Cu is soluble in Ag_3Sn, while the additional copper usu-

ally precipitates as Cu_3Sn, the ε phase of the copper-tin system, although amounts of Cu_6Sn_5, the η' phase, may also occur. The low-copper particles are mostly lathe cut irregular, although spherical atomized particles are also used. The amalgamation reaction for a low-copper amalgam is:

$$Ag_3Sn\text{-}Cu_3Sn\text{-}Zn + Hg \rightarrow$$
$$Ag_{22}SnHg_{27} + Sn_8Hg +$$
$$Ag_3Sn\text{-}Cu_3Sn\text{-}Zn \text{ (unreacted)} \quad \text{(Eq 6)}$$

In Eq 6, Ag_3Sn with Cu_3Sn and zinc react with mercury to form two major reaction products of $Ag_{22}SnHg_{27}$ (the γ phase of the Ag-Hg system with dissolved tin and referred to as the γ_1 amalgam phase) and Sn_8Hg (the γ phase of the Sn-Hg system and referred to as the γ_2 amalgam phase) (Ref 108). Unreacted Ag_3Sn with Cu_3Sn and zinc particles are held together in a γ_1 matrix with γ_2 interspersed within the matrix. Typical distributions of the phases range up to about 30 wt% for γ, 60 to 80% for γ_1, 5 to 30% for γ_2, and up to about 3% for ε (Ref 109). Very minimal η' may also form. Zinc is generally distributed uniformly throughout material. Porosities are in all amalgam structures. As high as 6 to 7 vol% occur with some systems (Ref

Table 5   Compositions of selected dental amalgam alloys

Alloy	Composition, wt%			
	Ag	Sn	Cu	Zn
Low-copper				
Cresilver	75.0	24.6	0.1	0.3
Pure Lab	72.0	26.0	1.0	1.0
New True Dentalloy	72.8	26.2	2.4	1.0
Microalloy	69.0	26.6	3.5	0.9
Lustralloy	68.0	26.0	5.1	0.9
High-copper-dispersed				
Optalloy II	69.8	20.0	9.7	0.5
Dispersalloy	69.3	18.1	11.6	1.0
Cluster	69.8	16.2	13.5	0.5
Phasealloy	62.0	18.5	18.5	1.0
Cupralloy	63.5	16.9	19.5	0.2
High-copper-single				
Tytin	59.5	27.6	12.2	0
Indiloy	60.0	22.0	13.0	(5.0 ln)
Valiant	49.5	30.0	20.0	(0.5 Pd)
Cupralloy ESP	41.0	32.5	26.5	0
Sybraloy	40.0	31.2	28.8	0

Source: Ref 67

110). Interconnection of the γ_2 phase throughout the bulk may also occur (Ref 111). Transformation of the γAg-Hg (γ_1 amalgam phase) to the βAg-Hg phase (β_1 amalgam phase) can also occur with aging (Ref 112). However, because of the dissolved tin in the γ_1 structure, stability is increased. Figure 20 presents the microstructure of a polished low-copper amalgam.

High-Copper Amalgams. The alloy particles with the high-copper dispersed-phase type are blends of conventional particles with basically spherical silver-copper eutectic particles in the proportion of about 3 to 1, respectively. The dispersed particles can be composed of a variety of silver-copper compositions, with other alloying elements, and combined in varying proportions with the conventional particles.

The alloy particles with the single-particle high copper are compositions that can contain up to 30% Cu and more. The particles are mostly atomized into spherical shape.

The setting reaction for high-copper dispersed-phase amalgam is:

$$Ag_3Sn\text{-}Cu_3\,Sn\text{-}Zn + Ag\text{-}Sn + Hg \rightarrow$$
$$Ag_{22}SnHg_{27} + Cu_6Sn_5 +$$
$$Ag_3Sn\text{-}Cu_3Sn\text{-}Zn\ (unreacted) +$$
$$Ag\text{-}Cu\ (unreacted) \qquad (Eq\ 7)$$

and for high-copper single-particle amalgam is:

$$Ag_3Sn\text{-}Cu_3Sn\text{-}Zn \rightarrow$$
$$Ag_{22}SnHg_{27} + Cu_6Sn_5 +$$
$$Ag_3Sn\text{-}Cu_3Sn\text{-}Zn\ (unreacted) \qquad (Eq\ 8)$$

For dispersed-phase amalgam, γ initially reacts with mercury to form γ_1 and γ_2 phases, as with the low-copper amalgam. However, an additional reaction occurs between γ_2 and the silver-copper particles to form η' and additional γ_1. The η' phase forms reaction rings around the dispersed particles as well as islands of reaction phase within γ_1 matrix. Figures 21 and 22 present the microstructure of a dispersed-phase amalgam and EDS x-ray mapping for silver, mercury, tin, and copper, respectively.

For single-particle high-copper amalgam, reaction of the initially formed γ_2 phase occurs with the ε phase of the original alloy particles instead of with a dispersed particle to form the η' phase again. The γ_1 phase is likely to become tin enriched. Reaction zones around the original alloy particles, as well as products within the matrix, occur.

Figure 23 shows the microstructure of a polished, etched, and slightly repolished high-copper single-particle amalgam that shows primarily the distribution of the η' phase. The elimination of γ_2 phase and the subsequent formation of η' phase are time dependent and are dependent on the amalgam system (Ref 113). For fast-reacting amalgams, formation of η' may be complete within hours, while for slower reacting systems, η' may continue to form for months. The single-particle high-copper amalgams contain higher percentages of the η' phase and lower percentages of the γ_2 phase, although all high-copper amalgams contain minimal γ_2 relative to conventional amalgams. Porosities

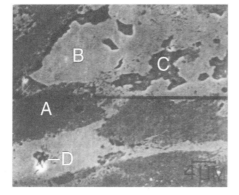

Fig. 20 SEM micrograph of polished, etched, and partially repolished low-copper amalgam (Minimax). A, γ; B, γ_1; C, γ_2; D, porosity

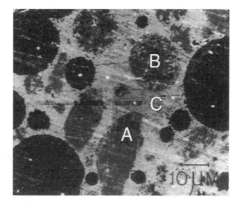

Fig. 21 SEM micrograph of polished, etched, and partially repolished high-copper dispersed-phase amalgam (Cupralloy). A, γ; B, Ag-Cu; C, γ_1. See also Fig. 22.

with the high-copper amalgams can be up to approximately 5 vol% and with a smaller size distribution than with the conventional type (Ref 110). The γ_1 to β_1 transformation can also occur to a limited extent. With the high-copper amalgams, both indium (5%) and palladium (0.5%) containing amalgams add specific characteristics to the amalgams and have gained limited use.

Crown and Bridge and Partial Denture Alloys

High-Nobility Alloys. Gold-base alloys for cast appliances have traditionally been based on the chemical compositional requirements of ANSI/ADA Specification No. 5, which covers gold dental casting alloys (Ref 114). This specification requires a minimum of 75 wt% Au plus platinum group metals. Alloys meeting the requirements of the specification became known as types I to IV (Table 6). This requirement has served to reject alloys that would have tarnished in the mouth. Some alloys that have complied with the compositional requirement were, however, found to tarnish in the mouth, while others with lower nobility were developed with very good tarnish resistance.

Composition of High-Nobility Alloys. The primary alloy elements of high-nobility alloys are gold, silver, and copper, along with additions of palladium, platinum, and zinc, as well as grain-refining elements, such as rubidium and iridium. Figure 24 shows the compositions

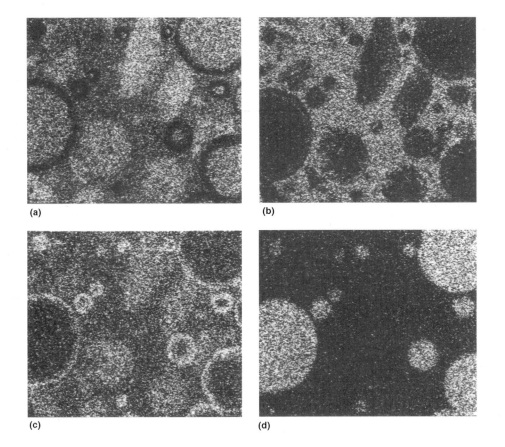

Fig. 22 Elemental maps obtained by energy-dispersive spectroscopy of the high-copper amalgam shown in Fig. 21. (a) EDS mapping for silver. (b) EDS mapping for mercury. (c) EDS mapping for tin. (d) EDS mapping for copper

for about 75 currently available dental casting alloys projected onto a pseudo (Au, Pd, Pt)-Ag-Cu ternary diagram. Actually, all of the compositions shown are referred to as low gold content alloys, which are covered in the following section. Also shown in Fig. 24, near the gold + platinum group metal apex, are dashed lines referring to the minimum nobility content of the four types (I to IV) of high-nobility alloys from the ANSI/ADA Specification No. 5. High-, medium-, and low-nobility alloys are currently used. High- and medium-nobility alloys refer to compositions with gold plus platinum group metal contents greater than 75 wt%, while the low-nobility alloys refer to compositions with less than 75 wt% Au plus platinum-group metals. Table 6 includes compositions for a number of high and low gold content alloys.

For the most part, properties of the high-nobility cast dental alloys follow similar patterns as those shown by the Au-Ag-Cu ternary alloys, although the additional alloying elements in the dental alloys have significant effects on properties. Because the high-nobility alloys have relatively small liquidus-solidus gaps, casting segregations, inhomogeneities, and coring effects are not major problems. Microstructurally, single-phase structures predominate because compositions fall within the single-phase region of the Au-Ag-Cu system. Grain refinement by the noble metal additions of ruthenium and iridium decreases grain sizes to 20 to 50 μm and increases strengths and elongations by about 30 and 15%, respectively (Ref 116).

Hardening Mechanisms of High-Nobility Alloys. Type III and IV cast alloys, which are

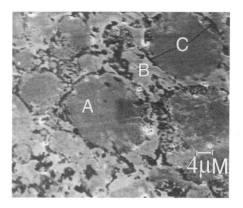

Fig. 23 SEM micrograph of polished, etched, and partially repolished high-copper amalgam (Sybraloy). A, alloy particles; B, γ_1; C, η

Table 6 Compositions of noble metal containing crown and bridge alloys

Alloy	Type	Nobility		Composition, wt%				
		at.%	wt%	Au	Pt	Pd	Ag	Cu + Zn
22K	I	83.1	91.7	91.7	...	—	5.6	2.7
NeyOro A-A	I	73.9	85.0	81.0	...	4.0	12.0	3.0
NeyOro A-1	II	64.3	80.0	78.0	...	2.0	13.0	7.0
NeyOro B-2	III	60.6	78.0	74.0	...	4.0	12.0	10.0
NeyOro G-3	IV	57.3	76.0	69.0	3.0	4.0	12.0	12.0
NeyOro No. 5	IV	48.2	68.0	64.0	2.0	2.0	19.0	13.0
NeyOro B-20	IV	47.3	65.0	62.0	...	3.0	26.0	9.0
Densilay	III	46.6	64.0	60.0	...	4.0	27.0	9.0
Sterngold 20	III	45.1	63.5	59.5	...	4.0	25.0	11.5
NeyOro CB	III	43.8	63.0	59.0	...	4.0	23.0	14.0
Midigold	III	34.6	52.0	48.5	...	3.5	35.0	13.0
Tiffany	IV	34.1	54.0	50.0	...	4.0	25.0	21.0
Pentron 20	III	32.2	40.0	20.0	...	20.0	40.0	20.0 ln + Zn
Sunrise	III	30.8	46.0	39.0	1.0	6.0	41.0	13.0
Paliney CB	III	30.5	39.0	15.0	1.0	23.0	44.0	17.0
Duallor	III	30.4	45.9	40.0	...	5.9	40.5	13.6
Neycast III	III	29.9	52.0	42.0	2.0	8.0	9.0	39.0
Albacast	III	24.4	25.0	...	...	25.0	70.0	5.0
Miracast	III	24.1	46.0	41.0	1.0	4.0	9.0	45.0
Ney 76	III	22.7	25.0	...	...	25.0	59.0	16.0
Econocast	III	18.3	36.0	26.0	...	10.0	...	64.0
Salivan	III	8.2	8.0	...	...	8.0	70.0	22.0 ln

Source: Ref 115

used for restorations subjected to high biting stresses, can be hardened by heat treatment. The primary hardening mechanism in gold dental alloys is by disorder-order superlattice transformations of the silver-copper system. The ordered domains of the silver-copper binary system also extend into the ternary phase Au-Ag-Cu regions. Typical heat treatment times and temperatures are 15 to 30 min at 350 to 375 °C (660 to 705 °F). Often, it is adequate to bench cool the casting in the investment after casting to gain hardness. Because of the complexity of the dental gold alloy compositions, the exact hardening mechanisms depend on the particular composition of the alloys. Table 7 presents a schematic of the age-hardening mechanisms and related microstructures occurring in gold dental alloys. Included are representations for high-gold alloys (HG), low-gold alloys (LG), Au-Ag-Pd-base alloys (GSP), and 18 karat and 14 karat gold alloys. Five types of phase transformations are found (Ref 117):

- The formation of the AuCu(I) ordered platelets and twinning characterized by a stair-step fashion
- The formation of the AuCu (II) superlattice with periodic antiphase domain structure
- The precipitation of the PdCu superlattice with face-centered tetragonal (fct) structure analogous to the AuCu(I)
- Spinodal decomposition giving rise to a modulated structure
- The formation of the lamellae structure developed from grain boundaries by discontinuous precipitation

Low-Nobility Alloys. Ever since the increases in the gold prices have taken place,

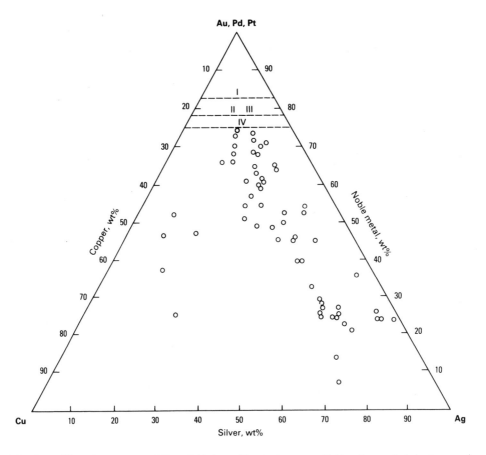

Fig. 24 Compositions of some commercially available low-gold-content crown and bridge alloys projected onto a pseudo noble metal (Au, Pt, Pd)-Ag-Cu ternary phase diagram. Also shown near the noble metal apex are minimum noble metal contents for types I, II and III, and IV conventional alloys required by ANSI/ADA Specification No. 5.

Table 7   Hardening mechanisms for some dental alloys

The hatched areas represent the hardness peaks on aging. (9/5) °C + 32 °F.

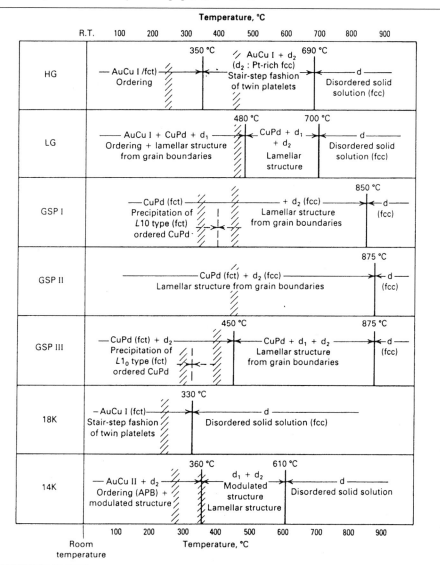

	Composition, wt%				
Alloy	Au	Pt	Pd	Ag	Cu
HG	68	11	6	6	9
LG	30	. . .	22	29	18
GSP-I	20.0	. . .	25.2	44.9	9.9
GSP-II	12.0	. . .	28.0	48.8	11.2
GSP-III	10.0	. . .	25.4	50.0	12.8
18K	75.0	. . .	. . .	8.7	16.3
14K	58.3	. . .	. . .	14.6	27.1

Source: Ref 117

new economy golds with lower gold contents have been introduced and have become popular. Figure 25 shows the trends in sales of dental casting alloys in the United States from 1976 to 1981. In a more recent survey of 488 dental laboratories, 46.5% of the responses indicated that only 0 to 25% of the crown and bridge alloys that they processed contained gold. Only 27.9% responded that 51% or more of their alloys contained gold (Ref 119).

Compositions of Low-Nobility Alloys. Low-noble metal alloys comprise a wide variety of compositions (Table 6). Gold-, palladium-, silver-, and copper-base alloys are used. Platinum and zinc contents are usually held to several weight percent maximum, if present. Microstructurally, the low gold content casting alloys are complex, and examination of phase diagrams of either the Au-Ag-Cu or Ag-Pd-Cu ternary systems indicates that the liquidus-solidus gaps between the various phases can be large (Ref 116). Therefore, coring and casting segregations occur upon solidification during casting. The alloys are characterized by dendritic structures combined with additional phases located within interdendritic positions. Both silver- and copper-rich segregations occur. The presence of gold, platinum, zinc, and other alloying elements further complicates the structures.

The addition of palladium and zinc to the Au-Ag-Cu alloy systems makes heat treatments to single-phase structures difficult. In silver-rich phases, the solubility limit for palladium and zinc is only about 1 to 2% at 500 °C (930 °F), while for copper-rich phases, solubilities are much higher—of the order of 10%. Therefore, precipitation of palladium- and zinc-rich phases occurs. Differences also occur in the gold contents between the phases with the copper-rich phases having the higher contents (Ref 120).

Silver-palladium-base alloys with additions of copper, gold, and zinc are also complex and contain multiple phases. Microstructurally, these alloys are characterized by silver-rich matrices interspersed with Pd-Cu-Zn enriched compounds. As many as three different Pd-Cu-Zn compounds have been detected in one alloy system. The Pd-Cu-Zn compounds are actually composed of two face-centered cubic (fcc) phases in addition to a body-centered cubic (bcc) $PdCu_xZn_x-1$ phase. In addition, the silver-rich matrixes are normally cored with silver-enriched dendritic arms and copper segregations in the interdendritic areas (Ref 121).

The hardening mechanisms associated with the low-nobility alloys are shown in Table 7. In addition to the gold-copper disorder-order transformations, ordering due to the palladium-copper superlattices is also usually involved because of replacement of some of the gold by palladium.

Silver-indium alloys with small additions of palladium or gold have also been used for crown and bridge applications. Figure 26 presents microstructures for a number of low-gold alloys.

Base Metal Alloys. Most of the base metal alloys for all metal cast crowns and bridges are composed of nickel-chromium alloys, although stainless steels are also used, particularly outside of the United States. Nickel-chromium alloys are also used for the construction of partial dentures. However, cobalt-chromium alloys far exceed any other alloy for use in this application. Titanium alloys are also being developed for dental applications. Table 8 presents the compositions for a number of base metal alloys intended for crown and bridge, partial denture, porcelain fused to metal, and implant applications.

Nickel-Chromium Alloys. The primary alloying element with the nickel-base alloys is chromium between about 10 and 20 wt%. Molybdenum up to about 10%; manganese and aluminum up to about 4% each; and silicon, beryllium, copper, and iron up to several percent each can also be added. The carbon con-

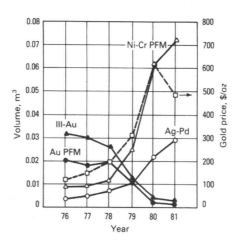

Fig. 25 Trends in alloy use along with the market price of gold. Source: Ref 118

tents range between about 0.05 and 0.4%. Elements such as gallium, titanium, niobium, tin, and cobalt can also be added. Because of differences in properties required for crown and bridge applications versus partial denture applications, minor modifications in compositions occur between nickel-chromium alloys intended for the two applications. This is reflected by the fact that crown and bridge nickel-chromium alloys contain higher percentages of iron, very minimal or no aluminum and carbon, and copper additions (Ref 131).

Chromium and molybdenum are added for corrosion resistance. In order to be effective, these elements must not be concentrated along grain boundaries. Chromium contents below about 10% deplete the interior of the grains leading to corrosion. Molybdenum protects

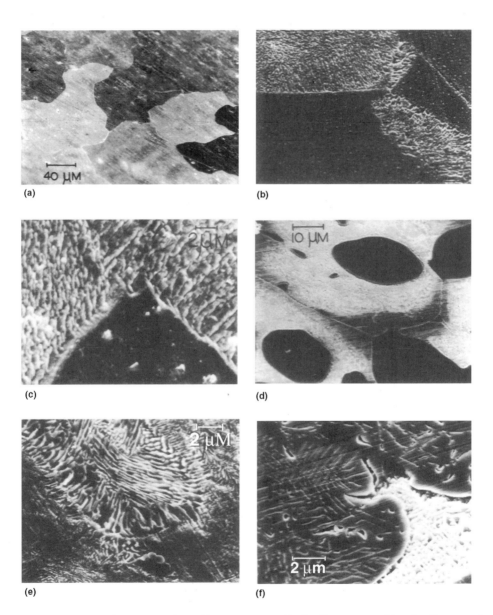

Fig. 26 SEM micrographs of etched as-cast low-gold-content crown and bridge alloys. (a) Sterngold 20. (b) Tiffany. (c) Midas. (d) Pentron 20. (e) Sunrise. (f) Econocast. See Table 6 for chemical compositions of these alloys.

against concentration cell corrosion, such as pitting and crevice corrosion, and is also a solid-solution hardener. Manganese and silicon are reducing agents, while aluminum also improves corrosion resistance and improves strength through its formation of intermetallic compounds with nickel. Silicon, like beryllium and gallium, lowers the melting temperature. Beryllium is also a solid-solution hardener and improves castability. Niobium, like molybdenum and iron, affects the coefficient of thermal expansion. Gallium is a stabilizer and improves corrosion resistance. The oxide-forming elements and the elements promoting good bond strength to porcelain are discussed in the section "Porcelain Fused to Metal Alloys" in this chapter.

Although the compositions for many of these alloys are similar, differences occur with regard to microstructure and properties. In comparing the microstructures of four different commercial nickel-chromium alloys, it was noted that one of the alloys had thin, elongated carbides

and intragranular precipitates adjacent to grain boundaries. A second alloy showed discontinuous spherical carbides, the third showed a continuous grain-boundary phase and cored dendrites, and the fourth showed a dendritic precipitate (Ref 132). In another alloy, the dark interdendritic carbides changed to a lamellar pattern at certain sites and were surrounded by dispersed carbide particles and the δ' phase of Ni_3Al (Ref 133). Heat treatments were shown to have drastic effects on the microstructures of several as-cast nickel-chromium alloys (Ref 134).

Cobalt-Chromium Alloys. The primary alloying element with the cobalt-base alloys is chromium between about 20 to 30%. Molybdenum is also present in amounts up to about 10%; small additions of elements such as silicon, manganese, iron, and nickel are sometimes also present. The carbon contents usually range between about 0.05 and 0.4% (Ref 131). This composition forms the basis for two additional generalized compositions. The first includes a

Table 8 Compositions of base metal wires, crown and bridge, porcelain fused to metal, partial denture, and implant alloys

Name	Co	Ni	Cr	Mo	Fe	Si	Mn	Cu	Al	C	Other	Ref
Wires												
18-8 Stainless steel	...	8–10	17–19	...	bal	...	2	...	...	0.08–0.2	...	122
Elgiloy	40	15	20	7	bal	...	2	...	...	0.15	...	122
Nitinol	1.4	48.6	...	...	...	...	...	...	...	...	50 Ti	123
β-titanium	...	...	...	11.5	...	...	...	...	...	...	bal Ti	124
Crown and bridge												
Howmedica III	0.3	67.5	19.7	4.2	0.1	3.0	1.2	1.8	...	0.1	2 Sn	125
Gemini II	...	79.9	12.4	2.0	0.1	0.1	0.1	0.1	2.8	0.2	2.1 Be	125
Dentillium	8.0	6.0	28.5	2.5	46.0	...	...	...	...	...	...	126
MS	...	4.7	...	...	3.0	...	0.7	71.8	19.8	...	...	68
Porcelain fused to metal												
Ceramalloy	0.01	69.9	19.9	5.6	0.1	1.0	0.01	...	...	0.2	2.9 B	125
Wiron S	0.02	70.6	15.7	4.5	0.2	1.5	3.2	...	3.8	0.1	...	125
Ultratek	+	81.0	11.4	2.0	...	...	0.02	+	2.2	...	Be	127
Partial denture												
Vitallium	62.5	...	30.0	5.0	1.0	0.5	0.5	...	...	0.5	...	126
Platinore	60.7	2.7	26.7	5.8	2.6	0.6	0.5	...	...	0.3	0.3 W, 0.1 Pt	126
Nobillium	62.0	...	32.0	5.0	...	0.35	...	0.04	...	0.35	0.05 Ga	128
Implant(a)												
Vitallium	61.1	0.3	31.6	4.4	0.6	0.6	0.7	...	...	...	...	129
Stellite 25	49.8	10.0	20.0	...	3.0	...	...	...	...	0.15	15 W	130
MP35N	35.0	35.0	20.0	10.0	...	...	...	...	...	...	...	130
Ticonium	15.4	54.3	24.6	4.3	0.7	0.5	0.03	0.03	0.02	...	...	129

(a) Titanium and titanium alloys also used. See text for details.

group of alloys that has been developed from the above basic composition, but with each modified by the addition of one or more elements in order to obtain a particular range of properties (Ref 135). Some of these modifying elements include gallium, zirconium, boron, tungsten, niobium, tantalum, and titanium.

The second generalized composition includes replacement-type alloys, with a major portion of the cobalt replaced by nickel and/or iron. The resulting composition is a cross between cobalt-base alloys and stainless steels. The effects of the individual elements on the properties of the alloys are similar to those already discussed for the nickel-chromium alloys. The alloys are hardened primarily by carbide formation. Therefore, the carbon content is of primary importance.

A number of carbides, including MC, M_6C, M_7C_3, and $M_{23}C_6$, have been detected in dental cobalt-chromium alloys (Ref 136). Solid-solution strengthening also occurs, as well as intermetallic compound formation strengthening, with a number of the modified alloy types. Certified alloys for partial dentures must contain a minimum cobalt-chromium-nickel content of 85% with a minimum of 20% Cr as required by ANSI/ADA Specification No. 14 for dental base metal casting alloys (Ref 137).

Microstructurally, the cobalt-chromium alloys are typified by a cored austenitic solid-solution matrix interspersed with isolated carbides, as shown in Fig. 27. However, depending on composition, the microstructures can vary considerably. In comparing the microstructures of a number of different cobalt-chromium alloys, the unmodified alloys with the basic composition given above exhibited large grains, with both large and small carbides being, respectively, either randomly dispersed or precipitated along grain boundaries (Ref 135). For the modified alloys containing additional alloying elements, the grain sizes were smaller than for the unmodified materials, with the carbides dispersed within the grains rather than being precipitated along grain boundaries.

The microstructures for modified cobalt-chromium alloys were analyzed in greater detail (Ref 138). For one typical alloy, the underlying matrix had the highest cobalt concentration with lowest chromium and molybdenum concentrations. The numerous continuous precipitates located along grain boundaries were moderately high in cobalt and low in chromium and molybdenum. The dark areas within the grain interiors contained high carbon, moderately high chromium and molybdenum, and low cobalt. Dispersed precipitates located within the matrix had high chromium and molybdenum contents and low cobalt.

An extensive project was undertaken regarding the development of a new dental superalloy system (Ref 139). The outcome of the project indicated that a cobalt-base alloy with desirable properties for dental applications could be made from a 40Co-30Ni-30Cr matrix. The alloy is strengthened by the precipitation of coherent intermetallic compounds of tantalum. Alloys that are stronger and more ductile than conventional dental alloys were obtainable. The results were reinvestigated, and it was again concluded that tantalum does improve the properties somewhat (Ref 140).

Stainless Steel Alloys. Some stainless steels are available for crown and bridge applications. One example is the alloy Dentillium, listed in Table 8. This alloy, as well as its modified version for partial denture applications, is an iron-base composition with 24 to 28% Cr, 6 to 8% Co, 4 to 6% Ni, and 2.5% Mo. Microstructurally, two phases exist (Ref 138). The

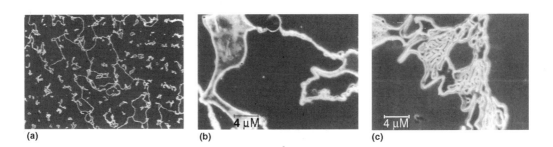

(a)   (b) 4 µM   (c) 4 µM

Fig. 27 SEM micrographs of etched cobalt-chromium partial denture alloys. (a) and (b) Neoloy. (c) Nobillium

matrix is high in chromium, molybdenum, iron, and cobalt and is low in nickel, but the precipitates are high in nickel and reduced in chromium, molybdenum, iron, and cobalt. Stainless steel preformed crowns are also occasionally used for temporary restorations.

Titanium-Base Alloys. Cast titanium alloys have shown potential for crown and bridge and partial denture applications, as well as for porcelain bonding. Because titanium alloys have high melting temperatures, casting of these alloys has not been possible until recently in the dental laboratory. The introduction of a lower-melting titanium alloy has made this requirement achievable (Ref 141). The first alloy to be successfully cast had a composition of 82Ti-13Cu-4.5Ni with a melting temperature of 1330 °C (2426 °F). The introduction of an argon/electric arc vertical centrifugal casting machine and a vacuum-argon electric arc pressure casting machine made the casting of the higher melting point titanium alloys also achievable. Pure titanium and Ti-6Al-4V have been successfully cast by these latter methods (Ref 142).

Copper-Aluminum Alloys. The copper-aluminum restorative alloys have elicited renewed interest because of their similarity in appearance to the yellow gold alloys and because of the volatility of gold prices. The compositions include copper base, with about 10 to 20% Al, and up to approximately 10% iron-manganese nickel (Table 8). The as-cast etched structures are dendritic.

Alloy Color. Color is a surface characteristic that is related to alloy composition. Although color by itself has no affect on biocompatibility and the properties of the alloy, it has become equated with quality for many people, including some professionals. Alloy color remains an important issue. The white golds are held by many to be inferior to the yellow golds. The significance of yellow color as an indicator of alloy quality is so strong that a number of nonnoble yellow alloys, such as copper-aluminum, that resemble gold alloys in appearance and lack tarnish resistance have become available.

Yellowness in dental gold alloys is imparted by the gold and copper. Absence of yellowness is no assurance that the alloy is lacking gold or copper content. Color can be a misleading indicator of composition. For example, some dental gold alloys for porcelain fused to metal restorations contain more than 80% Au, yet yellowness is absent because of the strong whitening effect of palladium and platinum. Detailed information on alloy color and the characterization of dental alloys by colorimetry can be found in Ref 105 and 143 to 149.

Factors Related to Casting. Dental alloys must be cast into thin sections and intricate shapes in order to produce the margins and curvatures on restorations and to provide an accurately fitting casting. The castability of dental alloys is evaluated by the ability to be cast into shapes, such as wedges, spirals, rods of various shapes, and mesh grids of various sizes. The casting accuracy is usually evaluated by the degree of fit a finished casting possesses with a master die.

Many factors determine the castability of alloys. Some of these include the casting temperature and surface tension of the molten alloy, as well as many variables associated with the casting technique, some of which include wax pattern preparation, position of the pattern in the casting ring, techniques used in alloy heating, and centrifugal casting force. Some factors affecting casting accuracy include the thermal contraction of the alloy as a result of going from liquid to room temperature, the effectiveness of investment material to compensate for the thermal contraction of the alloy, anisotropic contractions, and the roughness of the casting.

There are indications that the base metal castings produce inferior fits for crown and bridge uses as compared to castings made from conventional gold alloys (Ref 150). Low-gold alloys with about 50% Au generated fits that were satisfactory. Part of the problem with the base metal alloys may be the use of casting techniques that were developed for the gold alloys.

Casting porosity is another important factor in the casting process. Although casting technique variables affect porosity contents, alloy composition can also affect porosity. One way in which composition affects porosity is the generation of internal shrinkage pores between microstructural phases in complex multiphase alloys. This microporosity weakens alloys, makes finishing and polishing more difficult, and is a prime factor in tarnishing. Palladium in alloys is susceptible to occluding gases from the melt. Therefore, palladium-containing alloys have the potential for becoming affected mechanically through embrittlement.

Porcelain Fused to Metal Alloys

Stringent demands are placed on the alloy system meant to be used as a substrate for the baking on or firing of a porcelain veneer. The thermal expansion coefficients of alloy and porcelain must be matched so that the porcelain will not crack and break away from the alloy as the temperature is cooled from firing temperature to room temperature. Thermal expansion coefficients of porcelains are in the range of 14×10^{-6} to 15×10^{-6} in./in. °C. Selection of an alloy with a slightly larger coefficient by about 0.05% is recommended so that the alloy will be under slight compression.

The alloy must be high melting so that it can withstand the firing temperatures involved with the porcelain. However, the temperature must not be excessively high so that conventional dental equipment can still be used. A temperature of 1300 to 1350 °C (2370 to 2460 °F) is about maximum. The porcelain firing procedures require an alloy with high hardness, strength, and modulus so that thin sections of the alloy substrate can support the porcelain, especially at the firing temperatures.

High mechanical properties are also required for resisting sag of long span bridge unit assemblies during firing. The alloy should also have the ability to absorb the thermal contraction stresses due to any mismatch in expansion coefficients as well as occlusal stresses without plastic deformation. Therefore, too high of a modulus for a material with an insufficient yield strength is contraindicated, although too high of an elastic deformation is also contraindicated. High bond strengths are required so that the porcelain veneers remain attached to the alloy. The alloy system must also be chemically compatible with the porcelain. Alloying elements must not discolor porcelain, yet must have tarnish and corrosion resistance to the fluids in the oral environment. The compositions for a number of porcelain fused to metal (PFM) alloys are presented in Table 9.

In order to promote and form high bond strengths between porcelain and alloy, the alloy must have the ability to form soluble oxides that are compatible with the porcelain. At the firing temperature, the porcelain should spread or wet the surface of the alloy. Therefore, both mechanical and chemical interactions are involved in this process. In order to promote chemical interactions, specific oxide-forming elements, such as tin, indium, or gallium, are added to the alloy in low concentrations. The addition of iron, nickel, cobalt, copper, and zinc provide the means for hardening.

Alloy color with the PFM alloys is not as demanding as with the crown and bridge alloys because the alloy is masked by the porcelain veneer. However, the margins between metal and porcelain can still be seen. This consideration still makes the yellow alloys more aesthetically pleasing, especially for anterior restorations. White alloys have the effect of producing a grayish color.

The fabrication of the PFM restoration consists of a complex set of processes. After casting, the alloy substrate is subjected to a preoxidation heat treatment to achieve the optimal surface oxides that are important for porcelain bonding. As many as three or more different porcelain firings follow. These include a thin opaque layer adjacent to the alloy, followed by body porcelain layers, including both dentin and enamel porcelain buildups. The opaque layer should mask the color of the alloy from interfering with the appearance of the porcelain. The body porcelain layers build up the restoration to the desired occlusion. The alloy-porcelain systems are slowly cooled from firing temperatures

Table 9   Compositions of noble metal porcelain fused to metal alloys

Alloy	Composition, wt%					Ref
	Au	Pt	Pd	Ag	Other	
Ceramco	87.5	4.2	6.7	0.9	0.3Fe, 0.4Sn	151
Degudent	84.8	7.9	4.6	1.3	1.3In, 0.1Ir	152
Vivostar	54.2	. . .	25.4	15.7	4.6Sn	153
Cameo	51.4	. . .	29.5	12.1	6.8In	153
P-D	59.4	. . .	36.4	. . .	4.0Ga	154
P-G	19.9	0.9	39.0	35.9	3Ni, 1.2Ga	154
JP92	. . .	. . .	60.5	32.0	7.5In	155
A 36	1.8	. . .	77.8	. . .	10.4Ga, 10Cu	156
Orion Star	. . .	. . .	78.0	. . .	In, Sn, Cu, Ga, Co	. . .

to accommodate dimensional changes occurring in both alloy and porcelain. Therefore, the alloy substrates are subjected to a number of temperature cycles during processing that affect their microstructure and properties. The slow cooling cycles also permit the formation of the compounds important for hardening of alloys.

Noble Metal PFM Alloys. The evolution of alloys for the PFM restoration has generated at least four different noble alloy systems. These are classified as Au-Pt-Pd, Au-Pd with and without silver, Ag-Pd, and high-palladium content alloys (Ref 116, 140, 157, 158).

Gold-Platinum-Palladium PFM Alloys. The compositions of alloys included within this group are in the range of 80 to 90% Au, 5 to 15% Pt, 0 to 10% Pd, and 0 to 5% Ag, along with about 1% each of tin and indium. Other additions may include up to about 1% each of iron, cobalt, zinc, and copper. Platinum and palladium additions increase melting temperature and decrease thermal expansion coefficients, with platinum having the added effect of hardening the alloy. Iron is the principal hardening agent. Iron promotes the formation of an ordered iron-platinum type intermetallic phase that forms between 850 and 1050 °C (1560 and 1920 °F) upon cooling from the firing temperature (Ref 116). The ordered phase is finely dispersed throughout matrix. Iron, along with tin and indium, promotes bonding to porcelain by diffusing into the porcelain up to about 60 μm at the firing temperature. Tin and indium also promote solid-solution strengthening. Alloys within this group range in color from light yellow to yellow.

Even though these alloys have many advantages, their high cost and low sag resistances have necessitated the development of additional alloy systems. Unless they are used in thick sections, for example, 3×3 mm (0.12×0.12 in.), plastic deformation of long spans will occur during firing.

Gold-Palladium and Gold-Palladium-Silver PFM Alloys. Gold-palladium with and without silver alloys were developed as alternatives to the costly Au-Pt-Pd alloys. The Au-Pd-Ag system was one of the first alternative systems. Up to 15% Ag and 30% Pd replaced all of the platinum and a large fraction of the gold from the Au-Pt-Pd system, which resulted in substantial cost savings. The Au-Pd-Ag alloys possessed better mechanical properties for the PFM restoration. Because gold-palladium, gold-silver, and palladium-silver are all solid-solution alloys, the ternary Au-Pd-Ag system also forms a series of solid-solution alloys over the entire compositional ranges. Therefore, the matrices of the Au-Pd-Ag dental alloys are single phase. Up to 5% Sn is added, which hardens the alloy by forming compounds with palladium that are dispersed throughout matrix. Tin is also an oxide former and bonding agent with porcelain. Because platinum was avoided, there was no need to incorporate iron for hardening. Their shortcoming was the ability of silver from the alloy to vaporize, diffuse, and combine with the porcelain at the firing temperature, thus inducing color changes, mostly greenish, along the alloy-porcelain margin. Sodium-containing porcelains were more susceptible to this color change.

The development of the silver-free gold-palladium alloys eliminated the discoloration of the porcelain. Their compositions cover a wide range: 50 to 85% Au, 10 to 40% Pd, 0 to 5% Sn, and 0 to 5% In, along with possible additions from zinc, gallium, and other elements. The alloy matrix is based on the gold-palladium binary system, which is of the solid-solution type. Hardening is due to Pd-(In, Sn, Ga, Zn) complexes that disperse throughout the matrix. Microstructurally, a fine network of gold-rich regions are entwined by second-phase particles of Pd-(Sn, In, Ga, and Zn). Their color is only a pale yellow, unlike some of the deeper yellow Au-Pt-Pd alloys. However, about a 30 to 40% cost savings is obtained. Their mechanical properties are superior, which means good sag resistance at the firing temperatures. The only disadvantage with these alloys is their lower thermal expansion coefficients when used with some of the higher-expanding porcelains.

Some newer gold-palladium alloys have up to 5% Ag, which is much lower than the 15% contents used with the original Au-Pd-Ag alloys. This results in better thermal expansion matches with porcelain and avoids the discoloration problem with porcelain because of the lower silver concentrations. The gold-palladium alloys have gained a large percentage of the PFM alloy market.

Palladium-Silver PFM Alloys. These alloys were developed out of the need to reduce the cost of the PFM restoration even more than from those fabricated from gold-palladium alloys. Compositions range from 50 to 60% Pd, 25 to 35% Ag, 5 to 10% Sn, 0 to 5% In, and up to 2% Zn. The silver and palladium contents are just about reversed in magnitude as compared to those compositions used with the silver-palladium crown and bridge alloys discussed earlier in this article.

The microstructures of the alloys are based on the palladium-silver solid-solution system. Instead of using copper to harden the alloys, hardening occurs through compounds formed between palladium and tin, indium, zinc, and others. Hardening rates are high, which indicates nondiffusional reactions. It is likely that hardening occurs by ordering processes that form by spinodal decomposition (Ref 116). Oxides are imparted to the alloy surface because of the oxide-forming ability of indium, tin, and zinc alloying additions. This promotes high bond strengths. The mechanical properties of the palladium-silver alloys, along with the high-palladium alloys discussed in the paragraphs that follow, are superior to those of any other system, excluding the nickel-chromium alloys. As with the Au-Pd-Ag alloys, the chief disadvantage is the ability of silver to discolor porcelains during firing. In order to overcome this problem, various methods have been used, including coupling agents composed of porcelains or colloidal gold.

High-Palladium PFM. These alloys represent the most recent developments in alloys for PFM restorations (Ref 159–164). Their compositions are 75 to 85% Pd with 0 to 15% Cu, 0 to 10% Ga, 0 to 8% In, 0 to 5% Co, 0 to 5% Sn, and 0 to 2% Au. The alloys are based on either the Pd-Cu-Ga or the Pd-Co-Ga ternary systems. Regardless of the high copper contents, these alloys do not induce porcelain discoloration and bonding problems. Many of these alloys have better workability than other types of PFM alloys, while retaining high hardnesses. The hardness is dependent on the formation of intermetallic compounds with palladium upon cooling from the firing temperature. The alloy forms strong bonds with porcelain because of the alloy oxidizer content. Oxides form with palladium and the alloying additives. However, palladium oxide (PdO) forms only during heating and cooling because of the relatively low decomposition temperature for the oxide. The oxide-forming ability of the added oxidizers is dependent on alloy composition, temperature, and time. Indium, gallium, and cobalt oxidize preferentially, while copper and tin show nonpreferential oxidation. Cobalt suppressed the oxida-

tion for copper and tin in one alloy system (Ref 160).

The palladium-gallium eutectic dominates the alloy systems. Additions of both indium and copper reduce the solid solubility of gallium so that the eutectic forms at lower gallium contents (Ref 154). Microstructurally, as-cast structures are dendritic, with moderate compositional variations occurring due to coring. The interdendritic regions contain higher amounts of alloying elements. For a Pd-Cu-Ga alloy, the interdendritic precipitates are fcc with the composition of $Pd_3Ga_xCu_{1-x}$ (Ref 164). Upon cooling below 500 °C (930 °F), an ordered fct structure forms rapidly. This lattice straining produces the high hardnesses and yield strengths characteristic of these materials.

Base metal PFM alloys are primarily composed of the nickel-chromium alloys. Cobalt-chromium alloys are also used, but they constitute only a very small percentage of base metal use for PFM. Titanium-base alloys are currently being developed for PFM usage.

The nickel-chromium PFM alloys are very similar, if not the same, as the compositions of the nickel-chromium alloys used for partial dentures, which are discussed in this article. One distinction in the compositions, however, is the absence of carbon with the PFM compositions (Ref 131). The microstructures for two alloy systems are presented in Fig. 28.

The mechanical properties of the nickel-chromium alloys are excellent for the PFM restoration. The high strengths, moduli, yield strengths, and hardnesses are used to advantage with PFM and partial dentures. Thinner alloy sections can be made from nickel-chromium alloys than from the noble metal alloys. The flexibilities of long span partial denture frameworks are only one-half those for the high gold-content alloys. Additionally, the sag resistances of the nickel-chromium alloys at the porcelain firing temperatures are superior to all of the noble metal alloys.

The bond strengths are seriously impaired by nonadherent or loosely attached oxides. A properly attached oxide is characterized by minute protrusions on the underside of the oxide layer at the alloy/oxide interface that extend into the alloy. For alloys containing additional microstructural phases, larger peg-shaped protrusions also occur on the underside of the oxide layer, improving oxide adherence (Ref 165). The oxide layer on nickel-chromium alloys contains nickel oxide (NiO) on the exterior of the oxide scale, chromium oxide (Cr_2O_3) at the interior covering the alloy, and nickel-chromium oxide ($NiCr_2O_4$) in between. The relative amounts of the oxides depend on the chromium concentration and alloying elements in the alloy, as well as temperature, time of oxidation, and pO_2 in atmosphere.

The bond strengths between alloy and porcelain are significantly affected by minor alloying elements. The additional alloying elements of molybdenum, aluminum, silicon, boron, titanium, beryllium, and manganese also form oxides of their own. An aluminum content of 5% is necessary for aluminum oxide (Al_2O_3) to form, while 3% Si is required to form silicon dioxide (SiO_2), which increases in concentration as the alloy/oxide interface is approached. Manganese forms manganese oxide (MnO) and manganese chromite ($MnCr_2O_4$), and these are mainly concentrated at the outermost part of the oxide. Even though molybdenum oxide (MoO) volatilizes above 600 °C (1110 °F), molybde-num is still found in the oxide layer close to the alloy/oxide interface with alloys containing more than 3% Mo. Beryllium, which improves the adherence of the oxide layer to the alloy, is also found concentrated near the alloy/oxide interface. Similarly, niobium is found in the oxide layer close to alloy. Tin does not diffuse throughout oxide (Ref 166).

The difficulties experienced with nickel-chromium alloys for dental applications have been at least partly related to their processing due to the use of casting techniques that had been well established for the lower-melting gold-base alloys. Because the nickel-chromium alloys melt between 1200 and 1400 °C (2190 and 2550 °F), as compared to the 850 to 1050 °C (1560 to 1922 °F) melting range for the gold-base alloys, additional casting shrinkages must be compensated for with the nickel-chromium alloys. This involves the use of phosphate or silicate-bonded investment materials as compared to the gypsum-bonded investments used with the gold-base alloys. Technique variables with

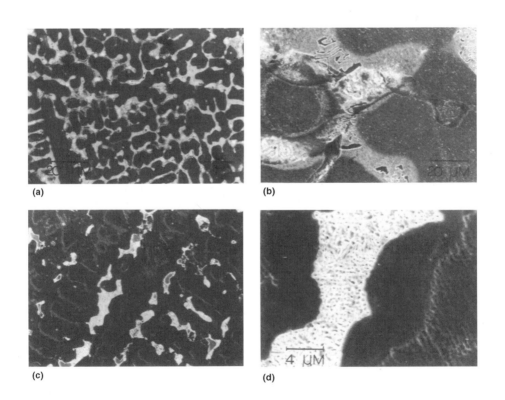

(a)

(b)

(c)

(d)

Fig. 28 SEM micrographs of etched nickel-chromium alloys for fusing with porcelain. (a) and (b) Ceramalloy. (c) and (d) Biobond

these higher-temperature investments are still being resolved. Also, the use of the gas-air torch for alloy melting, which is very popular in the dental field, cannot be used to melt nickel-chromium alloys.

Another disadvantage often cited with the harder nickel-chromium alloys as compared to the softer gold alloys is their increased finishing costs. This factor, though, should be more than offset by the decreased cost of the alloy. Even though casting accuracy may be improved with improvements in casting techniques, there may still be differences in castabilities between the different alloys. The ability to cast thin sections is a prime requirement with the dental technique.

Other PFM Alloy Systems. The compositions of cobalt-chromium alloys for porcelain fused to metal usually have nickel, tungsten, and molybdenum as major alloying elements. Tungsten and molybdenum are high-temperature strengtheners and therefore increase sag resistances. Tantalum and ruthenium can also be added in minor amounts. The carbon is also reduced or eliminated with PFM alloys (Ref 131). The carbon monoxide gases generated during firing of porcelain are likely to cause porosities in the interface and in porcelain. Carbon along the interface also interferes with porcelain wetting alloy during firing.

Alloy oxidation and alloy-porcelain compatibility must be better controlled in order for success to be achieved with porcelain fused to titanium alloy restorations. Titanium oxidations occurring at the currently used firing temperatures of about 1000 °C (1830 °F) must be decreased in order to achieve satisfactory alloy-porcelain bonding. The use of low firing temperatures has reduced alloy oxidations and porcelain-alloy concentrations. Newly formulated porcelains have been used with only about one-half the coefficient of thermal expansion and with firing temperatures as low as 550 °C (1020 °F) (Ref 167). Pure titanium and Ti-6Al-4V are candidate metal substrates for PFM restorations.

Wrought Alloys for Wires

Property Requirements with Orthodontic Biomechanics. Orthodontic wires (frequently used round sizes are 0.3 to 0.7 mm, or 0.012 to 0.028 in., in diameter) constitute a large percentage of the wrought alloys used in dentistry.

The wires currently in use include stainless steels, Co-Cr-Ni Elgiloy-type alloys, nickel-titanium Nitinol-type alloys, and β-titanium. The stainless steel and Elgiloy wires have been used extensively with conventional orthodontic biomechanics. That is, the ability to move teeth was based to a large extent on the stiffnesses of the wire appliances. Materials with high yield strength to modulus of elasticity ratios were required. The energy released from the wires during springback corresponded to areas on stress-strain curves with large slopes.

With the newer orthodontic biomechanics methodologies, however, materials with lower yield strength to modulus of elasticity ratios are desired. Here the nickel-titanium and β-titanium wires are used. The released energy under stress-strain curves with lower slopes can be large because of the greater deflections involved. The designs associated with the newer orthodontic approaches also permit greater energies to be released with time. Certified orthodontic wires comply with the property requirements of ANSI/ADA Specification No. 32, which covers base wires for orthodontics (Ref 168).

Gold-base wires are currently used on a very limited basis; in the past, gold-base wires were used more extensively. One application, however, still relies on gold-base wires. This is for clasps on partial denture frameworks and bridges. Because of their greater ductility, clasps fabricated from gold-base alloys permit adjustments to be made with less possibility for clasp breakage. One disadvantage with this application is the need to subject the soldered bridge assembly to a heat treatment operation. The soldering leaves the gold wires in a softened condition. For this reason, base metal wires with better ductility than the cobalt-chromium frameworks but requiring no follow-up heat treatments have been used (Ref 169). Except for cast Co-Cr-Mo implant alloys, all additional implant alloys, including Co-Cr-W, modified cobalt-chromium, and titanium and its alloys, are used in the wrought form and are covered in the section "Implant Alloys" in this chapter.

Stainless Steel and Elgiloy Wires. The stainless steels used are usually the austenitic 18-8 type, although precipitation-hardening type steels have also been used. The springback of the 18-8 wires can be improved by a stress-relief heat treatment. A 400 °C (750 °F) treatment for 10 min of the as-received drawn wires generates significant improvements in spring-back (Ref 170). The Elgiloy wires are of the modified cobalt-chromium type. In addition to cobalt and chromium, other major alloying elements include nickel and iron. Aluminum, silicon, gallium, and copper are not added to the Elgiloy wires, as with the PFM cobalt-chromium alloys, because bonding agents with porcelain are not needed. Mechanical properties are controlled primarily through the carbon additions, which affect carbide formation. Although the operator has some control over the mechanical properties of the cobalt-chromium wires through heat treatments, the Elgiloy wires are supplied in different temper designations from soft to semiresilient to resilient.

Nitinol and β-Titanium Wires. Nitinol alloys have attracted interest because of their shape memory effects. Nitinol wires can almost be bent back on themselves without taking a permanent set. Even greater deformations by as much as 1.6 times can be achieved with newer superelastic nickel-titanium alloys (Ref 171). The composition of Nitinol is primarily the intermetallic compound of NiTi. The alloy is tough, resilient, and has a low modulus of elasticity. The alloy does not respond to heat treatments except for the normal homogenizing softening treatments of as-cast alloys. Cobalt is added in order to obtain critical temperatures that are useful for the shape memory effect.

Alpha-titanium (hexagonal close-packed structure) is the stable form of titanium at room temperature. By adding alloying elements to the high-temperature form of β-titanium (bcc structure), the β phase can also exist at room temperature, but in the metastable condition. The β stabilizers include molybdenum, vanadium, cobalt, tantalum, manganese, iron, chromium, nickel, cobalt, and copper. Beta-titanium is strengthened by cold working or by precipitating the phase. A variety of heat treatments can be used to alter the properties of the wires (Ref 124).

Permanent magnets are used for the fixation of dentures, bridgework, and for corrective therapy by controlling the movement of teeth. Either the attractive or repulsive forces between magnets with opposite or the same polarities have been used to advantage. For example, the repulsive forces have been used to correct crossbite and to realign teeth.

The new generation of rare-earth magnets provides large magnetic forces per unit volume of material, unlike the Alnico and other previously used magnets. Disk-shaped magnets 5 to 10 mm (0.2 to 0.4 in.) in diameter and 2 mm (0.08 in.) thick that are embedded in the properly designed appliance will often provide the forces necessary in dental biomechanic treatments. Some compositions that have proved useful in dental treatment include samarium cobalt ($SmCo_5$, Sm_2Co_5) and neodymium-iron-boron ($Nd_2Fe_{17}B$).

Soldering Alloys

Composition and Applications. Gold-base and silver-base solder alloys are used for the joining of separate alloy components (Table 10). High fusing temperature base alloy solders are also used for the joining of nickel-chromium and other alloys. In many cases, the term brazing would be more appropriate, but the term is seldom used in dentistry. The gold-containing solders are used almost exclusively in bridgework because of their superior tarnish and corrosion resistance. The use of nonnoble metal containing silver-base solders is mainly limited to the joining of stainless steel and cobalt-chromium wires in orthodontic appliances because of the impermanence of the appliances.

The joining by soldering of small units to form a large one-piece partial denture is employed in some processing techniques. This is

Table 10 Compositions of selected dental solders

Type	Composition, wt%						
	Au	Pd	Ag	Cu	Sn	In	Zn
Silver	...	...	52.6	22.2	7.1	...	14.1
Gold	45.0	...	20.6	28.4	4.3	...	2.9
	63.0	2.7	19.0	8.6	...	6.5	...

done to prevent framework distortions that may occur with large one-piece castings. The salvaging of large, poorly fitting castings by sectioning, repositioning, and soldering the pieces together also takes place. Both pre- and postsoldering techniques are used with PFM restorations. These imply that the soldering is carried out either prior to or after the porcelain has been baked onto the alloy substrate. Therefore, presoldering uses high fusing temperature solders, while postsoldering uses lower fusing temperature solders.

Gold-base solders are most often rated according to their fineness, that is, the gold content in weight percent related to a proportional number of units contained in 1000. Conventional gold-base crown and bridge alloys are seldom soldered together with solders having less than a 600 to 650 fineness. The soldering of gold-base wire clasps to cobalt-chromium partial dentures is another application for the higher-fineness solders. However, with the use of the low gold content crown and bridge alloys, lower-fineness solders are used. The lower-fineness solders are also occasionally used to solder the cobalt-chromium Elgiloy wires. The gold-base solders usually do not contain platinum or palladium, which increases melting temperatures. The important requirement to be satisfied during soldering is that the solders melt and flow at temperatures below the melting ranges of the parts to be joined.

The compositions of gold-base solders are largely Au-Ag-Cu alloys to which amounts of zinc, tin, indium, and others have been added to control melting temperatures and flow during melting. The silver-base solders are basically Ag-Cu-Zn alloys to which smaller amounts of tin have been added. The higher-fusing solders to be used with the high-fusing alloys are usually specially formulated for a particular alloy composition, because not all alloys have good soldering characteristics.

Microstructure of Solder-Alloy Joints. The microstructural appearance of the gold alloy-solder joints provides information as to their quality. A thin, distinct, continuous demarcation between the solder alloy and the casting alloy should exist, indicating that the solder has flown freely over the surface and that no mutual diffusion between the alloys has occurred. The junction region should be free of isolated and demarcated domains, indicative of the formation of new alloy phases. Obviously, porosity is

to be avoided. However, microporosity among the phases in solder may be unavoidable. As with the cooling that occurs with all alloys, differences in the thermal expansion coefficient among phases can generate microporosity. The presence of a distinct layer of columnar dendrites within the solder starting at the solder/alloy interface and projecting into the solder bulk is assurance that there has been no tendency of the alloy surface to melt (Ref 172, 173). The solidified solder tends to match the grain size of the parent alloy by epitaxial nucleation of the solder by the casting alloy. The microstructural characteristics of low gold content casting alloys interfaced by soldering affect the microstructural characteristics of the solidified solder (Ref 172, 173).

Microstructurally, a silver-base solder is multiphasal. Both silver and copper-zinc rich areas occur, which is in contrast to some of the higher-fineness gold-base solders that are single phase.

Implant Alloys

Applications and Compositions. Dental implants, which are used for supporting and attaching crowns, bridges, and partial and full dentures, can be of the endosseous and subperiosteal types. The endosseous implants pass into or through the mandibular or maxillary arch bones, while the subperiosteal implants are positioned directly on top of or below the mandibular or maxillary bones, respectively. Endosseous implants are usually selected for size and type from implants already made, while the subperiosteal implants are usually custom made for the particular case. Therefore, both cast and wrought forms of implants are used. Commercially pure titanium and Ti-6Al-4V are the most commonly used implant materials. Cobalt-base castings are most often used for subperiosteal systems (i.e., implants that contact the exterior bone surfaces). Wrought cobalt alloys have also been utilized, but to a much lesser degree.

Cast versus Wrought Cobalt-Chromium Alloys. Castable cobalt-chromium alloys are similar to Vitallium and Haynes Stellite-21 alloys, while the wrought forms are similar to surgical Vitallium and Haynes Stellite-25 alloys. Table 8 includes compositions for some of these implant alloys. Two important distinctions exist between the cast and wrought forms (Ref 174). The casting alloy contains 5% Mo, while the wrought form contains 14 to 16% W. Molybdenum is added as a hardening agent, an oxide former, and to increase crevice and pitting corrosion resistance. Tungsten is added as a hardener and as an oxide former.

Because the wrought form can be either cold or hot worked, the alloy needs additional protection against deterioration during working. Carbides provide strengthening only up to 880 °C (1615 °F). Tungsten overcomes much of the loss in strength at higher temperatures by being a source of solid-solution strengthening above 1100 °C (2010 °F). The carbon content in the castable alloy is also higher than in the wrought form (0.35% to 0.05 to 0.15%). Carbide precipitations occur in the Co-Cr-Mo castable alloy, which presents a high resistance to wear. It is one of the materials of choice for applications involving moving parts.

Microstructurally, extreme differences exist between the cast and worked forms. The as-cast and annealed structures consist of distinct grains and grain boundaries interspersed with precipitated phases, similar to the micrographs shown in Fig. 27 for partial denture alloys. The cold-rolled, annealed, and hot-worked structures show a very fine grain structure oriented in the direction of working. For both structures, however, the matrix was fcc and contained carbide particles. The large chemical inhomogeneities across the surface of the alloys were indicated by the large changes in the x-ray intensities for cobalt, chromium, and molybdenum in traversing across the surfaces.

Modified cobalt-chromium alloys contain higher nickel contents. One wrought alloy included in this category is MP35N (35Co-35Ni-20Cr-10Mo). Microstructurally, the alloy takes the character of cobalt-chromium alloys. However, no carbides are formed because carbon has not been added to the alloy.

Porous Surfaces. Alloy powders of the same composition as the implants have been sintered onto the surfaces of the implants for generating bone ingrowth to obtain better retention between the implant and the bone. Examples of porous coated implants are shown in chapter 10, "Biomaterials for Dental Applications."

Tarnish and Corrosion under Simulated or Accelerated Conditions

Low-Copper Amalgams. The Sn_8Hg (γ_2) phase shown in Fig. 20 is electrochemically the most active phase in conventional amalgam. Upon exposure to an electrolyte, the tin oxide (SnO) in couple becomes operative. The formed SnO may or may not protect the γ_2 phase from further corrosion. Depending on environmental conditions, the tin from the γ_2 phase will either be protected by a film of SnO or consumed by additional corrosion reactions.

In the case of an artificial saliva, the γ_2-tin becomes protected. This is shown in Fig. 29 on the anodic polarization curve as the current peak at about –0.7 V versus SCE, which relates in potential to the SnO/Sn couple. With increasing potential, the film protects the amalgam, as shown by the presence of a limiting or passivating current. The film will remain passivating until the potential of another redox reaction is reached that is controlling and nonpassivating. This is the situation that occurs in Cl⁻ solution when the corrosion potential for the amalgam approaches and surpasses the redox potential for a reaction that produces $SnOCl \cdot H_2O$.

If this condition is satisfied, the SnO passivating film breaks down, exposing freely corroding γ_2-tin to the electrolyte. Nonprotective products of the form $SnOHCl \cdot H_2O$ precipitate. This is represented on the polarization curve in Fig. 29 as the sharp increase in current at about –0.1 V. Because the interconnection of the γ_2 phase, the interior γ_2 can also become corroded. Figure 30 shows the devastating effect that corrosion of the γ_2 phase has on the microstructure of a conventional amalgam, while Fig. 31 shows typical tin-containing products that precipitate on the surface.

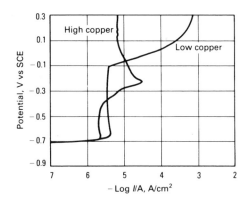

Fig. 29 Anodic polarization at 0.03 V/min of both low-copper (Microalloy) and high-copper (Sybraloy) amalgams in artificial saliva. Source: Ref 67

High-Copper Amalgams. Corrosion of high-copper amalgams by γ_2-phase corrosion will not occur because of its almost complete absence from the microstructure. Although possessing better corrosion resistance than the γ_2-phase, the $Cu_6Sn_5(\eta')$ phase will be the least-resistant phase in the microstructure (Fig. 21, 22). Upon exposure to solution, any corrodable tin within the material first forms a protective SnO film indicated on the anodic polarization curve in Fig. 29 as the small current peak at about –0.7 V. Upon attaining a steady-state corrosion potential in chloride solution, high-copper amalgam is likely to surpass redox poten-

tials for couples of $CuCl_2/Cu$, $Cu(OH)_2$, Cu_2O/Cu, and $CuCl_2 \cdot 3Cu(OH)_2/Cu$. Under these conditions, both soluble and insoluble corrosion products will form. This is indicated on the polarization curve as a small anodic current peak at about –0.25 V.

Microstructurally, if the copper from the η' phase becomes exhausted by corrosion, copper corrosion from the silver-copper and γ particles may also follow. Freed by copper corrosion, tin also becomes corroded. Corrosion of the γ_1-tin decreases the stability of the γ_1 phase, which is likely to be transformed into the β_1 phase. Unlike low-copper amalgam, the interior of high-copper amalgam is not likely to become affected by corrosion, because of the noninterconnection of any of the phases. Figure 32 shows a corroded high-copper dispersed-phase amalgam, emphasizing the reaction zones of the η' phase, the interior of the silver-copper particles, the γ particles, and the matrix.

Tarnish of Gold Alloys. Because tarnish is by definition the surface discoloration of a metallic material by the formation of a thin film of oxide or corrosion product, the quantification of dental alloy tarnish by assessing color changes on surfaces is most appropriate. By determining the color of an alloy before and after exposure to a test solution, the degree of discoloration can be obtained by quantitative colorimetry techniques, which are described in Ref 105 and 144 to 149. The use of quantitative colorimetry in conjunction with SIMS for determining the effects of alloy nobility (in atomic

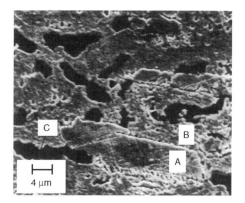

Fig. 30 SEM micrograph of corroded (10 µA/cm²) low-copper amalgam (New True Dentalloy) in 0.2% NaCl after removal of corrosion products by ultrasonics. A, alloy particles; B, matrix; C, regions formerly occupied by γ_2 phase

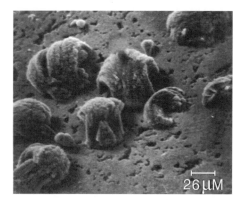

Fig. 31 SEM micrograph of low-copper amalgam (New True Dentalloy) after immersion in artificial saliva. The clumps of corrosion products contain tin. Source: Ref 175

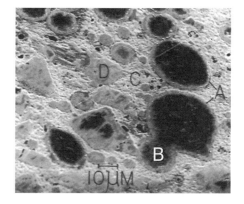

Fig. 32 SEM micrograph of corroded (5 µA/cm²/d) high-copper amalgam (cluster) in 0.2% NaCl solution. Note the definition of the η' rings (A), Ag-Cu particles (B), matrix (C), and η' particles (D).

percent) and sulfide concentration on color changes in gold crown and bridge alloys is detailed in Ref 176.

Effect of Microstructure on Tarnishing Behavior. The devastating effect of microgalvanic coupling on tarnishing behavior is shown by a comparison of solid-solution-annealed and as-cast structures (Fig. 33). The as-cast alloys, composed of two-phase structures, consistently showed greater color change or tarnish (Ref 146).

Single-phase as-cast Au-Ag-Cu alloys with gold contents between 50 and 84 wt% were observed microstructurally to tarnish in Na_2S solutions by localized microgalvanic cells. The characteristics of the various tarnished surfaces included a uniformly speckled appearance, dendritic attack, matrix attack, grain-boundary dependent attack, and grain-boundary attack. Silver-rich areas discolored preferentially because of the operation of the silver-rich areas as anodes and the surrounding copper-rich areas as cathodes. The uniformly speckled appearance occurred with high-silver low-copper contents, while the grain orientation dependent appearance occurred with low-silver high-copper contents. The dendritic and matrix attack

occurred with alloys containing intermediate silver and copper contents (Ref 96).

For Au-Ag-Cu-Pd alloys with gold contents between 35 and 73 wt%, the tarnishability in oxygenated 2% Na_2S is shown to be affected by altering the microstructure through heat treatment. Tarnishing occurred on multiphase structures annealed at 500 °C (930 °F), but did not occur on single-phase structures annealed at 700 °C (1290 °F). Silver-, copper-, and palladium-rich phases were precipitated. Some alloys, though, showed only silver- and copper-rich phases. In these cases, the palladium tended to follow the copper-rich phase. Splitting of the matrix into thin lamellae of alternating silver and copper enrichments occurred. The silver-rich phases in all materials were attacked by the sulfide and were responsible for the tarnish. Age hardening by AuCu(I)-ordered precipitates increased the tendency of the silver-rich lamellae to tarnish (Ref 177).

In sulfide solutions, silver sulfide (Ag_2S) is the principle product of tarnish, although copper sulfides (Cu_2S and CuS) also form. These products are produced by the operation of microgalvanic cells set up between silver-rich and copper-rich lamellae. The addition of palladium to Au-Ag-Cu alloys considerably reduces the rate of tarnishing by slowing down the formation of a layer of silver and copper sulfides on the surface. This has been shown to be due to the enrichment of palladium and gold on the surface of the alloy when exposed to the atmosphere prior to sulfide exposure (Ref 178). The rate of diffusion from the bulk to the surface is hindered by the palladium enrichment. The active sites on the alloy surface for the sulfidation reaction are selectively blocked by the palladium atoms (Ref 178).

Figure 26 presents chemically etched microstructures for a number of different casting alloys. All structures are multiphase, except for Sterngold 20 and Midas. After the surfaces were repolished and exposed for 3 days to a 0.016% Na_2S solution with a rotating tarnish tester (15 s exposure/min), the surfaces were again examined by scanning electron microscopy (SEM). Some of the results are presented in Fig. 34, which shows that tarnishing for all alloys took the form of dark patches over the alloy surfaces.

Effect of the Silver/Copper Ratio. The silver/copper ratio is an important aspect in affecting the tarnish and corrosion resistance of gold

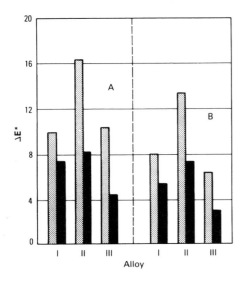

Fig. 33 Color change vector ΔE^* for three low-gold alloys (I, Miracast; II, Sunrise; III, Tiffany) in both the as-cast (left bar for each alloy) and solutionized at 750 °C (1380 °F) (right bar for each alloy) conditions after exposure for 3 days to artificial saliva (A) or 0.5% Na_2S solution (B). Source: Ref 146

dental alloys. A comparison of Midacast to Neycast III and Miracast (see Table 6) shows that all three alloys have about the same nobility but vastly different Ag/Cu ratios (based on weight percent), ranging from 41/7.4 for Midacast to 10.3/37.9 and 9.8/37.7 for Neycast and Miracast, respectively (Ref 177). A comparison of their polarization behavior in a sulfide solution shows the Midacast exhibits increases in current density up to 10 μA/cm^2 at –0.3 V, while Neycast III and Miracast exhibit a current density of ~1 μA/cm^2 extending to positive potentials. Therefore, high silver content relative to low copper content in low gold alloys can have detrimental effects on tarnishing and corrosion. For Forticast (the composition also given in Table 6), unacceptable levels of tarnish would occur if the silver/copper ratio were changed (Ref 158). For some low-gold alloys, the best resistance to tarnishing has been obtained by using ratios between 1.2 and 1.4 and a palladium content of 9 wt%.

Effect of the Palladium/Gold Ratio. Increasing the palladium content in gold alloys increases the tarnish resistance. However, in Au-Ag-Cu-Pd alloys, this effect is greater. The palladium/gold ratio is just as important as the silver/copper ratio. In Au-Ag-Cu alloys without palladium, the degree of tarnish (subjective test: 0 = least and 8 = most) was evaluated to be between 6.5 and 8 for all silver/copper ratios (1:3, 1:2, 2:3, 1:1, 3:2, 2:1 3:1) (Ref 101). However, in alloys having palladium/gold ratios of 1:12, the degree of tarnish diminished to between 2 and 3.

Tarnishing and Corrosion Compared. Figure 35 shows reflection loss versus nobility and weight loss versus nobility for the same 15 gold alloys. Tarnishing was by immersion for 3 days in 0.1 M Na$_2$S, while corrosion was by immersion in 0.1 M lactic acid. As is evident, a number of alloys that appear not to have been affected by corrosion are, however, largely affected by tarnishing (Ref 179).

Corrosion of Gold Alloys. Electrochemical polarization has been applied to the corrosion evaluation of gold dental alloys. High nobility alloys exhibited low current densities over a wide range in potentials in Ringer's solution, but low nobility alloys exhibited increased current densities and decreased breakdown potentials (Ref 180). Very small current peaks on the anodic polarization curves for some gold alloys in artificial saliva were detected and interpreted to be due to the dissolution of alloying components (Ref 181).

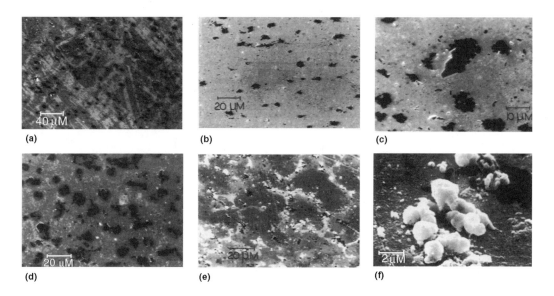

(a) (b) (c)

(d) (e) (f)

Fig. 34 SEM micrographs of low-gold alloys after 72 h of alternate-immersion tarnishing in artificial saliva containing 0.016% Na$_2$S. (a) Sterngold 20. (b) Tiffany. (c) Pentron 20. (d) Sunrise. (e) and (f) Econocast. See Table 6 for chemical compositions. Source: Ref 176

A comparison of the anodic polarization of noble alloys in artificial saliva with and without sulfide indicated that without sulfide the electrochemistry is governed mainly by chloride ions. The alloys passivate in a state with very low current densities, which makes detection of differences among the alloys difficult. With sulfide added to the artificial saliva, a preferential sulfidation of the less noble alloy component is induced. The sulfidation is characterized by a critical potential and limiting current density, both of which may be dependent on composition (Ref 182).

The corrosion susceptibilities for silver and copper in various gold alloys were quantified by an analysis of both forward and reverse polarization scans (Ref 183). Both silver and copper demonstrated characteristic current peaks during either oxidation or reduction. The heights of the current peaks were taken to be a measure of the amount of corrodible silver and copper in the alloys. In a similar technique, the integrated current from the polarization curves within a potential range of –0.3 V versus SCE to +0.3 V was taken to be a measure for the corrodable species (Ref 184). Figure 36 presents a rank ordering of eight as-cast gold alloys in regard to nobility plotted versus their integrated anodic currents, while Fig. 37 shows the effect of heat treatment state on the polarization corrosion index for a low gold content alloy.

Silver-Palladium Alloys. Silver is prone to tarnishing by sulfur and is prone to corrosion by chloride. The addition of palladium to silver generates alloys with much better resistance to tarnishing and silver corrosion. In 1-to-7 diluted Ringer's solution and 0.1% NaCl, alloys with more than 40% Pd showed passive anodic polarization behavior (Ref 185). In sulfur-saturated air, the amount of sulfur deposited onto the surfaces of silver-palladium alloys was minimal for compositions with ≥40 wt% Pd (Ref 182). In artificial saliva, two transitions in the corrosion currents occurred with palladium content. The first occurred at about 22% Pd, where the current decreased from 6 to 1 μA. The second transition occurred at about 29% Pd, where the current decreased to about 0.4 μA and then remained fairly constant throughout the rest of the compositional range (Ref 186). Figure 38 shows the color change vectors for the pure metals and alloys from the silver-palladium system

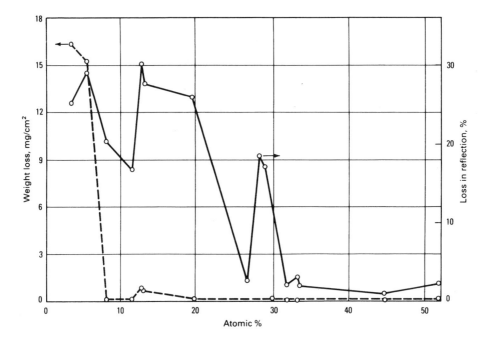

Fig. 35 Effect of nobility (in atomic percent) on tarnish (percent loss in reflection after 3 days in 0.1% Na₂S) and corrosion (weight loss after 7 days in aerated 0.1 M lactic acid plus 0.1 M NaCl at 37 °C or 99 °F) of 15 gold alloys. Source: Ref 179

after tarnishing in artificial saliva with 0.5% Na$_2$S. Compositions 50Pd-50Ag and 75Pd-25Ag showed the best tarnish resistance (Ref 187).

Corrosion behavior and tarnishing behavior usually must be viewed independently. That is, corrosion is not an indicator for tarnishing, and vice versa. Alloy nobility dominates corrosion behavior, while alloy nobility, composition, and microstructure, in conjunction with environment, influence tarnishing behavior.

Microstructurally, the silver-palladium alloys tarnish by chlorides and/or sulfides becoming deposited over the silver-rich matrix, while the palladium-rich precipitates display resistance to chlorides and sulfides. With forward and reverse scan polarization, the amounts of corrodable silver and copper in silver-palladium alloys were characterized by comparing the relative current magnitudes for reduction peaks. Microstructurally, the alloys were composed of a corrosion-resistant copper- and palladium-rich phase and a nonresistant silver-rich phase. Increased tarnish and corrosion of the silver-rich phase component occurred by microgalvanic coupling (Ref 188). Manipulation of the microstructural features through heat treatments produced structures with varying proportions of the tarnish-resistant and tarnish-prone phases. Age hardening increased the proportion of the tarnish- and corrosion-prone phases (Ref 189, 190).

High-Palladium Ceramic Alloys. Alloys with up to 80% Pd and additions of copper, gallium, tin, indium, gold, and others were shown to exhibit good saline corrosion resistance in the potential range and Cl$^-$ ion concentration associated with oral use. Anodic polarization

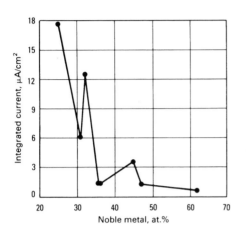

Fig. 36 Integrated anodic currents between –0.3 V versus SCE and +0.3 V (at 0.06 V/min) for eight gold alloys in deaerated 1% NaCl plotted against the atomic nobility. Source: Ref 146

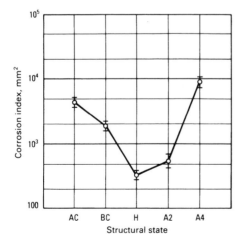

Fig. 37 Corrosion index (area in mm^2 under polarization curve between –1.0 V versus SCE and +0.4 V at 0.6 V/min) versus the heat treatment state of Midigold, a low-gold-content alloy. AC, as-cast; BC, bench cool; H, homogenized; A2, aged for 2 h at 350 °C (660 °F); A4, aged for 4 h at 350 °C (660 °F). Source: Ref 73

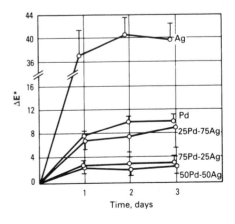

Fig. 38 Color change vector ΔE^* for pure silver, palladium, and three Ag-Pd binary compositions after exposure to Na$_2$S solutions. Source: Ref 187

showed passive behavior until breakdown occurred, which was well above potential magnitudes occurring intraorally (Ref 163). For similar compositions and palladium-base compositions containing cobalt, spontaneous passivation or active-passive behavior occurred in chloride solutions. Differences among the polarization profiles for the various palladium-base alloys were detected, but any differences corresponded to high potentials generally above the biodental range (Ref 161).

The effects of adding copper and gallium to palladium were determined by modeling alloy composition and corresponding electrochemical behavior to a linear regression and equation. The resultant coefficients accounted for the individual elemental effects on corrosion potential and anodic Tafel constants. Elements that increased the nobility of the corrosion potential also increased the rate of corrosion. This was attributed to anodic protection occurring at the surface of the alloys (Ref 162).

Nickel-Chromium Alloys. The tarnish resistance and corrosion resistance of these alloys result from balancing the composition with regard to the passivating elements chromium, molybdenum, manganese, and silicon. Alloys containing increased amounts of molybdenum and manganese exhibited increased passivation. Increasing the chromium content too much (above 20%) can precipitate an additional phase and alter the corrosion resistance. By using polarization methods, 3 different behaviors were observed with 12 nickel-chromium alloys with varying compositions in deaerated and aerated artificial saliva (Ref 191). Some alloys were constantly passive, others were either active/passive or passive according to the aeration condition of the electrolyte, and still others (<16% Cr without molybdenum) were constantly active and corroding.

Corrosion potentials for nickel-chromium alloys in artificial saliva were low, ranging between about –0.2 V and –0.8 V versus SCE. Breakdown potentials varied, depending on composition. For alloys with less than 16% Cr and no molybdenum, breakdown potentials as low as –0.2 V occurred. For compositions with higher chromium contents and with molybdenum and various manganese contents, breakdown potentials as high as +0.6 V also occurred.

Pitting attack occurs with these alloys because they rely on protective surface oxide films for imparting protection. From electro-chemical and immersion tests, the resistance of nickel-chromium alloys to pitting attack was found to be good in solutions with Cl^- concentrations equivalent to that found in saliva. Only at higher Cl^- concentrations are pitting and tarnishing likely to occur (Ref 192).

Cobalt-Chromium Alloys. Compared to the nickel-chromium alloys, the cobalt-chromium alloys for partial denture and implant prosthesis exhibit superior tarnish and corrosion resistance. Cobalt-chromium alloys exhibit passive behavior to potentials of at least +0.5 V (Ref 70, 193), but the nickel-chromium alloys exhibit much greater variations in behavior. For some of the nickel-chromium alloys, breakdown potentials can be as low as –0.2 V (Ref 191, 193). In spite of the excellent corrosion resistance of cobalt-chromium alloys, allergic reactions to cobalt, chromium, and nickel contained in appliances made from these alloys are known to have occurred (see the section "Allergic Hypersensitive Reactions" in this chapter).

Titanium Alloys. Titanium and titanium alloys, like the cobalt-chromium alloys, have proved to be resistant to tarnish and corrosion. The anodic polarization for pure titanium and its alloys indicates passivities over at least several volts in overvoltage (Ref 70, 193). This demonstrates the tenacity and protectiveness of the titanium oxide films formed on these materials.

With regard to the newer casting titanium alloys for crown and bridgework and partial dentures, good corrosion resistance is still preserved (Ref 141). Concerns must be raised because the casting alloys contain higher percentages of alloying elements, with the potential for elucidating diminished chemical stabilities.

Nitinol, containing about 50% Ni and 50% Ti, does not exhibit the same high corrosion resistance as alloys with 80 to 90% Ti, and higher.

Wrought Orthodontic Wires. A comparison of their anodic polarization curves (Fig. 39) shows that both β-titanium and Elgiloy exhibit resistance to corrosion in artificial saliva. No breakdown in passivity occurred within the potential ranges employed (+0.8 V). With Nitinol and stainless steel wires, breakdown occurred at +0.2 and 0.05 V, respectively. Nitinol and stainless steel also exhibited current increases upon potential reversals at +0.8 V, an indication of the susceptibility to pitting corrosion. Breakdown potentials differed by as much as 0.6 V between different brands of stainless steel wires. Variations in the polarization characteristics of stainless steel have been related to microstructure (Ref 70) and to surface preparation and finish (Ref 71). Microstructurally, the Nitinol wires were observed to suffer pitting attack after polarization tests (Ref 195).

Silver and Gold Solders. A corroded silver soldered-stainless steel joint is shown in Fig. 40. Microstructurally, silver solders are composed of two phases: silver- and copper-zinc rich segregations (Ref 196). The copper-zinc regions are the least resistant to corrosion. These solders corrode by microgalvanic coupling, either by cells set up between the two microstructural phases or between solder and the parts they join. Figure 41 shows the copper-zinc phase of a silver solder attacked by corrosion. In addition to the release of copper and zinc into the surrounding environment, metallic ions from the wires themselves were also shown to be leached into the wires (Ref 25). The leaching of nickel and chromium from stainless steel wires occurred with greater intensity than from the wires of the cobalt-chromium type.

Figure 42 shows the polarization curves for both silver and gold (450 fine) solders. The silver solder is characterized by active behavior, as indicated by the low corrosion potential of –1.2 V versus SCE in 0.16 M NaCl on the anodic polarization traverse and the numerous current peaks related to redox reactions with the elements constituting the solder. Therefore, zinc, tin, copper, and even silver products are likely to be precipitated or become dissolved in solution.

The polarization curve for gold solder indicates intense activity by the sharp current density peak at +0.25 V. Because the solder con-

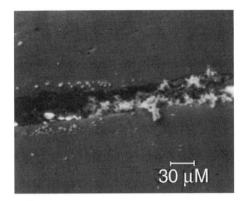

Fig. 40 SEM micrograph of a corroded stainless steel-silver soldered joint after immersion in a 1% H_2O_2 solution. Source: Ref 196

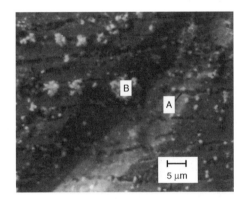

Fig. 41 SEM micrograph of a corroded silver solder in 1% NaCl (held at –0.05 V versus SCE) showing the destruction of the copper-zinc-rich phase (A) and the accumulation of products (B) that contain copper, zinc, and chlorine. Source: Ref 196

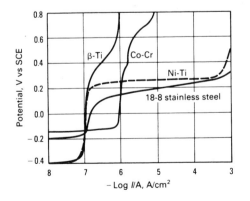

Fig. 39 Anodic polarization at 0.03 V/min of four orthodontic wires in artificial saliva. Source: Ref 194

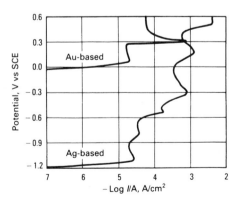

Fig. 42 Anodic polarization at 0.03 V/min of silver and gold (450 fine) solders in 1% NaCl solution. Source: Ref 196

tains silver, copper, and zinc, in addition to gold, this peak is probably due to the corrosion of one of these elements. Figure 43 shows the gold solder after the polarization test. Corrosion has delineated the basic microstructure of the solder alloy. Chlorine was detected with the white appearing phase.

Silver-Indium Alloys. These alloys rely on the unusual properties of indium oxide for providing tarnish and corrosion control. Small amounts of noble metals, such as palladium, may also be added in an attempt to improve corrosion resistance. Anodic polarization of a silver-indium alloy in artificial saliva indicated only a very narrow potential range of about 0.1 V of reduced current densities. The tarnish resistance of these alloys appears to be accept-

able, but the long-term corrosion resistance has not been established (Ref 197).

Copper-Aluminum Alloys. A comparison of the released copper in human saliva from a dental copper-aluminum alloy to that from a high-copper amalgam is shown in Fig. 44. The amalgam released more copper over a 45-day interval. No aluminum, iron, manganese, or nickel was detected. Figures 45(a) to (c) show micrographs from an *in vivo* restoration at various magnifications. Large amounts of organic matter were absorbed onto the surface, as well as light powdery corrosion products composed of copper oxides (Ref 68).

Rare-Earth Permanent Magnets. The anodic polarization of $SmCo_5$, Sm_2Co_{17}, and $Nd_2Fe_{14}B$ in artificial saliva indicates active

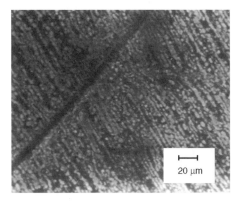

Fig. 43 SEM micrograph of a corroded (polarized to +0.5 V versus SCE) gold solder (450 solder) in 1% NaCl. The light areas contain chlorine. Source: Ref 196

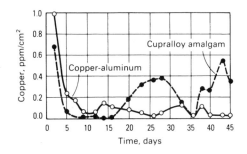

Fig. 44 Released copper into human saliva from a copper-aluminum crown and bridge alloy (MS) and a high-copper amalgam (Cupralloy) plotted against time for up to 45 days. Source: Ref 68

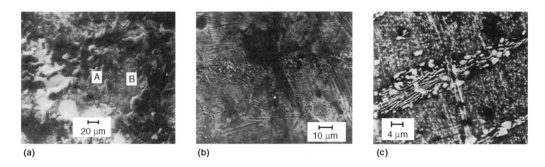

(a)　　　　　　　　　(b)　　　　　　　　　(c)

Fig. 45 SEM micrographs of the copper-aluminum restoration shown in Fig. 18 at higher magnifications. In (a), both accumulated plaque (A) and corrosion products (B) occur. (b) Higher-magnification view of the areas identified by (B) contain copper. The light-appearing areas are probably copper oxides. (c) Still higher magnification of the products shown in (b). Here the copper oxides are deposited over the dark copper-rich microstructural phase. Source: Ref 68

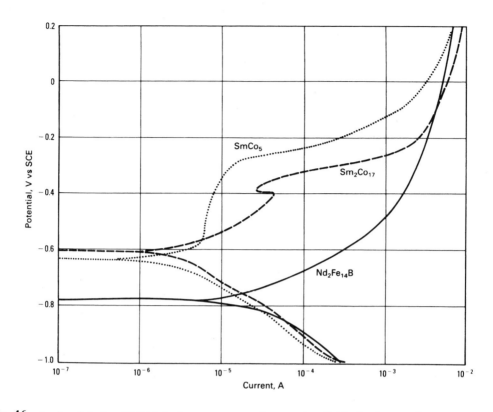

Fig. 46 Anodic polarization at 0.03 V/min of permanent rare-earth magnets in artificial saliva. Source: Ref 198

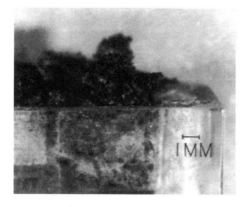

Fig. 47 Photograph of an orthodontic appliance containing a $Nd_2Fe_{14}B$ magnet after intraoral use for several weeks. Iron was identified in the corrosion products. Source: Ref 198

behavior (Fig. 46). Additional *in vitro* and *in vivo* tests have indicated their poor chemical stability. Scanning electron microscopy, energy dispersive spectroscopy, and secondary ion mass spectroscopy identified some of the products to be oxides and chlorides of samarium, in the case of samarium-cobalt materials, and of iron and neodymium with the Nd-Fe-B materials. Figure 47 shows an $Nd_2Fe_{17}B$ orthodontic bracket after several weeks of *in vivo* use. Abundant amounts of corrosion products occurred. In their present state, these materials are unacceptable for routine bioapplications. However, because of their extreme usefulness in providing relatively large magnetic forces from small volumes of material, special efforts are being made to apply surface coating technologies to the rare-earth magnets (Ref 198).

ACKNOWLEDGMENT

The information in this chapter is largely taken from H.J. Mueller, Tarnish and Corrosion of Dental Alloys, *Corrosion,* Vol 13, *Metals Handbook,* 9th ed., ASM International, 1987, p 1336–1366.

REFERENCES

1. *Dental Technician, Prosthetic,* Navpers 10685 c, U.S. Naval Dental School, Bureau of Naval Personnel, 1965, p 256
2. G. Ravasini, *Clinical Procedures for Partial Crowns, Inlays, Onlays, and Pontics. An Atlas,* Quintessence Publishing, 1985, p 136
3. K.L. Stewart, K.D. Rudd, and W.A. Kuebker, *Clinical Removable Partial Dentures,* C.V. Mosby, 1983, p 31, 230, 494
4. T.M. Graber and B.F. Swain, *Orthodontics: Current Principles and Techniques,* C.V. Mosby, 1985, p 385
5. D.C. Smith and D.F. Williams, *Biocompatibility of Dental Materials,* Vol 1–4, CRC Press, 1982
6. *Workshop on Biocompatibility of Metals in Dentristry,* Conference Proceedings, American Dental Association, 1984
7. *An International Workshop: Biocompatibility, Toxicity and Hypersensitivity to Alloy Systems Used in Dentistry, Proceedings,* The University of Michigan School of Dentistry, 1985
8. D.C. Smith, The Biocompatibility of Dental Materials, *Biocompatibility of Dental Materials,* Vol 1, D.C. Smith and D.F. Williams, Ed., CRC Press, 1982, p 11
9. D.C. Smith, Tissue Reaction to Noble and Base Metal Alloys, *Biocompatibility of Dental Materials,* Vol IV, D.C. Smith and D.F. Williams, Ed., CRC Press, 1982, p 55
10. A. Halse, Metal in Dentinal Tubles Beneath Amalgam Fillings in Human Teeth, *Arch. Oral Biol.,* Vol 20, 1975, p 87–88
11. K. Arvidson and R. Wroblewski, Migration of Metallic Ions from Screwposts into Dentin and Surrounding Tissues, *Scand. J. Dent. Res.,* Vol 86, 1978, p 200–203
12. W. Schriever and L.E. Diamond, Electromotive Forces and Electric Currents Caused by Metallic Dental Fillings, *J. Dent. Res.,* Vol 31, 1952, p 205–229
13. I. Kleinberg, Etiology of Dental Caries, *J. Can. Dent. Assn.,* Vol 12, 1979, p 661–668
14. I.D. Mandel, Dental Caries, *Am. Sci.,* Vol 67, 1979, p 680–688
15. E. Hals and A. Halse, Electron Probe Microanalysis of Secondary Carious Lesions Associated with Silver Amalgam Fillings, *Acta Odontol. Scand.,* Vol 33, 1975, p 149–160
16. N. Kurosahi and T. Fusayama, Penetration of Elements from Amalgam into Dentin, *J. Dent. Res.,* Vol 52, 1973, p 309–317
17. L.W.J. van der Linden and J. van Aken, The Origin of Localized Increased Radiopacity in the Dentin, *Oral Surg.,* Vol 35, 1973, p 862–871
18. B.L. Dahl, Hypersensitivity to Dental Materials, *Biocompatibility of Dental Materials,* Vol 1, D.C. Smith and D.F. Williams, Ed., CRC Press, 1982, p 177–1 85
19. E.W. Mitchell, Summary and Recommendations to the Workshop, *Workshop on Biocompatibility of Metals in Dentistry,* Conference Proceedings, American Dental Association, 1984
20. M. Bergan and O. Ginstrup, Dissolution Rate of Cadmium from Dental Gold Solder Alloys, *Acta Odontol. Scand.,* Vol 33, 1975, p 199–210
21. D.R. Zielke, J.M. Brady, and C.E. del Rio, Corrosion of Silver Cones in Bone: A Scanning Electron Microscope and Microprobe Analysis, *J. Endo.,* Vol 1, 1975, p 356–360
22. R.A. James, Host Response to Dental Implant Devices, *Bicompatibility of Dental Materials,* Vol IV, D.C. Smith and D.F. Williams, Ed., CRC Press, 1982, p 163–195
23. J.R. Natiella, Local Tissue Reaction/Carcinogenesis, *International Workshop on Bicompatibility, Toxicity, and Hypersensitivity to Alloy Systems Used in Dentistry,* Section 6, Conference Proceedings, University of Michigan School of Dentistry, 1985
24. R.S. Mateer and C.D. Reitz, Corrosion of Amalgam Restorations, *J. Dent. Res.,* Vol 49, 1970, p 399–407
25. M. Berge, N.R. Gjerdet, and E.S. Erichsen, Corrosion of Silver Soldered Orthodontic Wires, *Acta Odontol. Scand.,* Vol 40, 1982, p 75–79
26. B. Angmar-Mansson, K.-A. Omnell, and J. Rud, Root Fractures Due to Corrosion, *Odontol. Revy.,* Vol 20, 1969, p 245–265
27. D.C. Mears, Metals in Medicine and

Surgery, *Int. Met. Rev.,* Vol 22 (No. 218), 1977, p 119–155

28. J.R. Cahoon and L.D. Hill, Evaluation of a Precipitation Hardened Wrought Cobalt-Nickel-Chromium-Titanium Alloy for Surgical Implants, *J. Biomed. Mater. Res.,* Vol 12, 1978, p 805–821

29. T.C. Ruck and J.F. Fulton, *Medical Physiology and Biophysics,* 18th ed., W.B. Saunders, 1960

30. H.C. McCann, Inorganic Components of Salivary Secretions, *Art and Science of Dental Caries Research,* R.S. Harris, Ed., Academic Press, 1968, p 55–73

31. D.B. Ferguson, Salivary Glands and Saliva, *Applied Physiology of the Mouth,* C.L.B. Lavell, Ed., John Wright, 1975, p 145–179

32. H.J. Mueller, Binding of Corroded Ions to Human Saliva, *Biomaterials,* Vol 6, 1985, p 146–149

33. H.J. Mueller, Characterization of the Acquired Biofilms on Materials Exposed to Human Saliva, *Proteins at Interfaces,* T.A. Horbett and J. Brash, Ed., Advances in Chemistry Series, American Chemical Society, 1987

34. S.A. Ellison, The Identification of Salivary Components, *Saliva and Dental Caries,* I. Kleinberg, S.A. Ellison, and I.D. Mandell, Ed., *Sp. Supp. Microbiol. Abst.,* 1979, p 13–29

35. C.E. Ingersoll, Characterization of Tarnish, *J. Dent. Res.,* Vol 55, 1976, IADR No. 144

36. K. Barton, chapter 2, *Protection against Atmospheric Corrosion,* John Wiley & Sons, 1973

37. I.C. Schoonover and W. Souder, Corrosion of Dental Alloys, *J. Am. Dent. Assoc.,* Vol 28, 1941, p 1278–1291

38. J.C. Muhler and H.M. Swenson, Preparation of Synthetic Saliva from Direct Analysis of Human Saliva, *J. Dent. Res.,* Vol 26, 1947, p 474

39. D.A. Carter, T.K. Ross, and D.C. Smith. Some Corrosion Studies on Silver-Tin Amalgams, *Br. Corros. J.,* Vol 2, 1967, p 199–205

40. G. Tani and F. Zucci, Electrochemical Evaluation of the Corrosion Resistance of the Commonly Used Metals in Dental Prosthesis, *Minerva. Stomat.,* Vol 16, 1967, p 710–713

41. J.M. Meyer and J.N. Nally, Influence of Artificial Salivas on the Corrosion of Dental Alloys, *J. Dent. Res.,* Vol 54, 1975, IADR No. 76

42. B.W. Darvell, The Development of an Artificial Saliva for In-Vitro Amalgam Corrosion Studies, *J. Oral Rehab.,* Vol 5, 1978, p 41–49

43. M.L. Swartz, R.W. Phillips, and M.D. El Tannir, Tarnish of Certain Dental Alloys, *J. Dent. Res.,* Vol 37, 1958, p 837–847

44. F. Fusayama, T. Katayori, and S. Nomoto, Corrosion of Gold and Amalgam Placed in Contact with Each Other, *J. Dent. Res.,* Vol 42, 1963, p 1183–1197

45. C.E. Guthrow, L.B. Johnson, and K.R. Lawless, Corrosion of Dental Amalgam and Its Component Phases, *J. Dent. Res.,* Vol 46, 1967, p 1372–1381

46. F.V. Wald and F.H. Cocks, Investigation of Copper-Manganese-Nickel Alloys for Dental Purposes, *J. Dent. Res.,* Vol 50, 1971, p 44–59

47. M. Marek and R.F. Hockman, Corrosion Behavior of Amalgam Electrode in Artificial Saliva, *J. Dent. Res.,* Vol 51, 1972, IADR No. 63

48. J. Brugirard, R. Bargain, J.C. Dupuy, H. Mazille, and G. Monnier, Study of the Electrochemical Behavior of Gold Dental Alloys, *J. Dent. Res.,* Vol 52, 1973, p 828–836

49. *The National Foundry,* American Pharmaceutical Association, 1970, p 624

50. M. Marek and E. Topfl, Electrolytes for Corrosion Testing of Dental Alloys, *J. Dent. Res.,* Vol 65, 1986, IADR No. 1192

51. N.K. Sarkar and E.H. Greener, In Vitro Corrosion of Dental Amalgam, *J. Dent. Res.,* Vol 50, 1971, IADR No. 13

52. G.F. Finkelstein and E.H. Greener, In Vitro Polarization of Dental Amalgam in Human Saliva, *J. Oral. Rehab.,* Vol 4, p 355–368

53. G.F. Finkelstein and E.H. Greener, Role of Mucin and Albumin in Saline Polarization of Dental Amalgam, *J. Oral Rehab.,* Vol 5, 1978, p 95–110

54. H. Do Duc, P. Tissot, and J.-M. Meyer, Potential Sweep and Intensiostatic Pulse Studies of Sn, Sn_8Hg, and Dental Amalgam in Chloride Solution, *J. Oral Rehab.,* Vol 6, 1979, p 189–197

55. R.I. Holland, Effect of Pellicle on Galvanic Corrosion of Amalgam, *Scand. J. Dent. Res.,* Vol 92, 1984, p 93–96

56. H.J. Mueller, The Effects of a Human Salivary Dialysate upon Ionic Release and Electrochemical Corrosion of a Cu-Al Alloy, *J. Electrochem. Soc.,* Vol 134, 1987, p 555–580

57. A. Schulman, H.A.B. Linke, T.K. Vaidyanathan, Tarnish of Dental Alloys by Oral Microorganisms, *J. Dent. Res.,* Vol 63, 1984, IADR No. 55

58. M. Stern and E.D. Weisert, Experimental Observation on the Relation between Polarization Resistance and Corrosion Rate, *Proc. ASTM,* Vol 59, 1959, p 1280–1291

59. M. Marek, The Corrosion of Dental Materials, *Corrosion: Aqueous Processes and Passive Films,* Vol 23, *Treatise on Materials Science,* J.C. Scully, Ed., Academic Press, 1983, p 331–394

60. M. Bergman, O. Ginstrup, and B. Nilsson, Potentials of and Currents between Dental Metallic Restorations, *Scand. J. Dent. Res.,* Vol 90, 1982, p 404–408

61. K. Nilner, P.-O. Glantz, B. Zoger, On Intraoral Potential and Polarization Measurements of Metallic Restorations, *Acta Odontol. Scand.,* Vol 40, 1982, p 275–281

62. J.M. Mumford, Electrolytic Action in the Mouth and Its Relationship to Pain, *J. Dent. Res.,* Vol 36, 1957, p 632–640

63. C.P. Wang Chen and E.H. Greener, A Galvanic Study of Different Amalgams, *J. Oral Rehab.,* Vol 4, 1977, p 23–27

64. R. Soremark, G. Freedman, J. Goldin, and L. Gettleman, Structure and Microdistribution of Gold Alloys, *J. Dent. Res.,* Vol 45, 1966, p 1723–1735

65. D.B. Boyer, K. Chan, C.W. Svare, The Effect of Finishing on the Anodic Polarization of High-Copper Amalgams, *J. Oral Rehab.,* Vol 5, 1978, p 223–228

66. G. Palaghias, Oral Corrosion and Corrosion Inhibition Processes, *Swed. Dent. J.,* Supp 30, 1985

67. H.J. Mueller and A. Edahl, The Effect of Exposure Conditions upon the Release of Soluble Copper and Tin from Dental Amalgams, *Biomaterials,* Vol 5, 1984, p 194–200

68. H.J. Mueller and R.M. Barrie, Intraoral Corrosion of Copper-Aluminum Alloys, *J. Dent. Res.,* Vol 64, 1985, IADR No. 1753

69. G.N. Jenkins, *The Physiology and Biochemistry of the Mouth,* 4th ed., Blackwell, 1978, p 284–359

70. H.J. Mueller and E.H. Greener, Polarization Resistance of Surgical Materials in Ringer's Solution, *J. Biomed. Mater. Res.,* Vol 4, 1970, p 29–41

71. E.J. Sutow, S.R. Pollack, and E. Korostoff, An In Vitro Investigation of the Anodic Polarization and Capacitance Behavior of 316-L Stainless Steel, *J. Biomed. Mater. Res.,* Vol 10, 1976, p 671–693

72. H.J. Mueller, The Binding of Corroded Metallic Ions to Salivary-Type Proteins, *Biomaterials,* Vol 4, 1983, p 66–72

73. J.R. Strub, C. Eyer, and N.K. Sarkar, Microstructure and Corrosion of a Low-Gold Casting Alloy, *J. Dent. Res.,* Vol 63, 1984, IADR No. 793

74. M.P. Keenan, Effects of Gold Finishing on Plaque Retention, *J. Dent. Res.,* Vol 56, 1977, IADR No. 121(B)

75. C.W. Svare, G. Belton, and E. Korostoff, The Role of Organics in Metallic Passivation, *J. Biomed. Mater. Res.,* Vol 4, 1970, p 457–467

76. G.C.F. Clark and D.F. Williams, The Effects of Proteins on Metallic Passivation, *J. Biomed. Mater. Res.,* Vol 16, 1982, p 125–134

77. S.A. Brown and K. Merritt, Electrochemical Corrosion in Saline and Serum, *J. Biomed. Mater. Res.,* Vol 14, 1980, p 173–175

78. S.A. Brown and K. Merritt, Fretting Corrosion in Saline and Serum, *J. Biomed. Mater. Res.,* Vol 15, p 479–488

79. H.J. Mueller, The Effect of Electrical Signals upon the Adsorption of Plasma Proteins to a High Cu Alloy, *Biomaterials: Interfacial Phenomena and Applications,* S.L. Cooper and N.A. Peppas, Ed., ACS monograph series 199, American Chemical Society, 1982

80. R.C. Salvarezza, M.E.L. de Mele, H.H. Videla, and F.R. Goni, Electrochemical Behavior of Aluminum in Human Plasma, *J. Biomed. Mater. Res.,* Vol 19, 1985, p 1073–1084

81. H. Hero and L. Niemi, Tarnishing In Vivo of Ag-Pd-Cu-Zn, *J. Dent. Res.,* Vol 65, 1986, p 1303–1307

82. H. Do Duc and P. Tissot, Rotating Disc and Ring Disc Electrode Studies of Tin in

Neutral Phosphate Solution, *Corros. Sci.,* Vol 19, 1979, p 191–197

83. I.D. Mandel, Relation of Saliva and Plaque to Caries, *J. Dent. Res.,* Vol 53, 1974, p 246

84. T. Ericson, K.M. Pruitt, H. Arwin, and I. Lunstrom, Ellipsometric Studies of Film Formation on Tooth Enamel and Hydrophilic Silicon Surfaces, *Acta Odontol. Scand.,* Vol 40, 1982, p 197–201

85. R.E. Baier and P.-O. Glantz, Characterization of Oral in Vivo Films Formed on Different Types of Solid Surfaces, *Acta Odontol. Scand.,* Vol 36, 1978, p 289–301

86. K. Skjorland, Auger Analysis of Integuments Formed on Different Dental Filling Materials in Vivo, *Acta Odontol. Scand.,* Vol 40, 1982, p 129–134

87. K. Hannesson Eggen and G. Rolla, Gel Filtration, Ion Exchange Chromatography and Chemical Analysis of Macromolecules Present in Acquired Enamel Pellicle (2-hr), *Scand. J. Dent. Res.,* Vol 90, 1982, p 182–188

88. A. Bennick, G. Chau, R. Goodlin, S. Abrams, D. Tustian, and G. Mandapallimattam, The Role of Human Salivary Acidic Proline-Rich Proteins in the Formation of Acquired Dental Pellicle in Vivo and Their Fate after Adsorption to the Human Enamel Surface, *Arch. Oral Biol.,* Vol 28, 1983, p 19–27

89. T. Sonju and P.-O. Glantz, Chemical Composition of Salivary Integuments Formed in Vitro on Solids with Some Established Surface Characteristics, *Arch. Oral Biol.,* Vol 20, 1975, p 687–691

90. D.I. Hay, The Adsorption of Salivary Proteins by Hydroxyapatite and Enamel, *Arch. Oral Biol.,* Vol 12, 1967, p 937–946

91. G. Rolla, Formation of Dental Integuments—Basic Chemical Considerations, *Swed. Dent. J.,* Vol 1, 1977, p 241–251

92. A.C. Juriaanse, M. Booij, J. Arends, and J.J. Ten Bosch, The Adsorption in Vivo of Purified Salivary Proteins on Bovine Dental Enamel, *Arch. Oral Biol.,* Vol 26, 1981, p 91–96

93. H.J. Mueller, Differential Scanning Calorimetry of Adsorbed Protein Films, *Transactions of the 13th Annual Meeting Society of the Biomaterials,* 1987

94. R.D. Norman, R.V. Mehra, and M.L. Schwartz, The Effects of Restorative Materials on Plaque Composition, *J. Dent. Res.,* Vol 50, 1971, IADR No. 162

95. J.J. Tuccillo and J.P. Nielsen, Microprobe Analysis of an in Vivo Discoloration, *J. Prosthet. Dent.,* Vol 31, 1974, p 285–289

96. J.J. Tuccillo and J.P. Nielson, Observation of Onset of Sulfide Tarnish on Gold-Base Alloys, *J. Prosthet. Dent.,* Vol 25, 1971, p 629–637

97. R.P. Lubovich, R.E. Kovarik, and D.L. Kinser, A Quantitative and Subjective Characterization of Tarnishing in Low-Gold Alloys, *J. Prosthet. Dent.,* Vol 42, 1979, p 534–538

98. G.W. Marshall, N.K. Sarkar, and E.H. Greener, Detection of Oxygen in Corrosion Products of Dental Amalgam, *J. Dent. Res.,* Vol 54, 1975, p 904

99. H. Otani, W.A. Jesser, and H.G.F. Wilsdorf, The in Vivo and the in Vitro Corrosion Products of Dental Amalgam, *J. Biomed. Mater. Res.,* Vol 7, 1973, p 523–539

100. A.B. Burse, M.L. Swartz, R.W. Phillips, and R.W. Oykema, Comparison of the in Vivo and in Vitro Tarnish of Three Gold Alloys, *J. Biomed. Mater. Res.,* Vol 6, 1972, p 267–277

101. B.R. Laing, S.H. Bernier, Z. Giday, and K. Asgar, Tarnish and Corrosion of Noble Metal Alloys, *J. Prosthet. Dent.,* Vol 48, 1982, p 245–252

102. H. Hero and J. Valderhaug, Tarnishing in Vivo and in Vitro of a Low-Gold Alloy Related to Its Structure, *J. Dent. Res.,* Vol 64, 1985, p 139–143

103. H. Hero and R.B. Jorgensen, Tarnishing of a Low-Gold Alloy in Different Structural States, *J. Dent. Res.,* Vol 62, 1983 p 371–376

104. L. Gettlemen, R.F. Cocks, L.A. Darmiento, P.A. Levine, S. Wright, and D. Nathanson, Measurement of in Vivo Corrosion Rates in Baboons and Correlation with in Vivo Tests. *J. Dent. Res.,* Vol 59, 1980, p 689–707

105. L. Gettleman, C. Amman, and N.K. Sarkar, Quantitative in Vivo and in Vitro Measurement of Tarnish. *J. Dent. Res.,* Vol 58, 1979, IADR No. 969

106. Revised American Dental Association Specification No. 1 for Alloy for Amalgam, *J. Am. Dent. Assoc.,* Vol 95, 1977, p 614–617

107. Addendum to ANSI/ADA Specification

No. 1 for Alloy for Amalgam, *J. Am. Dent. Assoc.,* Vol 100, 1980, p 246

108. D.B. Mahler and J.D. Adey, Microprobe Analysis of Three High Copper Amalgams, *J. Dent. Res.,* Vol 63, 1984, p 921–925

109. J.W. Edie, D.B. Boyer, and K.C. Chjan, Estimation of the Phase Distribution in Dental Amalgams with Electron Microprobe, *J. Dent. Res.,* Vol 57, 1978, p 277–282

110. J. Leitao. Surface Roughness and Porosity of Dental Amalgam, *Acta Odontol. Scand.,* Vol 40, 1982, p 9–16

111. R.W. Bryant, Gamma-2 Phase in Conventional Amalgam-Discrete Clumps or Continuous Network—A Review, *Aust. Dent. J.,* Vol 29, 1984, p 163–167

112. L.B. Johnson, X-Ray Diffraction Evidence for the Presence of β(Ag-Hg) in Dental Amalgam, *J. Biomed. Mater. Res.,* Vol 1, 1967, p 285–297

113. S.J. Marshall and G.W. Marshall, Jr., Time-Dependent Phase Changes in Cu-Rich Amalgams, *J. Biomed. Mater. Res.,* Vol 13, 1979, p 395–406

114. Revised ANSI/ADA Specification No. 5 For Dental Casting Gold Alloy, *J. Am. Dent. Assoc.,* Vol 104, 1981, p 70

115. J.P. Moffa, Alternative Dental Casting Alloys, *Dent. Clin. N. Am.,* Vol 27, 1983, p 194–200

116. R.M. German, Precious-Metal Dental Casting Alloys, *Int. Met. Rev.,* Vol 27, 1982, p 260–288

117. K. Yasuda and K. Hisatsune, The Development of Dental Alloys Conserving Precious Metals: Improving Corrosion Resistance by Controlled Aging, *Int. Dent. J.,* Vol 33, 1983

118. D.L. Smith, Dental Casting Alloys, Technical and Economic Considerations in the USA, *Int. Dent. J.,* Vol 33, 1983, p 25–34

119. S.A. Aquilino and T.D. Taylor, Prosthodontic Laboratory Survey, *J. Prosthet. Dent.,* Vol 53, 1984, p 879–885

120. H. Hero, Tarnishing and Structures of Some Annealed Dental Low-Gold Alloys, *J. Dent. Res.,* Vol 63, 1984, p 926–931

121. L. Niemi and H. Hero, Structure, Corrosion, and Tarnishing of Ag-Pd-Cu Alloys, *J. Dent. Res.,* Vol 64, 1985, p 1163–1169

122. R.C. Craig, H.J. Skesnick, and F.A. Peyton, Application of 17-7 Precipitation Hardenable Stainless Steel in Dentistry, *J. Dent. Res.,* Vol 44, 1965, p 587–595

123. S. Civjan, E.F. Huget, and L.B. de Simon, Effects of Laboratory Procedures on 55-Nitinol, *J. Dent. Res.,* Vol 52, 1973, IADR No. 51

124. A.J. Goldberg and C.J. Burstone, An Evaluation of Beta-Stabilized Titanium Alloys for Use in Orthodontic Appliances, *J. Dent. Res.,* Vol 57, 1978, p 593–600

125. E.F. Huget and S.G. Vermilyea, Base Metal Dental and Surgical Alloys, *Biocompatibility of Dental Materials,* Vol IV, D.C. Smith and D.F. Williams, Ed., CRC Press, 1982, p 37–49

126. H.F. Morris and K. Asgar, Physical Properties and Microstructure of Four New Paertial Denture Alloys, *J. Dent. Res.,* Vol 57, 1978, IADR No. 218

127. A.T. Kuhn, The Corrosion of Metals and Alloys Used in Dentistry, *Restoration of the Partially Dentate Mouth,* J.F. Bates, D.J. Neill, and H.W. Preiskel, Ed., Quintessence Publishing, 1984, p 160–175

128. K. Asgar and F.C. Allan, Microstructure and Physical Properties of Alloys for Partial Denture Castings, *J. Dent. Res.,* Vol 47, 1968, p 189–197

129. S. Civjan, E.F. Huget, W.L. Erhard, and G.J. Vaccaro, Characterization of Surgical Casting Alloys, *J. Dent. Res.,* Vol 50, 1971, IADR No. 584

130. T.M. Devine and J. Wulff, Cast vs Wrought Cobalt-Chromium Surgical Implant Alloys, *J. Biomed. Mater. Res.,* Vol 9, 1975, p 151–167

131. R.G. Craig (Chm), Section One Report, *International Workshop on Biocompatibility, Toxicity, and Hypersensitivity to Alloy Systems Used in Dentistry,* Conference Proceedings, University of Michigan School of Dentistry, 1985

132. E.F. Huget and S.G. Vermilyea, Base Metal Dental and Surgical Alloys, *Biocompatibility of Dental Materials,* Vol IV, D.C. Smith and D.F. Williams, Ed., CRC Press, 1982, p 34–49

133. T.G. Goodall, The Metallography of Heat Treatment Effects in a Nickel-Base Casting Alloy, *Aust. Dent. J.,* Vol 24, 1879, p 235–237

134. S. Winkler, H.F. Morris, and J.M. Monteiro, Changes in Mechanical Properties and Microstructure Following Heat Treat-

ment of a Nickel-Chromium Alloy, *J. Prosthet. Dent.,* Vol 52, 1984, p 821–827

135. K. Asgar and F.C. Allan, Microstructure and Physical Properties of Alloys of Partial Denture Castings, *J. Dent. Res.,* Vol 47, 1968, p 189–197

136. K. Asgar and F.A. Peyton, Effect of Microstructure on the Physical Properties of Cobalt-Base Alloys, *J. Dent. Res.,* Vol 40, 1961, p 63–72

137. Revised ANSI/ADA Specification No. 14, Dental Base Metal Casting Alloys, *J. Am. Dent. Assoc.,* Vol 105, 1982, p 686–687

138. H.F. Morris and K. Asgar, Physical Properties and Microstructure of Four New Commercial Partial Denture Alloys, *J. Prosthet. Dent.,* Vol 33, 1975, p 36–46

139. H. Mohammed and K. Asgar, A New Dental Superalloy System, *J. Dent. Res.,* Vol 53, 1973, p 7–14

140. J.F. Bates and A.G. Knapton, Metal and Alloys in Dentistry, *Int. Met. Rev.,* Vol 22 (No. 215), 1977, p 39–60

141. R.M. Waterstrat, N.W. Rupp, and O. Franklin, Production of a Cast Titanium-Base Partial Denture, *J. Dent. Res.,* Vol 57A, 1978, IADR No. 717

142. M. Taira, J.B. Moser, and E.H. Greener, Mechanical Properties of Cast Ti Alloys for Dental Uses, *J. Dent. Res.,* Vol 65, 1986, IADR No. 603

143. E.F.I. Roberts and K.M. Clarke, The Colour Characteristics of Gold Alloys, *Gold Bull.,* Vol 9, 1979, p 9–19

144. R.M. German, M.M. Guzowski, and D.C. Wright, Color and Color Stability as Alloy Design Criterion, *J. Met.,* Vol 32, 1980, p 20–27

145. D.J.L. Treacy and R.M. German, Chemical Stability of Gold Dental Alloys, *Gold Bull.,* Vol 17, 1984, p 46–54

146. P.P. Coroso, Jr., R.M. German, and H.D. Simmons, Jr., Tarnish Evaluation of Gold-Based Dental Alloys, *J. Dent. Res.,* Vol 64, 1965

147. R.M. German, The Role of Microstructure in the Tarnish of Low Gold Alloys, *Metallography,* Vol 14, 1981, p 253–266

148. R.M. German, D.C. Wright, and R.F. Gallant, in Vitro Tarnish Measurements on Fixed Prosthodontic Alloys, *J. Prosthet. Dent.,* Vol 47, 1982, p 399–406

149. D.C. Wright and R.M. German, Quantification of Color and Tarnish Resistance of Dental Alloys, *J. Dent. Res.,* Vol 58A, 1979, IADR No. 975

150. D.A. Nitkin and K. Asgar, Evaluation of Alternative Alloys to Type III Gold for Use in Fixed Prosthodontics, *J. Am. Dent. Assoc.,* Vol 93, 1976, p 622–629

151. S. Civjan, E.F. Huget, and J. Marsden, Characterization of Two High-Fusing Gold Alloys, *J. Dent. Res.,* Vol 51, 1972, IADR No. 222

152. J.F. Bates and A.G. Knapton, Metal and Alloys in Dentistry, *Int. Met. Rev.,* Vol 22, 1982, p 39–60

153. S. Civjan, E.F. Huget, N.N. Dvivedi, and H.E. Cosner, Jr., Characterization of Two Au-Pd-Ag Alloys, *J. Dent. Res.,* Vol 52, 1973, IADR No. 46

154. E.F. Huget, S.G. Vermilyea, and J.M. Vilca, Studies on White Crown-and-Bridge Alloys, *J. Dent. Res.,* Vol 57, 1978, IADR No. 722

155. P.F. Mezger, M.M.A. Vrijhoef, and E.H. Greener, Corrosion Resistance of Three High Palladium Alloys, *Dent. Mater.,* Vol 1, 1985, p 177–179

156. M.M.A. Vrijhoef and J.M. van der Zel, Oxidation of Two High-Palladium PFM Alloys, *Dent. Mater.,* Vol 1, 1985, p 214–218

157. R.L. Bertolotti, Selection of Alloys for Today's Crown and Fixed Partial Denture Restorations, *J. Am. Dent. Assoc.,* Vol 108, 1984, p 959–966

158. J.J. Tuccillo, Compositional and Functional Characteristics of Precious Metal Alloys for Dental Restorations, *Alternatives to Gold Alloys in Dentistry,* T.M. Valega, Ed., Conference Proceedings, DHEW Publication (NIH) 77-1227, Department of Health, Education, and Welfare, 1977

159. P.J. Cascone, Phase Relations of the Palladium-Base, Copper, Gallium, Indium Alloy System, *J. Dent. Res.,* Vol 63, 1984, IADR No. 563

160. M.M.A. Vrijhoef, Oxidation of Two High-Palladium PFM Alloys, *Dent. Mater.,* Vol 1, 1985, p 214–18

161. N. Sumithra, T.K. Vaidyanathan, S. Sastri, and A. Prasad, Chloride Corrosion of Recent Commercial Pd-Based Alloys, *J. Dent. Res.,* Vol 62, 1983, IADR No. 346

162. S.M. Paradiso, Corrosion Evaluation of Pd-Cu-Ga, *J. Dent. Res.,* Vol 43, 1984, IADR No. 43

163. P.R. Mezger, M.M.A. Vrijhoef, and E.H. Greener, Corrosion Resistance of Three High-Palladium Alloys, *Dent. Mater.,* Vol 1, 1985, p 177–180

164. A. Oden and H. Hero, The Relationship Between Hardness and Structure of Pd-Cu-Ga Alloys, *J. Dent. Res.,* Vol 65, 1986, p 75–79

165. J.R. Mackert, Jr., E.E. Parry, and C.W. Fairhurst, Oxide Metal Interface Morphology Related to Oxide Adherence, *J. Dent. Res.,* Vol 63, 1984, IADR No. 405

166. G. Baron, Auger Chemical Analysis of Oxides on Ni-Cr Alloys, *J. Dent. Res.,* Vol 63, 1984, p 76–80

167. D.L. Menis, J.B. Moser, and E.H. Greener, Experimental Porcelain Compositions for Application to Cast Titanium, *J. Dent. Res.,* Vol 65, 1986, IADR No. 1565

168. ANSI/ADA Specification No. 32, New American Dental Association Specification No. 32 for Orthodontic Wires Not Containing Precious Metals, *J. Am. Dent. Assoc.,* Vol 95, 1977, p 1169–71

169. P.J. Brockhurst, Base Metal Wires for Gold Alloy Soldering to Cast Cobalt-Chromium Alloy Partial Dentures, *Aust. Dent. J.,* Vol 15, 1970, p 499–506

170. M.R. Marcotte, Optimum Time and Temperature for Stress Relief Heat Treatment of Stainless Steel Wire, *J. Dent. Res.,* Vol 52, 1973, p 1171–1175

171. C.J. Burstone and J.Y. Morton, Chinese NiTi Wire—A New Orthodontic Wire, *Am. J. Ortho.,* Vol 87, 1985, p 445–452

172. M. Bergman, Combinations of Gold Alloys in Soldered Joints, *Swed. Dent. J.,* Vol 1, 1977, p 99–106

173. C.E. Janus, D.F. Taylor, and G.A. Holland, A Microstructural Study of Soldered Connectors of Low-Gold Casting Alloys, *J. Prosthet. Dent.,* Vol 50, 1983, p 657–663

174. T.M. Devine and J. Wulff, Cast vs Wrought Cobalt-Chromium Surgical Implant Alloys, *J. Biomed. Mater. Res.,* Vol 9, 1975, p 151–167

175. H.J. Mueller and B.C. Marker, Effect of PO_4^{2-} and Cl^- upon Product Deposition on NTD and Cupralloy, *J. Dent. Res.,* Vol 59, IADR No. 279, 1980

176. H.J. Mueller, SIMS and Colorimetry of In-Vitro Sulfided Crown and Bridge Alloys, *Fifth International Symposium on New Spectroscopic Methods for Biomedical Research,* Battelle Laboratories and University of Washington, 1986

177. H. Hero, Tarnishing and Structures of Some Annealed Dental Low-Gold Alloys, *J. Dent. Res.,* Vol 63, 1984, p 926–931

178. E. Suoninen and H. Hero, Effect of Palladium on Sulfide Tarnishing of Noble Metal Alloys, *J. Biomed. Mater. Res.,* Vol 19, 1985, p 917–934

179. R. Kropp, Application of Corrosion and Tarnish Tests to Different Dental Alloys, *J. Dent. Res.,* Vol 65, 1986, IADR No. 197

180. T.K. Vaidyanathan and A. Prasad, in Vitro Corrosion and Tarnish Characteristics of Typical Dental Gold Compositions, *J. Biomed. Mater. Res.,* Vol 15, 1981, p 191–201

181. J. Brugirard, Baigain, J.C. Dupuy, H. Mazille, and G. Monnier, Study of the Electrochemical Behavior of Gold Dental Alloys, *J. Dent. Res.,* 1973, p 838–836

182. W. Popp, H. Kaiser, H. Kaesche, W. Bramer, and F. Sperner, Electrochemical Behavior of Noble Metal Dental Alloys in Different Artificial Saliva Solutions, *Proceedings of the 8th International Congress of Metallic Corrosion,* Vol 1, DECHEMA, 1981, p 76–81

183. N.K. Sarkar, R.A. Fuys, and J.W. Stanford, The Chloride Corrosion Behavior of Silver-Base Casting Alloys, *J. Dent. Res.,* Vol 58, 1979, p 1572–1577

184. D.C. Wright, R.M. German, and R.F. Gallant, Copper and Silver Corrosion Activity in Crown and Bridge Alloys, *J. Dent. Res.,* Vol 60, 1981, p 809–814

185. T.K. Vaidyanathan and A. Prasad, In Vitro Corrosion and Tarnish Analysis of Ag-Pd Binary System, *J. Dent. Res.,* Vol 60, 1981, p 707–715

186. N. Ishizaki, Corrosion Resistance of Ag-Pd Alloy System in Artificial Saliva: An Electrochemical Study, *J. Osaka Dent. Univ.,* Vol 3, 1969, p 121–133

187. L.A. O'Brien and R.M. German, Compositional Effects on Pd-Ag Dental Alloys, *J. Dent. Res.,* Vol 63, 1984, IADR No. 44

188. N.K. Sarkar, R.A. Fuys, and J.W. Stanford, The Chloride Behavior of Silver-Base Casting Alloys, *J. Dent. Res.,* Vol 58, 1979, p 1572–1577

189. L. Niemi and R.I. Holland, Tarnish and

Corrosion of a Commercial Dental Ag-Pd-Cu-Au Casting Alloy, *J. Dent. Res.,* Vol 63, 1984, p 1014–1018

190. L. Niemi and H. Hero, Structure, Corrosion, and Tarnishing of Ag-Pd-Cu Alloys, *J. Dent. Res.,* Vol 64, 1985, p 1163–1169

191. J.M. Meyer, Corrosion Resistance of Ni-Cr Dental Casting Alloys, *Corros. Sci.,* Vol 17, 1977, p 971–982

192. R.J. Hodges, The Corrosion Resistance of Gold and Base Metal Alloys, *Alternatives to Gold Alloys in Dentistry,* T.M. Valega, Ed., DHEW Publication (NIH) 77-1227, Department of Health, Education, and Welfare, 1977

193. N.K. Sarkar and E.H. Greener, In Vitro Corrosion Resistance of New Dental Alloys, *Biomater. Med. Dev. Art. Org.,* Vol 1, 1973, p 121–129

194. H.J. Mueller and C.P. Chen, Properties of a Fe-Cr-Mo Wire, *J. Dent.,* Vol 11, 1983, p 71–79

195. N.K. Sarkar, W. Redmond, B. Schwaninger, and A.J. Goldberg, The Chloride Corrosion Behavior of Four Orthodontic Wires, *J. Oral Rehab.,* Vol 10, 1983, p 121–128

196. H.J. Mueller, Silver and Gold Solders—Analysis Due to Corrosion, *Quint. Int.,* Vol 37, 1981, p 327–337

197. D.L. Johnson, V.W. Rinne, and L.L. Bleich, Polarization-Corrosion Behavior of Commercial Gold- and Silver-Base Casting Alloys in Fusayama Solution, *J. Dent. Res.,* Vol 62, 1983, p 1221–1225

198. A.D. Vardimon and H.J. Mueller, In Vitro and in Vivo Corrosion of Permanent Magnets in Orthodontic Therapy, *J. Dent. Res.,* Vol 64, 1985, IADR No. 89

CHAPTER 12

Friction and Wear of Dental Materials

FRICTION AND WEAR are not basic properties of materials but rather represent the response of a material pair in a certain environment to imposed forces, which tend to produce relative motion between the paired materials. Friction and wear behavior is therefore subject to the considerations of the testing geometry, the characteristics of the relative motion, the contact pressure between the surfaces, the temperature, the stiffness and vibrational properties of the supporting structures, the presence or absence of third bodies, the duration of contact, the chemistry of the environment in and around the interface, and lubrication (the presence of a lubricating film, such as saliva, separates surfaces during relative motion and reduces frictional forces and wear).

Several factors make the friction and wear of dental biomaterials unique (Ref 1). Most importantly, wear can produce biologically active particles, which can excite an inflammatory response. The wear process can also produce shape changes that can affect function. For example, wear in the oral cavity is characterized by the loss of the original anatomical form of the material. Wear of tooth structure and restorative materials may result from mechanical, physiological, or pathological conditions. Normal chewing (mastication) may cause attrition (physiologic wear) of tooth structures or materials, particularly in populations that consume unprocessed foods. Bruxism (see subsequent discussion) is an example of a pathological form of wear in which opposing surfaces slide against each other. If improperly performed, toothbrushing may cause an abrasive form of wear.

Human and hard dental tissues (enamel, dentin, and cementum), restorative materials

(metals, ceramics, composites, and polymers), and dental instruments (burs, curettes, and endodontic files) used to abrade tooth structure are all subject to friction and wear processes. Table 1 summarizes some typical dental materials susceptible to wear. Table 2 presents typical mechanical properties of these same materials. More detailed information on the characteristics of these materials can be found in Chapter 10, "Biomaterials for Dental Applications."

This chapter reviews the friction and wear of various dental materials that have been studied by fundamental wear measurements, simulated service wear measurements, and clinical measurements (Ref 2, 3). Correlations of properties such as hardness, fracture toughness, and wear are described, and wear mechanisms such as sliding or adhesive wear, two-body abrasion, three-body abrasion, erosion, and fatigue are identified.

Human Dental Tissues

The destruction of hard dental tissues by wear is categorized conveniently as physiologic wear, pathologic wear, prophylactic wear, and finishing procedure wear (Ref 4). In all of these types, the actual wear situation may vary considerably because of different substrates, opposing wear surfaces, lubrication systems involved, and third-body abrasives. An overview of different circumstances is provided in Table 3.

Physiologic Wear

Physiologic wear, or attrition (Ref 5), is caused by processes involving sliding contact wear, contact wear (impact without sliding), and noncontact wear from food abrasion alone.

Sliding contact wear produces the most prominent effects during normal masticatory function. An example of severe attrition is shown in Fig. 1. Attrition occurs because of function (Ref 6) and occurs only where the opposing teeth come into contact (Ref 7), so it can be distinguished from erosion (see the discussion of "Pathologic Wear" given subsequently).

Attrition in primitive man was often severe (with pulpal exposure), owing to the nature of the aboriginal diet of tough meat and sandy, fibrous plants, as studies on both skeletal and living representatives of aboriginal populations have attested (Ref 8–10).

Fundamental research on the degree and types of attrition found in the teeth of ancient, primitive, and modern populations has dealt mainly with the wear planes produced on molar surfaces (Ref 11–13) and with the effects of attrition on facial height (Ref 14–17) and on the position of the temporomandibular joint (Ref 16, 18). It is apparent that not all people wear on their teeth the same way. The patterns produced are frequently characteristic of ethnic variations.

Improved tooth care and dietary habits have lessened considerably the occurrence of attrition in modern populations. For additional information on the effects of food, degree of function, and age on attrition, see Ref 19 to 25.

Pathologic Wear

This cause of wear can be particularly destructive to individual teeth or the entire dentition. Xerostomia and bruxism are the most frequently reported pathologic causes of wear.

Xerostomia. This condition results in dryness of the oral cavity and causes brittleness of the teeth. It has been observed in women during and after menopause (Ref 26). Investigation of causes of abnormal tooth wear must take salivary factors into consideration (Ref 27, 28). Mucin-based saliva substitutes lubricate with values comparable to whole human saliva, whereas substitutes based on carboxymethylcellulose do not appear to lubricate well (Ref 29).

Bruxism. This condition is a nonfunctional mandibular movement that is manifested by occasional or habitual grinding or clenching of the teeth (Ref 30). The major effects of severe bruxism can be tooth wear and accelerated alveolar bone loss. An example of occlusal wear resulting from bruxism is shown in Fig. 2. This abnormal wear rapidly removes the cusps of teeth. Wear takes place mainly on incisal edges of upper and lower anterior teeth. With time, edges become highly polished and flattened. In the posterior teeth, wear appears as small saucerlike excavations.

Table 1 Simplified composition or microstructure of some typical dental materials susceptible to wear and friction

Material	Simplified composition or microstructure
Alloys	
Alloy crown	Au-Ag-Cu (single phase), Au-Pd, Ni-Cr
Amalgam (admixed)	Ag_2Hg_3, Cu_6Sn_5, Ag_3Sn-Cu_3Sn-Zn (unreacted), Ag-Cu (unreacted)
Amalgam (unicompositional)	Ag_2Hg_3, Cu_6Sn_5, Ag_3Sn-Cu_3Sn-Zn (unreacted)
Endodontic instruments	Stainless steel, carbon steel
Orthodontic wire	Austenitic stainless steel, Ni-Ti-Co, Ti-Mo-Zr-Sn
Ceramics	
Cements	
Zinc oxide-eugenol	Zinc eugenolate and zinc oxide (unreacted)
Zinc phosphate	Zinc phosphate and zinc oxide (unreacted)
Glass-ceramic inlays and crowns	Glass with crystalline alumina or fluoride-mica glass ceramic
Gypsum dies	$CaSO_4 \cdot 2H_2O$
Porcelain (PFM)	Potassium-sodium aluminosilicate glasses
Porcelain denture teeth	Quartz particles in a glass matrix
Polymers	
Cements	
Glass ionomer	Acrylic or maleic acid copolymer and calcium aluminosilicate matrix with aluminosilicate glass (unreacted) or silver-glass cermet (unreacted)
Zinc polyacrylate	Acrylic polymer and zinc oxide (unreacted)
Composites (hybrid)	Aromatic or urethane diacrylate matrix with silanated filler (quartz, borosilicate glass, lithium aluminum silicate, barium aluminum silicate, or colloidal silica)
Composites (microfilled)	Aromatic or urethane diacrylate matrix with colloidal silica
Denture acrylics	Polymethyl methacrylate (PMMA) with pre-polymerized PMMA or rubber-reinforced acrylic beads
Pit and fissure sealants	Aromatic or urethane diacrylate matrix with silanated filler
Plastic denture teeth	Polymethyl methacrylate matrix and beads

PFM, porcelain fused to metal. Source: Ref 1

Erosion. This condition is the chemical weakening of human enamel resulting from acid decalcification. The pH affects the rate of decalcification for uncleaned, cleaned, and mechanically abraded enamel (Ref 31). Chemical decalcification may be caused by environmental pollutants contaminating the air and/or saliva of patients. Accelerated wear is observed in people employed in occupations (for example, mining, or sulfuric acid production) where an unusual or severe atmospheric environment exists (Ref 32).

Unusual Habits. People who grasp needles or nails with their teeth or smoke pipes may also exhibit localized pathologic wear.

Prophylactic Wear

Toothbrush and Dentifrice. Oral hygiene is necessary for maintaining a healthy mouth and for social acceptance. The emphasis in the study of wear of the dentition by toothbrush and dentifrice has been the elimination of overly abrasive dentifrice components. Cervical abrasion resulting from improper and excessive toothbrush and dentifrice use is shown in Fig. 3.

The primary function of a dentifrice is to clean and polish the surfaces of the teeth accessible with a toothbrush. During cleaning, extraneous debris and deposits need to be removed from the tooth surface. These deposits listed in order of increasing difficulty of removal are (Ref 33):

- Food debris
- Plaque (a soft, mainly bacterial film)
- Acquired pellicle (a proteinaceous film of salivary origin)
- Calculus

The ideal abrasive should exhibit a maximum cleaning efficiency with minimum tooth abra-

Table 2 Typical properties of dental materials

Materials	Knoop hardness, kg/mm²	Yield strength		Ultimate tensile strength		Ultimate compressive strength	
		MPa	ksi	MPa	ksi	MPa	ksi
Alloys							
Alloy crown (Au-Ag-Cu)	125 (HV)	220	32	425	62	. . .	. . .
Amalgam			. . .				
Admixed	. . .	. . .	. . .	40	5.8	340	49
Unicompositional	. . .	. . .	. . .	50	7.3	450	65
Orthodontic wires							
Stainless steel	540	1500	218	2000	290	. . .	. . .
Ni-Ti-Co	. . .	340	49	. . .	. . .	. . .	. . .
Ti-Mo-Zr-Sn	. . .	960	139	. . .	. . .	. . .	. . .
Ceramics							
Cements							
Zinc oxide-eugenol	. . .	. . .	. . .	5	0.7	40	5.8
Zinc phosphate	40	. . .	. . .	14	2.0	170	25
Human teeth							
Dentin	70	170	25	50	7.3	300	44
Enamel	340	350	51	10	1.5	380	55
Glass-ceramic inlays	360	. . .	. . .	. . .	. . .	. . .	. . .
Gypsum dies	65	. . .	. . .	8	1.2	80	11.6
Porcelain (PFM)	460	. . .	. . .	25	3.6	150	22
Porcelain denture teeth	460	. . .	. . .	. . .	. . .	. . .	
Polymers							
Cements							
Glass ionomer	. . .	. . .	. . .	4	0.6	125	18
Zinc polyacrylate	. . .	. . .	. . .	10	1.5	70	10.2
Composites							
Hybrid	55	. . .	. . .	50	7.3	275	40
Microfilled	30	. . .	. . .	40	5.8	290	42
Denture acrylics	20	25	3.6	50	7.3	75	10.9
Pit and fissure sealant	25	. . .	. . .	30	4.4	170	25
Plastic denture teeth	20	55	8	. . .	. . .	76	11.0

PFM, porcelain fused to metal. Source: Ref 1

sion. In addition, a dentifrice should polish the teeth. Highly polished teeth are not only aesthetically desirable, but they may also be less receptive to the retention of deposits (Ref 34).

Typical dentifrice abrasives include: calcium carbonate, dibasic calcium phosphate dihydrate, anhydrous dibasic calcium phosphate, tricalcium phosphate, calcium sulfate, calcium pyrophosphate, insoluble sodium metaphosphate, and hydrated alumina (Ref 35).

Selection of a dentifrice by a dentist for a patient should be based on: (1) degree of staining, (2) force exerted on the brush, (3) method of brushing, and (4) amount of exposed dentin and cementum. The Council on Dental Therapeutics of the American Dental Association published information on the abrasivity of dentifrices in 1970 (Ref 36).

Prophylactic Paste. A dental prophylactic paste should be sufficiently abrasive to remove effectively exogenous stains, pellicle, materia alba, and oral debris from the tooth surface without causing undue abrasion to the enamel, dentin, or cementum. Polymeric materials, such as denture base and artificial tooth resins, composite restorations, and pit and fissure sealants, are particularly susceptible to abrasion because of their low hardness. The undesirable results of wear can be a reduction in anatomic contours and increased surface roughness.

Abrasives in commercial prophylactic pastes include: recrystallized kaolinite, silicon dioxide, calcined magnesium silicate, diatomaceous silicon dioxide, pumice, sodium-potassium-aluminum silicate, and zirconium silicate (Ref 37).

Cutting, Finishing, and Polishing Wear

Tooth structure and restorative dental materials are routinely reshaped and smoothened using special instruments for cutting and finishing. A highly polished surface is then produced by treatment with polishing pastes containing alumina or diamond abrasive particles less than 1 μm in size.

Wear Studies

Traditional wear theory divides observed wear into categories of adhesive wear, abrasive wear, corrosive wear, and surface fatigue wear (Ref 1). Adhesive wear is characterized by the formation and disruption of microjunctions. Abrasive wear involves a soft surface in contact with a harder surface. In this type of wear, particles are pulled off of one surface and adhere to the other during sliding. There can be two types of abrasive wear: two- and three-body abrasion (wear). This type of wear can be minimized if

Table 3 Classification of wear situations in dentistry

Intraoral wear event	Type of wear	Lubricant	Substrate	Opponent	Abrasive
Physiologic causes of wear					
Noncontact wear	3-body	Saliva/food	Tooth/restoration	. . .	Food
Direct contact wear	2-body	Saliva	Tooth/restoration	Tooth/restoration	. . .
Sliding contact wear	2-body	Saliva	Tooth/restoration	Tooth/restoration	. . .
Pathologic causes of wear					
Bruxism	2-body	Saliva	Tooth/restoration	Tooth/restoration	. . .
Xerostomia	2-body	. . .	Tooth/restoration	Tooth/restoration	. . .
Erosion	. . .	Saliva	Tooth/restoration	. . .	. . .
Unusual habits	2-body	Saliva	Tooth/restoration	Foreign body	. . .
Prophylactic causes of wear					
Toothbrush and dentifrice	3-body	Water	Tooth/restoration	Toothbrush	Dentifrice
Prophylactic pastes	3-body	Water	Tooth/restoration	Polishing cup	Pumice
Scaling and cleaning instruments	2-body	Saliva	Tooth/restoration	Instrument	. . .
Cutting, finishing, polishing					
Cutting burrs/diamonds	2-body	Water	Tooth/restoration	Burr	. . .
Finishing burrs	2-body	Water	Tooth/restoration	Burr	. . .
Polishing pastes	3-body	Water	Tooth/restoration	Polishing cup	Abrasive slurry

surfaces are smooth and hard and if particles are kept off the surface. Corrosive wear is secondary to physical removal of a protective layer and is therefore related to the chemical activity of the wear surfaces. The sliding action of the surfaces removes any surface barriers and causes accelerated wear. In surface fatigue wear, stresses are produced by asperities or free particles, leading to the formation of surface or subsurface cracks. Particles break off under cyclic loading and sliding.

Unfortunately, predictions of these wear models depend on the materials behaving in a relatively brittle fashion. Most dental materials under intraoral circumstances do not behave in this way; therefore, it is difficult to rank dental materials performance. Most wear tests have not faithfully predicted clinical performance.

Wear information on dental materials has been collected from fundamental studies with simple laboratory tests, simulation studies with customized machines, and clinical studies. Unfortunately, the fundamental laboratory tests and the simulation studies have not had much success in correlating with observed clinical wear.

Fundamental Laboratory Studies

In a single-pass sliding technique, fluorapatite single crystals served as a simple model system for human enamel, which is composed of hydroxyapatite. The wear and friction of fluorapatite single crystals under conditions of single- and multiple-pass sliding with a diamond hemisphere (360 μm in diameter) can be evaluated by interpretation of tangential force, track width, and surface failure classification data (Ref 38–40). A failure classification scale (Fig. 4) includes:

- *Class 1:* entirely ductile
- *Class 2:* mostly ductile with some tensile cracking
- *Class 3:* essentially tensile cracking
- *Class 4:* mostly tensile cracking with chevrons (chipping)
- *Class 5:* chevrons

Examples of classes 1, 3, and 5 are shown in Fig. 5.

The failure of fluorapatite at a 0.1 N (0.02 lbf) load for single-pass sliding in the <2110> direction is essentially ductile and progresses toward brittle failure as the load is increased (Ref 41). At 0.5 N (0.11 lbf) loads and higher, failure is characterized by chevron formation. Track width follows an exponential function, whereas

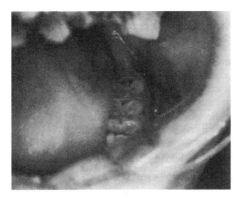

Fig. 1 Severe occlusal wear resulting from dental attrition. Source: Ref 4

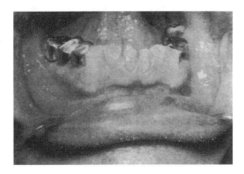

Fig. 2 Occlusal wear resulting from bruxism. Source: Ref 4

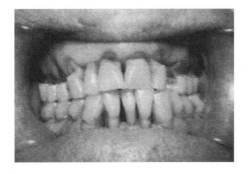

Fig. 3 Cervical abrasion resulting from excessive toothbrush and dentifrice use. Source: Ref 4

the tangential force (friction) increases linearly with normal load (Ref 41). The coefficient of friction is not a perfect indicator of wear. The track width data indicate that the principal mechanisms for the accommodation of strain are elastic deformation and cracking. Sliding in the <0110> direction results in slightly lower friction but substantially increased surface damage (Table 4).

The ductile-to-brittle transition for sliding of diamond on fluorapatite occurs at higher normal loads in air and dimethylformamide than in water (Table 4) (Ref 42). The lowering of the transition in water is explained on the basis of surface hardening as a result of the interaction of polar water molecules or their dissociation products and charged near-surface species. The interaction results in pinning of dislocations and a reduction in the ability of the lattice to accommodate strain by slip, thus effectively lowering the stress required to cause fracture.

Single-pass sliding by itself cannot completely describe the wear of fluorapatite single crystals (Ref 43). Wear tracks for a single and double pass on the same track in the opposite direction under a 0.7 N (0.16 lbf) load are shown in Fig. 6. The effect of sliding a second

pass across a wear track is shown in Fig. 7. When both tracks are made under a 0.5 N (0.11 lbf) load, catastrophic failure occurs at the intersection of the tracks. Considerable care is necessary in extrapolating single-pass wear data to repetitive wear measurements.

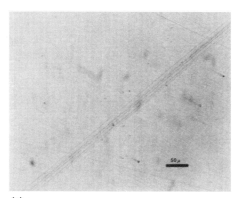

(a)

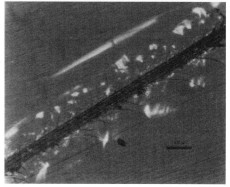

(b)

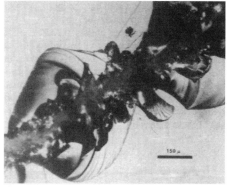

(c)

Fig. 5 Examples of surface failure of fluorapatite single crystals. (a) Class 1. (b) Class 3. (c) Class 5. Source: Ref 40

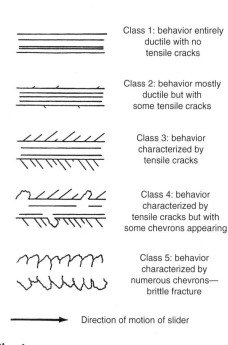

Class 1: behavior entirely ductile with no tensile cracks

Class 2: behavior mostly ductile but with some tensile cracks

Class 3: behavior characterized by tensile cracks

Class 4: behavior characterized by tensile cracks but with some chevrons appearing

Class 5: behavior characterized by numerous chevrons— brittle fracture

Direction of motion of slider

Fig. 4 Failure classification scale. Source: Ref 40

The frictional behavior and surface failure of human enamel has been studied by sliding with a diamond hemisphere (360 μm in diameter) in water (Ref 44, 45). Similar tests have been carried out on a sintered hydroxyapatite ceramic, which approximates the properties of human enamel (Ref 46). Table 5 compares the properties of these materials.

Simulation Studies

Chewing Machines. An early attempt to study attrition used a machine capable of simulating the actions of the human mandible during chewing to produce a variety of wear patterns (Ref 47). Much more sophisticated chewing machines have been developed to examine dental composite wear and are discussed later.

Brushing Machines (Dentifrices). Three main methods used to determine the loss of hard tooth tissue from brushing are: (1) measuring the amount of tooth tissue abraded from an irradiated tooth by the concentration of radioactive phosphorus in the wear debris (Ref 36, 48–51), (2) determining the change in profile of samples (Ref 52), and (3) measuring the change in reflectance of the surface of tooth structure (Ref 53).

Dentifrices used in 1942 were compared to a calcium carbonate standard (Ref 54, 55). Abrasion was found to occur 25 times faster on

Table 4 Influence of sliding direction and environment on friction and wear properties of fluorapatite single crystals for single-pass sliding on the basal plane

Condition	Coefficient of friction (β)	Ductile-to-brittle transition load N	Ductile-to-brittle transition load lbf
<2110> direction in air	0.22	0.75	0.17
<0110> direction in air	0.19	0.15	0.03
<2110> direction in water	0.24	0.18	0.04
<2110> direction in dimethylformamide	0.24	0.62	0.14

Source: Ref 41, 42

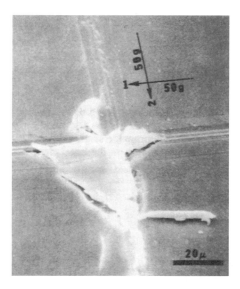

Fig. 7 Intersecting wear tracks on a fluorapatite single crystal under a 0.5 N (0.11 lbf) load. Source: Ref 43

Table 5 Properties of a sintered hydroxyapatite ceramic compared with human enamel

Property	HAP-60K-1200C	Human enamel
Compressive strength, MPa (ksi)	380 (55)	400 (58)
Young's modulus, GPa (psi × 10^6)	120 (17.4)	80 (11.6)
Knoop hardness, kg/mm²	450	340
Density, g/cm³	3.1	2.96
Coefficient of friction	0.24	0.36
Linear coefficient of thermal expansion, 10^{-6}/°C	9.2–11.8	11.4

Source: Ref 46

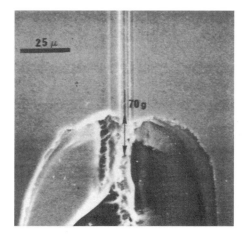

Fig. 6 Wear tracks on a fluorapatite single crystal for a single and double pass on the same track in the opposite direction under a 0.7 N (0.16 lbf) load. Source: Ref 43

dentin and 35 times faster on cementum than on the enamel tips of cusps. Abrasive power (percent abrasion of a calcium carbonate control) increases linearly with particle size (Ref 56, 57). On the other hand, the polishing ratio of zirconium silicate increases with decreasing particle size, and particle size distribution is important (Ref 53). Increasing the load on the brush also increases enamel and dentin abrasion scores (Ref 50, 58).

The radiotracer method can measure wear rates of dental tissues by as few as one or two strokes of a brush on dentin with commercial dentifrices. Use of this method has led to the observation that wear of dental tissues is proportional to penetration hardness if hard abrasives are used (Ref 49).

Brushing Machines (Toothbrush). A number of studies have attempted to determine the influence of the toothbrush and its variables on the wear of dental tissues. Plastic toothbrush bristles have little abrasive or polishing power (Ref 59–62). Other studies have compared automatic versus hand toothbrushes (Ref 63–65). In general, the mechanical toothbrushes produce less abrasion of hard tooth tissue than simulated manual brushing, but the forces associated with manual brushing are usually larger.

Many variables of toothbrushes and dentifrices have been examined with brushing machines. These include (Ref 4):

- *Dentifrice properties:* hardness, particle size, and particle distribution of the abrasive, and composition and concentration of remaining components
- *Toothbrush properties:* geometry, hardness, stiffness, and number of bristles
- *Substrate properties:* orientation, hardness, surface preparation
- *Testing conditions:* brush load, stroke length, stroke rate, number of strokes, and presence of saliva

Machines for Prophylaxis. Products containing quartz and pumice show higher cleansing values but generally result in greater abrasion to enamel and dentin (Ref 66). Abrasion of dentin by a pumice slurry is approximately 20 times greater than abrasion of enamel under standardized conditions (Ref 67). Increases in treatment time, load, and cup speed cause linear increases in abrasion of irradiated human enamel and dentin (Ref 68). Commercial prod-ucts containing calcined magnesium silicate and sodium-potassium-aluminum silicate show best polishing with low abrasivity (Ref 37). No clinical study has yet correlated the degree of abrasivity with any destructive effect on hard and soft tissues. American Dental Association Specification No. 37 includes a suggested abrasivity test that uses a radiotracer technique (Ref 69).

Cutting Machines. Cutting of human enamel by a high-speed diamond stone is enhanced by use of a solution of glycerol, ethanol, and water (2:1:2) when compared to cutting with water alone (Ref 70). Such a chemomechanical effect is also observed in the cutting of amalgam with diamonds and carbide burs and the cutting of composites with carbide burs. Cutting of hydroxyapatite blocks with autoclaved tungsten carbide burs is enhanced if the burs are dipped in sodium nitrate or commercial anticorrosive dips before autoclaving (Ref 71).

Clinical Studies

Clinical studies collect physiologic wear data produced by: (1) sliding contacts or direct contact alone (occlusal-contact-area wear) and (2) noncontact wear (contact-free wear), which is related to food abrasion. To effectively examine these events, pathologic and prophylactic wear must be absent or controlled. In addition to the restorative treatment variables in clinical studies, there are also intraoral variables and patient factors that complicate clinical results and interpretations.

Occlusal-contact-area wear of human enamel has been measured with a computerized three-dimensional measuring technique on tooth replicas over a period of four years (Ref 72). The steady-state wear rates at enamel occlusal contact areas are approximately 29 µm/year for molars and approximately 15 µm/year for premolars. These data agree with earlier reports of 33 µm/year (Ref 73) and 41 µm/year (Ref 74).

Observations of orthodontic patients with arrested carious lesions indicate that functional wear and toothbrushing are responsible for the arrestment by disturbance and removal of bacterial deposits (Ref 75). Changes in surface enamel morphology after acid etching are also the result of abrasion rather than the precipitation of mineral from saliva (Ref 62).

Enamel undergoes physiologic wear but is routinely redeposited by nucleation and growth of new hydroxyapatite from the calcium phosphate present in saliva. This process helps to compensate for losses that occur during physiologic, prophylactic, and polishing wear. Dentifrice abrasivity of enamel as measured in vivo by a cellulose acetate replication technique is much lower than abrasion caused by pumice or zirconium silicate (Ref 76).

Dental Amalgam

Dental amalgam is an alloy that results when mercury is mixed with an alloy containing silver, tin, copper, and sometimes zinc (Table 1). Before it hardens, the freshly mixed mass of amalgam can be packed into a cavity prepared in a tooth. Amalgams are usually limited to replacement of tooth tissue in the posterior teeth and often function in stress-bearing areas susceptible to occlusal wear. Some properties of dental amalgams are listed in Table 2.

Fundamental Laboratory Studies

Abrasion Tests. Two-body abrasion of dental amalgam has been measured using a Taber abrader (Ref 77), a silicon carbide two-body abrasion test (Ref 78), and a pin-on-disk test (Ref 79). With the Taber abrader, smearing of amalgam and clogging of the abrader wheel cause inconsistent ranking with clinical observations; clogging of the abrasive surface is avoided by abrading at a low load over a fresh abrasive surface on each pass. Ranking of amalgam and composite restorative materials with two-body abrasion tests is in better agreement with clinical observations than that done with three-body abrasion tests. Two-body abrasion test results on some typical dental amalgam alloys are given in Table 6. As indicated by

Table 6   Material loss on abrasion of dental amalgams

Material	Material loss, 10^{-4} mm³/mm of travel(a)	
	24 h	1 month
Spher-a-Caps	7.0	7.0
New True Dentalloy	6.5	6.3
Dispersalloy	5.6	4.9

(a) Load: 0.17 MPa (0.025 ksi). Source: Ref 2

these results, a dispersed high-copper amalgam (Dispersalloy, Johnson & Johnson) exhibited better resistance to silicon carbide two-body abrasion than spherical low-copper amalgams.

The pin-on-disk test (Ref 79) uses a cylindrical sample of enamel to rub on a rotating disk of amalgam. Measurements of wear rate are possible, but transfer of material from the disk to the pin confuses interpretation of the results.

Single-Pass Sliding. The wear of dental amalgam also has been studied by single- and double-pass sliding with a diamond hemisphere (360 µm in diameter) (Ref 80). The dispersed high-copper amalgam has the lowest values of tangential force and track width. The mode of surface failure under single- and double-pass sliding is ductile, with no evidence of subsurface failure. Smearing of phases for both spherical and dispersed amalgams during sliding does occur, but the dispersed amalgam is more resistant to smearing. Cracks that occur at higher loads propagate around the stronger phases. Wear is determined by resistance to penetration and by a ductile mode of surface failure over the load range tested.

Friction of dental amalgam is altered when any transfer of material from one member of the pair to the other member occurs (Ref 81). For example, when gold or dental composite slide against amalgam, amalgam material is transferred to the gold or composite surface, and the friction then becomes that of amalgam on amalgam.

Fracture toughness, critical strain energy release rate, and critical stress-intensity factor have been determined for several types of dental amalgams (Ref 82). Data are consistent with surface failure observed in single-pass wear studies.

An equation developed from single-pass studies (Ref 83) has been derived that relates the sliding frictional force (F) to normal load (N), fracture toughness, modulus of elasticity, yield strength, and slider diameter in the form of $F = KN^n$ (Table 7). The observed friction is caused primarily by plowing or deformation during single-pass sliding.

Simulation Studies

Amalgam abrasion from dentifrices in brushing machines has been studied by profilometry and laser reflection techniques, which both indicate that amalgam wears approximately 10 times more rapidly than gold alloys under the same conditions of simulated brushing with normal dentifrices (Ref 84).

Clinical Studies

The physiologic wear rates of amalgam are 6 to 15 μm/year in contact-free areas and 28 to 58 μm/year in occlusal contact areas (Ref 85). This wear may be compensated by continual amalgam expansion that produces occlusal extrusion. Therefore, the rate of attrition of amalgam is usually not considered to be a clinical problem.

Amalgam degrades at the tooth-restoration interface by a process called marginal fracture, which is the result of electrochemical corrosion in the presence of direct-contact stresses (Ref 86). Direct-contact areas on amalgams that are not stabilized by contacts on enamel may also produce noticeable facets.

Composite Restorative Materials

Composite restorative materials consist of a cross-linked polymer matrix that is chemically bonded by coupling agents to the surfaces of dispersed silica-based filler particles (Table 1). Composite restorations have the appearance of natural tooth tissue and can be placed directly into a cavity preparation for in situ hardening. They are recommended for restorations where occlusal stress is minimal and appearance is crucial. Composites are also available for lim-

ited posterior use in areas of occlusal stress, but they are less durable than amalgam (Ref 87). Some properties are listed in Table 2.

Wear resistance of composite restorations is important for clinical longevity, esthetics, and resistance to dental plaque. The need for markedly improved wear resistance has been emphasized by literature reviews (Ref 88–91). The reason that wear-resistant composites have not been developed is primarily because of the lack of understanding of the mechanisms of clinical wear. This problem is confounded by the lack of reliable and consistent clinical wear data.

Fundamental Laboratory Studies

The problem with all wear theories has been the lack of correlation of clinical wear results with laboratory properties. Mechanical properties do correlate with filler types and loading levels (Ref 92–97), but they do not predict clinical performance. To bridge the gap, a wide range of tests have been performed. Some of these are described as follows.

Abrasion Tests. Taber abrasion (Ref 81), single-pass sliding on abrasive papers (Ref 98), pin and plate (Ref 99), pin and disk (Ref 100), metallographic polishing (Ref 101), toothbrushing (Ref 102), and oscillating wear (Ref 103) tests have shown very little or no success in explaining intraoral wear. With the Taber abrader, smearing of resin and clogging of the abrader wheel produced apparently better resis-

Table 7 Friction of dental materials as described by various properties including fracture toughness

Material	Modulus of elasticity		Yield strength		Fracture toughness, J/m^2	n	K
	GPa	psi × 10^6	MPa	ksi			
Amalgams							
Spherical, low-copper	12.9	1.87	142	20.6	117	1.17	0.211
Lathe-cut, low-copper	12.8	1.86	119	17.3	247	1.31	0.146
Admixed, high-copper	17.7	2.57	130	18.9	104	1.25	0.124
Composite	7.8	1.13	135	19.6	182	1.23	0.190
Unfilled resin							
Acrylic	2.0	0.29	104	15.1	382	1.54	0.141
Diacrylate	1.8	0.26	65	9.4	402	1.19	0.338

Source: Ref 83

tance for unfilled resins than for composites; these results are inconsistent in ranking with clinical observations.

A silicon carbide two-body abrasion test was developed to avoid clogging effects (Ref 78). This test provided some agreement with early clinical studies, but its primary usefulness was to examine the relative effects of different formulation variables.

Improvements in the durability of composites depend on a thorough understanding of the wear behavior of the resin matrix (Ref 104). The resin with the lowest value of two-body abrasion also showed the lowest coefficient of friction and the most ductile behavior during single-pass sliding (Table 8). Abrasion resistance was improved by finishing the cured surface before testing (Ref 105). Reduced wear of large-particle composites was related to the increased size (relative to the abrasive), increased hardness, and increased volume fraction of the filler particles (Ref 106, 107).

Pin-on-disk testers were popular, at least in part, because subsurface damage detected during microdefect analysis of a few composites recovered from in vivo service was apparently the same as the structure observed in composites subjected to pin-on-disk wear using stainless steel sliders (Ref 108).

Two-body pin-on-disk abrasion of composite veneering resins was shown to be much higher for rubbing contact against porcelain versus enamel, gold, or the same veneering resin (Ref 109). Combinations of composite with composite, silver-reinforced glass ionomer, or porcelain wore excessively (Ref 110).

The enthusiasm for abrasion testing produced a large amount of data, but actual clinical wear mechanisms often proved to be quite different.

Single-Pass Sliding. The wear of composites also has been studied by single- and double-pass sliding with a diamond hemisphere (360 μm in diameter) (Ref 111, 112). The surface failure for unfilled diacrylate resins was more severe than that observed for an unfilled acrylic resin. Addition of nonsilanated filler to the diacrylate resin increased resistance to penetration but did not dramatically change the mode of failure (Fig. 8). Diacrylate resins that contained silanated filler (commercial composites) were ductile in failure during sliding and showed the higher resistance to penetration. Damage was more severe for double-pass than for single-pass sliding. Single-pass data did not, however, provide an estimate of volume lost on repetitive wear of composites.

Aging and Chemical Softening. The surface degradation of composites caused by accelerated aging in a weathering chamber was characterized by erosion of the resin matrices and exposure of filler particles (Ref 113). Differences in surface roughness and profile indicated that the aged composites were eroded at different rates. Surface crazing (Fig. 9) was observed for some aged composites. Surface degradation also resulted in color changes, particularly for large-particle composites but much less so for microfilled composites (Ref 114).

Single-pass sliding wear of aged, chemically cured, large-particle composites resulted in smaller track widths, lower tangential forces, easier dislodging of material, and more severe

Table 8 Material loss on abrasion and single-pass wear characteristics of dimethacrylate resins

Material	Material loss, 10^{-4} mm^3/mm of travel(a)	Coefficient of friction (β)	Ductile-to-brittle transition load	
			N	lbf
Tetraethylene glycoldimethacrylate	22.0	0.45	7.0	1.57
Bisphenol A-bis ethylmethacrylate	17.7	0.61	5.0	1.12
Bisphenol A-bis (2-hydroxy-propyl)methacrylate + ethylene glycol-dimethacrylate (1:1)	15.5	0.35	>10	>2.25
Bisphenol A-bis ethylmethacrylate + octafluoro-1-pentyl-methacrylate (9:3)	19.1	0.61	4.0	0.90
Bisphenol A-bis ethylmethacrylate + octafluoro-1-pentyl-methacrylate (3:9)	32.2	1.48	3.0	0.67

(a) Load: 0.18 MPa (0.026 ksi). Source: Ref 104

surface failure at lower normal loads than that of unaged composites (Ref 115). Ductile-to-brittle transitions occurred at lower normal loads (Table 9), and changes in morphology became more severe (Fig. 10) with increased aging (Ref 116).

Preconditioning composites in food-simulating liquids (heptane and several ethanol/water solutions) has been shown to decrease the hardness with a corresponding increase in pin-on-disk wear (Ref 117). Swelling of the polymer matrix and surface damage occurs during preconditioning. Increasing the degree of cure of the matrix polymer may inhibit diffusion of penetrants, and additional cross linking may reduce swelling and damage by solvents. Evidence of erosion has also been observed under in vivo conditions (Ref 118).

Fracture toughness, critical strain energy release rate (G_{Ic}), and critical stress-intensity factor (K_{Ic}) have been determined for experimental and commercial composites (Ref 119). The commercial composite was less resistant to crack initiation and had a higher K_{Ic} than its unfilled diacrylate resin. Data were consistent with surface failure observed in single-pass wear studies of these resins.

Correlating Abrasion with Hardness and Tensile Data. Hardness and tensile strength of large-particle composites were not related to measured in vitro abrasion rates (Ref 120). However, clinical abrasion of microfilled composites and unfilled resins appeared related to indentation hardness (Ref 121).

Simulation Studies

Most simulation studies evaluate physiologic wear. Few studies have dealt with prophylactic wear. Microfilled composites subjected to brushing abrasion with a dentifrice wore 5 to 10 times faster than large-particle composites (Ref 122). Abrasion slowed once the resin-rich layer of a composite was lost or when the composite was postcured by heat.

A limited study was reported in which composites were abraded by an artificial food bolus (Ref 123). Composites were placed along the edge of a rotating disk immersed in a millet seed suspension and ground against a stainless steel

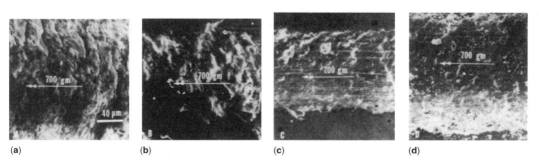

(a) (b) (c) (d)

Fig. 8 Scanning electron micrographs of double-pass wear scars made under a normal load of 7 N (1.6 lbf) of (a) unfilled diacrylate resin, (b) unfilled acrylic, (c) diacrylate resin with silanated filler, and (d) diacrylate resin with nonsilanated filler. Source: Ref 112

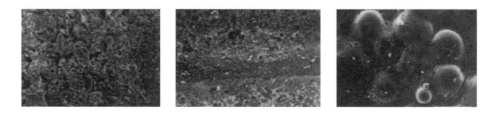

Fig. 9 Scanning electron micrographs of composites aged for 900 h showing surface crazing. Source: Ref 113

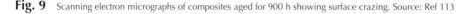

wheel. Although not perfect, the ranking of composites agreed with clinical studies.

Chewing machines have been developed to simulate the full range of intraoral wear events

Table 9 **Influence of increased aging on single-pass wear transitions of composites under conditions of accelerated aging**

Material	Ductile-to-brittle transition load, N (lbf)		
	Unaged	300 h	900 h
Large-particle composite			
Concise	2.8 (0.63)	1.8 (0.40)	1.5 (0.34)
Microfilled composite			
Finesse	8.0 (1.80)	3.3 (0.74)	3.0 (0.67)
Isopast	4.3 (1.0)	4.3 (1.0)	4.3 (1.0)
Silar	7.0 (1.57)	6.0 (1.35)	2.0 (0.45)

Concise and Silar, 3M Co. Source: Ref 116

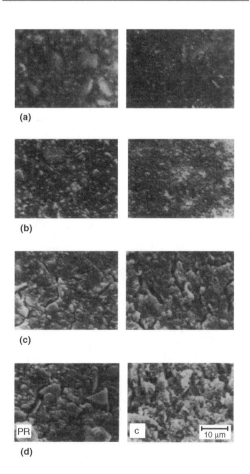

(a)

(b)

(c)

(d)

Fig. 10 Scanning electron micrographs of surface morphology of two large-particle composites aged at (a) 0, (b) 300, (c) 600, and (d) 900 h. Source: Ref 116

(Ref 124). The results have only shown a limited agreement with clinical studies.

Clinical Studies

Many direct clinical evaluations of wear rely on the United States Public Health Service (USPHS) criteria for classifying the loss of anatomical form of posterior restorations (Ref 125). Unfortunately, the USPHS criteria alone are not sufficient to detect early loss of material in posterior composites (Ref 126–131). Because of the crudeness of the USPHS scale, there was considerable impetus in the early 1980s to develop more precise indirect measurement techniques.

The first indirect method to become popular was designated the Leinfelder technique. It measured the loss of material using a stone cast poured from a clinical impression of the restoration to compare it to a series of calibrated stone casts (Ref 126, 130, 132). Other similar indirect cast methods have tried to refine the Leinfelder approach (Ref 133–135). Unfortunately, because of operational differences, these scales have been shown to underestimate actual wear by 50%.

The major advantage of indirect methods employing stone casts and evaluators is their inexpensive nature. All other methods, particularly computer digitization, are remarkably costly and thus impractical for even small clinical studies.

Electroplated or epoxy-resin replicas of restorations have been prepared from impressions and studied by optical, scanning electron, or reflex microscopy; by Moiré techniques; or with computer digitization (Ref 86, 136). Wear has also been measured by monitoring the recession of resin on the surfaces of prominent filler particles by scanning electron microscopy of sequences of impressions of a restoration (Ref 137).

A less-complicated method of clinically evaluating restorations is to place them into denture teeth in a removable denture (Ref 138–142). The dentures permit direct measurements of the samples by profilometry or three-dimensional computerized surface digitization.

Because of the large number of uncontrollable clinical variables involved in these studies, there is a broad distribution of results at each recall. The results are different for molars and premolars. Differences in operators and techniques among clinical studies are often so great that the results are not comparable at all. The reported results are often misrepresented as wear rates rather than total wear. Wear does not occur in a linear fashion.

Published wear rates for composites are 12 to 79 μm/year in contact-free areas and 39 to 135 μm/year in occlusal contact areas (Ref 85). For autocured (Ref 143) and ultraviolet-light-polymerized (Ref 144, 145) composites, wear has been shown to occur at decreasing rates after the first 3 years (Fig. 11). This same pattern of decreasing wear has now been reported for several newer visible-light-cured composites (Ref 146–148). For one composite, approximately 74% of the total wear over a 3 year period occurred during the first year, followed by 19% in the second year, and 6% in the third year. This pattern is less obvious if the first 6 months of data are excluded. The wear rate for the next few years may appear almost constant (Ref 149). The rate reported for a few microfilled composites appeared to be nearly linear (Ref 85, 150), but early wear may have been hidden by beveling of the restoration margins. Wear rates for posterior composites have been reported to drop to very low values after 5 to 8 years (Ref 145, 147, 148). Because of this overall decreasing rate of wear, it is hazardous to project long-term wear rates from any short period of time.

Wear of posterior conventional composites involves exfoliation of the filler particles as the resin matrix is continually worn away (Ref 147, 151). This process gives the appearance of a restoration submerging below the surface (Fig.

12). The wear is reduced in the hybrid composites by reducing the mean filler particle size from a range of 30 to 50 μm to a range of 3 to 5 μm and by increasing the amount of filler from 75 to 86 wt% (Ref 128). The use of softer barium glass (HK 400) to replace quartz filler (HK 600) in the particle size range of 10 to 20 μm also results in better wear resistance, although the glass particles themselves show evidence of wear.

Other factors leading to breakdown include the degradation of the silane coupling agent, which can cause microcracking of the resin (Ref 152), and the large mismatch in coefficient of thermal expansion between filler and resin (Ref 86, 118). Maximizing filler particle-to-particle contacts does not improve wear resistance (Ref 153). Resistance to wear is higher for unfinished composites than for those finished conventionally with a finishing bur and white stone, suggesting that finishing at least initially mechanically weakens the surface (Ref 154).

Another problem for clinical research is that different evaluation systems record different wear events. For the most part, the indirect method relies on relief occurring at margins to create contrasts that can be compared to standards. This method does not measure wear elsewhere on the occlusal surface. It is not clear

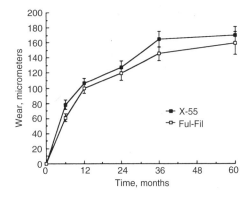

Fig. 11 Decreasing clinical wear rate of composites with time. Source: Ref 148

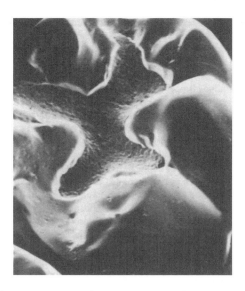

Fig. 12 Scanning electron micrograph of a composite restoration (Concise) with severe occlusal wear after a 7 year period. 10×. Source: Ref 88

where on the restoration direct clinical evaluation measures wear, but it seems most likely to be at the marginal areas. Profiling methods measure the general occlusal surface very well but are least accurate at the margins (Ref 155, 156).

A further complication of clinical research studies is that there has always been the wide distribution of wear values for individual restorations at any recall period. After 3 years, the wear ratings for composites vary from 0 to 350 µm (Ref 148).

In an attempt to understand this variation, the factors contributing to intraoral wear have been collected into categories for statistical analysis (Ref 157). The categories include factors involving cavity preparation, restoration, manipulation, intraoral location, and the patient. Although not all of these factors are yet well known, it has been possible to identify the major ones.

Intraoral location is the most important factor. First molars wear more than second molars, second premolars, and first premolars, in that order. Restoration width is also important. There are minor effects from arch, gender, and complexity of the restoration. Differences in formulations of materials have secondary effects (Ref 158). Understanding these effects, it is possible to normalize differences among clinical studies to pool the clinical data for posterior composites and correct these variations to an ideal clinical population using Weibull analysis (Ref 159).

Numerous theories of wear have been proposed for dental composites based on their microstructures and resistance to microfracture. The analysis typically is presented in terms of the filler, coupling agent, or resin matrix being the weakest link (Fig. 13). The percent conversion of monomer to polymer during curing (Ref 160–167), the depth of curing (Ref 168–174), the glass transition temperature of the polymer (Ref 175, 176), and the strength of the polymer (Ref 177–182) have all been proposed as reasons that the matrix might be most susceptible to microfracturing and thus wear. Problems with coupling agent effectiveness and hydrolysis have been proposed as possible weak links (Ref 152). It has been hypothesized that the surfaces of composites absorb chemicals from food and become predisposed to microfracture, thus permitting wear (Ref 108, 117). Different wear mechanisms have been theorized for different composite types (Ref 149). None of these mechanisms has been established, and none of the explanations is predictive.

A key observation was made by examination of local patterns of wear on composite surfaces (Ref 121, 138). Wear of resin seemed to occur only when separation of filler particles was greater than approximately 0.1 µm. It was proposed that abrasion was caused principally by abrasive particles in the food bolus and that the smallest effective particles were larger than 0.1 to 0.2 µm. Therefore, composites with interparticle spacings less than that dimension were microscopically protected against wear. No information has been available about the size, amount, or abrasivity of the wear-producing particles in food, but they are assumed to be significantly harder than the matrix, softer than the filler, and larger than 0.1 to 0.2 µm. For microfills and many hybrids containing ≥20 vol% of 0.4 µm microfiller particles, the computed average filler particle separation is <0.2 µm. This theory readily explains the apparent resistance to wear of those composites in vivo. Theoretical calculations of microfiller levels required for microprotection indicate that only a few percent are required. However, assuming that microfiller tends to be agglomerated, levels of 45 to 50% are necessary.

An extension of this argument has been that macroscopic protection would also exist for small cavity preparations. Increased exposure of the preparation walls shelters the adjacent composite and causes a decrease in the clinical wear rate. Most of the observed wear patterns and decreasing wear rates appear to be explainable on the basis of these two protection mechanisms alone (Fig. 14).

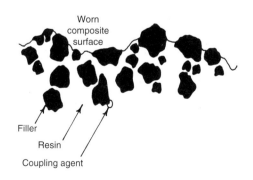

Fig. 13 Schematic of worn composite restoration indicating possible weak links

On this basis, most modern wear-resistant composites include high filler levels with sufficient microfiller to reduce the interparticle spacings to relatively low values. Improvements in coupling agents, strength of the resin matrix, and hydrophobicity may contribute to wear resistance as well.

Pit and Fissure Sealants

Pit and fissure sealants consist mainly of a polymer matrix with minor amounts of dispersed filler particles, primarily for coloration (Table 1). Sealants are designed to be more fluid than composites so they will penetrate the pits, fissures, and etched areas of enamel to produce macroscopic and microscopic mechanical retention. The purpose of sealants is to penetrate all cracks, pits, and fissures on the occlusal sur-faces of deciduous or permanent teeth at risk to dental caries, to seal these areas, and to provide effective protection against caries-producing bacteria. Some properties of sealants are listed in Table 2.

Fundamental Laboratory Studies

Two-body abrasion of sealants has been measured using a silicon carbide two-body abrasion test (Ref 183). Weight-loss data range from 22×10^{-4} to 24×10^{-4} mm^3/mm of travel, which is characteristic of wear of diacrylate resins with little or no filler. The addition of 40 wt% quartz to a sealer did not affect its resistance to two-body abrasion.

The wear of sealants also has been studied by single-pass sliding with a diamond hemisphere (360 μm in diameter) (Ref 183). The sealant with 40 wt% quartz was more resistant to pene-

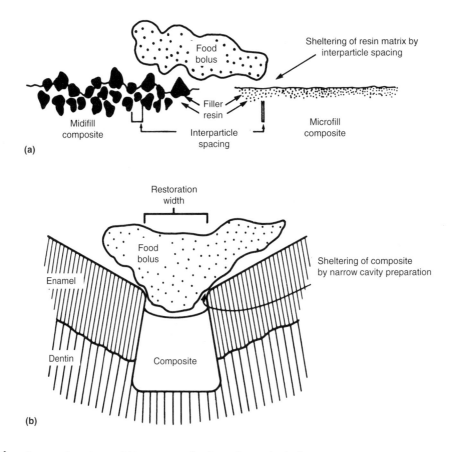

Fig. 14 Schematic of (a) micro- and (b) macroprotection theory. See text for details.

tration and showed less surface damage from single-pass sliding than two unfilled diacrylate sealants.

Clinical Studies

Direct clinical observations of 205 restorations after 4 years has shown that physiologic wear of sealants in the non-stress-bearing areas of pits and fissures is only slight (7%) (Ref 184). Wear on other occlusal surface areas where sealant may be applied inadvertently is apparently irrelevant, because these areas are naturally self-cleansing by abrasion from food. Therefore, the wear of sealants in that regard is clinically unimportant.

Dental Cements

Various modified zinc oxide-eugenol and zinc polyacrylate dental cements are used for temporary fillings (Table 1). Glass ionomers and silver-reinforced glass ionomers may be used for certain permanent restorations not subject to high occlusal forces. Representative mechanical properties of cements are listed in Table 2.

Fundamental Laboratory Studies

Two-body abrasion of temporary filling materials has been measured using a silicon carbide two-body abrasion test (Ref 185). The materials are ranked in an order that agrees with clinical observations. Two zinc polyacrylate cements (base consistency) had rates of abrasion much lower than modified zinc oxide-eugenol cements (Table 10).

The two-body abrasion of early glass ionomer cements used for class V restorations is similar to that of modified composites (Table 11) (Ref 186). Pin-on-disk wear of silver-reinforced glass ionomer restorative materials is less than that for conventional glass ionomers (Ref 187). Incorporation of silver appears to provide lubrication; however, the incidence of catastrophic failure during sliding is only reduced slightly.

Clinical Studies

Clinical investigations of glass ionomer restorations show increasing surface roughness and volume loss (Ref 188). In the absence of occlusal forces, glass ionomers demonstrate

some erosion, but a good internal bond is still maintained between the glass particles and the gel matrix (Ref 118).

Noble and Base-Metal Alloys

Numerous alloys based on gold-silver-copper, gold-palladium, or nickel-chromium are commercially available to make crowns to restore part or all of the coronal portion of a tooth. These alloys are used primarily in the posterior portion of the mouth where high strength is required and cosmetic appearance is secondary. They are presumed to be resistant to wear and have always been assumed to produce little or no wear of opponent teeth. Thus, very little research has been conducted. Crowns of porcelain fused to metal are often used to combine the aesthetics of porcelain with the strength and fit of a cast crown. In these situations, the

Table 10 Material loss on abrasion of dental cements used as temporary filling materials

Material	Material loss, 10^{-4} mm^3/mm of travel(a)
Zinc oxide-eugenol cements	
Tem Pak	29.1
B and T	22.9
IRM	18.6
EBAC	15.8
Zinc polyacrylate cements	
PCA Cement	5.0
Durelon	4.9

(a) Load: 0.036 MPa (0.005 ksi). Source: Ref 185

Table 11 Material loss on abrasion of class V restorative materials

Material	Material loss, 10^{-4} mm^3/mm of travel(a)
Glass ionomer cements	
ASPA	22.9
Fuji	17.0
Composites	
Cervident	14.7
Enamelite 500	19.5

(a) Load: 0.18 MPa (0.026 ksi). Source: Ref 186

abrasion characteristics of the metal alloy are supplanted by the properties of the porcelain.

Clinical Studies

From the limited data available, it appears that wear rates of gold alloys and porcelain are the same when opposing porcelain-fused-to-metal crowns, as shown in three patients with known bruxing and wear problems (Ref 189).

Porcelain and Plastic Denture Teeth

Porcelain or plastic denture teeth are fabricated at factories rather than in the dental office or dental laboratory. Their representative composition is reported in Table 1. Controversy continues among dentists as to the greater benefits of porcelain versus plastic teeth for prosthetic appliances (complete dentures, partial dentures). Shortly after plastic teeth were introduced (circa 1940), research reports condemning the choice of acrylic teeth for dentures also started appearing (Ref 190, 191). Since that time, acrylic teeth have been substantially improved and are now the prosthetic tooth material of choice for many dentists.

Fundamental Laboratory Studies

Two-body abrasion of acrylic teeth against sandblasted glass or with a Taber abrader has demonstrated that acrylic wears much faster than 22 carat gold, porcelain, and enamel, but only approximately 5% more rapidly than dentin (Ref 81, 192, 193). Under intermittent sliding, the rougher the porcelain, the more rapid was the wear of opposing gold and enamel (Ref 194).

The frictional behavior and surface failure of acrylic and porcelain denture teeth have been studied by single- and double-pass sliding with a diamond hemisphere (360 μm in diameter) in water and saliva (Ref 195, 196). Coefficients of friction are higher for acrylic teeth than for porcelain teeth (Table 12). Acrylic teeth show ductile behavior under sliding, with ductile-to-brittle transitions occurring at approximately 5 N (0.11 lbf). Porcelain teeth show brittle behavior under sliding, with ductile-to-brittle transitions occurring between 1.5 and 2.5 N (0.34 and 0.56 lbf). Differences in wear from sliding in water or saliva are not significant. Acrylic teeth show greater deviations from a Hertzian model.

The friction of various prosthetic tooth materials varies from wet to dry conditions (Ref 81, 197). When the materials in the two-body pair both involve polar bonding, the presence of water or other polar liquids increases the friction. However, when one of the solids involves nonpolar bonding, water either has no effect or acts as a mild lubricant. Lower loads on acrylic surfaces produce lower friction as a result of the ductile behavior of acrylic. The friction coefficient of acrylic/porcelain combinations (β = 0.30) is less than acrylic/acrylic (β = 0.37) and porcelain/porcelain (β = 0.51) combinations.

Simulation Studies

Chewing machines have traditionally been employed to evaluate abrasion resistance of prosthetic teeth. An articulator attached to a grinding machine was used as an early abrasion test (Ref 198). Dentures with full sets of acrylic teeth, porcelain teeth, or gold restorations were abraded against a denture with porcelain teeth in water, with and without an abrasive. Wear was measured as changes in vertical dimension of occlusion. Acrylic teeth showed heavy wear. Porcelain teeth withstood abrasion but were friable. Teeth with gold restorations wore severely when an abrasive was present. Similar tests with an instrument using a hemispherical pin on an elliptical disk (similar to a stomatognathic sys-

Table 12 Friction and wear properties of acrylic and porcelain denture teeth for single-pass sliding

Material	Coefficient of friction (β)	Ductile-to-brittle transition load	
		N	lbf
Acrylic teeth			
Dentsply			
Dentin	0.62	. . .	
Enamel	0.62	4.8	1.08
Myerson			
Dentin	0.55	. . .	
Enamel	0.54	5.6	1.26
Porcelain teeth			
Dentsply			
Dentin	0.24	. . .	
Enamel	0.24	2.6	0.58
Myerson			
Dentin	0.26	. . .	
Enamel	0.26	2.4	0.54

Source: Ref 195, 196

tem) showed that acrylic/acrylic and porcelain/acrylic combinations had less wear than porcelain/porcelain combinations (Ref 199).

The results of different pairs of wearing surfaces have not been consistent for all wear machines. Results from several chewing machines showed that acrylic/acrylic combinations produced less wear than acrylic/porcelain (Ref 200) and that wear decreased as contacting surface area of the acrylic teeth increased (Ref 201). In other wear machine tests, less wear was observed for porcelain/acrylic combinations than with acrylic/acrylic or porcelain/porcelain combinations (Ref 202, 203).

Occlusal wear studies using an artificial mouth and computerized profilometry to measure wear have shown that denture teeth made from a highly cross-linked copolymer with an interpenetrating polymer network (IPN) were more wear resistant than traditional acrylic resin teeth (Ref 204). The IPN denture teeth do not appear to produce measurable wear in contact with human teeth.

Clinical Studies

Acrylic teeth, when studied as a means of obtaining balanced functional occlusion in partial dentures, showed no tendency to wear over a period of 6 to 24 months (Ref 205). Abrasion of acrylic teeth has been observed clinically in dentures of 9 of 12 patients (Ref 206). A 5 year clinical appraisal of 114 denture patients with acrylic teeth showed a loss of occlusion in centric relation as a result of wear of acrylic posterior teeth (Ref 207). Porcelain teeth and variables such as bone loss or varying occlusal concepts were not evaluated. The results of a survey of 77 dentists were that porcelain/acrylic combinations appear to wear less than acrylic on acrylic (Ref 208).

Techniques involving removable sections of a fixed prosthesis along with replicas have been used to study wear in a male patient with extreme bruxing habits (Ref 209). Light-cured composite, gold alloy, porcelain, and heat-cured acrylic restorations generally wore more when opposed by porcelain or acrylic denture teeth (Table 13). Wear mechanisms observed included: combined tribochemical wear and fatigue for heat-cured acrylic, fatigue wear for light-cured composite and porcelain, and abrasion and fatigue wear for gold alloys. Wear of both porcelain and cross-linked resin teeth was mainly via fatigue. Abrasive wear occurred in

the presence of hard particles (Ref 210). Micro-filled composite resin teeth appeared to wear by fatigue and tribochemical wear (Ref 189).

The average vertical loss of denture teeth appears to be 0.1 mm (0.004 in.) or less per year for acrylic resin teeth (Ref 211, 212) and less for porcelain teeth (Ref 211). Clinical wear of a single acrylic tooth for one year has been measured from computer-generated data obtained from a reflex microscope and is 7.2 mm^3 (Ref 213).

Denture Acrylics

Denture bases are made primarily from polymethyl methacrylate, vinyl-acrylic, or rubber-reinforced acrylic polymers (Table 1). Their main use is to support plastic or porcelain artificial teeth. Some typical properties are listed in Table 2.

Fundamental Laboratory Studies

Two-body abrasion of heat-cured and self-cured acrylic denture resins correlates with scratch measurements and values of flexural modulus of elasticity (Ref 214). The abrasive wear rate of denture resins was much higher than that of composites, alloys, or teeth (Ref 215).

Dental Feldspathic Porcelain and Ceramics

Dental porcelain is primarily a glass with either some dispersed leucite or alumina crystals, or fluoride-mica crystals (Table 1). Porcelain has excellent aesthetic properties and resists wear extremely well. Some representative properties are reported in Table 2.

Table 13   Loss of materials in mm^3/month caused by acrylic or porcelain denture teeth on opposing restoration

Restorations	Opposing denture teeth	
	Acrylic	Porcelain
Heat-cured acrylic	3.9	8.3
Light-cured composite	1.9	5.4
Porcelain	1.0	1.1
Type III/IV gold alloy	0.6	1.2

Source: Ref 209

Fundamental Laboratory Studies

The frictional behavior and surface failure of dental feldspathic porcelain has been studied by single-pass sliding tests using a diamond hemisphere (360 μm in diameter) in air and water (Ref 216). The friction of as-glazed porcelain is higher and the surface damage is more extensive in water than in air (Table 14). Crack initiation within porcelain occurs at flaws such as scratches or residual pores, and these are propagated by elastic stresses associated with normal intraoral loads. The higher friction in bulk water is attributed to increased cracking and reduced amounts of recoverable elastic strain energy. Coating the porcelain with gold or chromium makes the friction independent of environment. Gold coating reduces the friction, but chromium coating does not. Chromium coating reduces the extent of damage from sliding compared to the as-glazed porcelain.

Simulation Studies

Simulated occlusal wear studies in an artificial mouth using enamel occluding on porcelain have demonstrated a high coefficient of wear for dental porcelain and suggest that an abrasive wear mechanism is involved (Ref 217).

Die Materials (Stone, Resin, and Metal)

The most common die material is calcium sulfate dihydrate (gypsum), but dies may be fabricated from epoxy resin or electroplated with silver or copper (Table 1). A dental die is a replica of the hard or soft tissues, or both, and must be strong and resistant to abrasion, because it is subjected to the stresses of carving and finishing a restoration. Some representative properties are listed in Table 2.

Fundamental Laboratory Studies

Two-body abrasion of stone, resin, and metal-plated dies is shown in Table 15. The metal-plated dies have the highest hardness and lowest loss in two-body abrasion. Although the dental stone is harder than the resins, the surface morphology of the stone (Fig. 15) makes it less abrasion resistant.

The surface failure of stone, resin, and metal-plated dies has been studied by single-pass sliding with a diamond hemisphere (360 μm in diameter) (Ref 218). The metal-plated dies are ductile up to a normal load of 10 N (2.25 lbf), whereas the resin and stone dies show brittle failure above 1 to 2 N (0.22 to 0.45 lbf).

Endodontic Instruments

Endodontic instruments such as files and reamers are manufactured from stainless steel or carbon steel wires by various combinations of machining and twisting (Table 1). These

Table 14   Friction and wear properties of dental feldspathic porcelain for single-pass sliding

Condition	Coefficient of friction (β)	Ductile-to-brittle transition load	
		N	lbf
As-glazed			
Air	0.18	5.9	1.33
Water	0.23	4.9	1.10
Gold coated			
Air	0.14	5.9	1.33
Water	0.14	4.9	1.10
Chromium coated			
Air	0.22	5.9	1.33
Water	0.22	5.9	1.33

Source: Ref 216

Table 15   Material loss on abrasion and surface hardness of dental die materials

Material	Material loss, 10^{-4} mm^3/mm of travel	Knoop surface hardness, kg/mm^2
Dental stone		
Duroc	14.8	54
Duroc with hardener	16.3	62
Resin		
Die-Met	2.8	25
Epoxydent	4.8	25
Metal		
Copper-plated	1.5	134
Silver-plated	0.9	128

Source: Ref 218

instruments are used to clean and shape the root canal before it is sealed.

Simulation Studies

The cutting mechanism of a reamer on dentin involves compression and chipping (Ref 219). Triangular reamers cut deeper than rectangular ones. The smaller the angle of the cutting edge, the greater the cutting ability (Ref 220).

Cutting in bovine bone as measured by a drill-press apparatus is more efficient with triangular than square reamers (Ref 221). Instruments appear to lose sharpness because of deformation or fracture of the blade.

Cutting in bovine bone or acrylic with a push-pull stroke in a linear motion also can be measured for various instruments (Ref 222, 223). Chips of acrylic appear to impair cutting efficiency. Reduced cutting efficiency has been observed with bovine bone.

Cutting ability of K-type stainless steel files was measured by depths of cut in polymethyl methacrylate on an instrument that controls the force on the files and the length and number of pull strokes (Ref 224). Variations in cutting are observed around the circumference of individual files and among files of the same size and brand (Ref 224, 225). Dry heat and salt sterilization has no effect on cutting ability of stainless steel files, but autoclave sterilization causes a reduction in their cutting ability (Ref 226). Sodium hypochlorite, hydrogen peroxide, and ethylene-diaminetetraacetic acid-urea peroxide irrigants cause a decrease in cutting ability, but a saline irrigant has no effect. Wear of K-type files under these conditions was not observed.

Cross-sectional design and flute design are more important variables in cutting than rake angle, wear resistance, capabilities for chip removal, and mode of use (Ref 227). Cutting efficiency of the tip of a file is better than the flute portion (Ref 228). In constricted canals (0.33 mm, or 0.013 in., in diameter), tip angles of files of 60 to 90° are most effective, whereas in larger canals (0.40 mm, or 0.016 in., in diameter), tip angles of files of 40 to 49° are most effective. The tip geometry, however, exerts a greater influence over cutting efficiency than tip length or angle. The pyramidal design is most efficient, whereas the conical tip is least efficient.

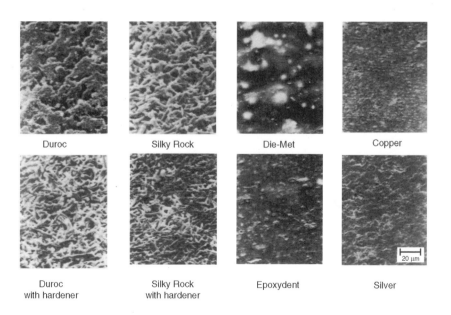

Duroc Silky Rock Die-Met Copper

Duroc with hardener Silky Rock with hardener Epoxydent Silver

Fig. 15 Scanning electron micrographs of stone, resin, and metal-plated dies. Source: Ref 218

Periodontal Instruments

High-quality cutting edges of periodontal instruments are essential for effective subgingival scaling and root planing in periodontal therapy. Cuttability is affected primarily by cutting forces, chip thickness ratios, chip form, and tool wear (Ref 229–231). Edge quality may be evaluated by the angle between the two edge-forming contiguous surfaces, the smoothness of the edge, edge sharpness or dullness, and the presence or absence of metallic projections (Ref 232).

A sharp curette is the most proficient means for removing calculus and for achieving an acceptable, smooth root surface in periodontal therapy (Ref 233). A dull instrument leaves behind smeared deposits on the root surface, and a damaged curette causes heavy scratches.

Fundamental Laboratory Studies

Laboratory cutting tests of whale bone indicate that high-speed steel results in more balanced chip formation than cemented carbide, better cutting forces than stainless steel and cemented carbide, less tool wear than stainless steel, and more ideal chip form than cemented carbide (Ref 231).

Simulation Studies

Root planing of extracted single-rooted teeth mounted in mannikin jaws indicates that stainless steel curettes show edge deformation after only 15 strokes (Ref 234). High-carbon steel curettes are more resistant to wear than stainless steel curettes (Ref 232).

Orthodontic Wires

Space closure and canine retraction in continuous arch wire techniques require sufficient force to overcome frictional forces between the bracket attached to the tooth and the arch wire (Fig. 16). Excessive wire/bracket friction may result in loss of anchorage or binding accompanied by little tooth movement. Factors that may influence friction are engagement of the arch wire in brackets that are out of alignment, ligatures pressing the arch wire against the base of the slot, active torque in rectangular wires, and

bodily tooth movement in which the tipping tendency is resisted by two-point contact between the bracket and arch wire (Ref 235).

Simulation Studies

Arch wire/bracket friction is affected by wire size, angulation, ligation force, bracket size, and wire type (Ref 236–238). Kinetic coefficients of friction of stainless steel, beta-titanium, nickel-titanium, and cobalt-chromium arch wires sliding on stainless steel or Teflon (E.I. DuPont de Nemours & Co., Inc.) polymer increase with normal load (Table 16) and increase in the presence of artificial saliva as compared to dry conditions (Ref 239). Stainless steel and beta-titanium wires show wear tracks after sliding under low normal loads (40 to 80 N, or 9.0 to 18.0 lbf).

There appears to be agreement that nickel-titanium wires have higher wire/bracket friction than stainless steel wires in zero torque/zero angulated brackets (Ref 240). At bracket angulations >3°, nickel-titanium wires have lower wire/bracket friction than stainless steel (Ref 238, 241). Under conditions of two-point contact, friction is inversely proportional to bracket

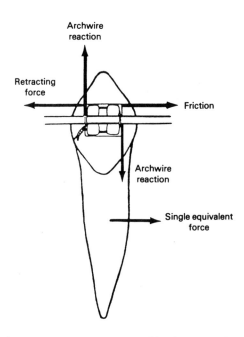

Fig. 16 Forces acting on a tooth/bracket system during translation. Source: Ref 235

Table 16 Coefficient of friction of orthodontic wire/material combinations for a normal load of 40 and 80 N (9.0 and 18.0 lbf) under wet conditions

Material	Coefficient of friction, 40 N (9.0 lbf)	Coefficient of friction, 80 N (18.0 lbf)
Stainless steel/stainless steel	0.035	0.085
Beta-titanium/stainless steel	0.025	0.122
Cobalt-chromium/stainless steel	0.041	0.122
Nickel-titanium/stainless steel	0.044	0.115
Stainless steel/Teflon	0.003	0.013

Source: Ref 239

width and is less for stainless steel wires than for nickel-titanium or beta-titanium wires (Ref 235). Surface roughness of nickel-titanium or beta-titanium wires may explain their relatively high friction (Ref 242).

ACKNOWLEDGMENT

The information in this chapter was largely taken from:

- J.M. Powers and S.C. Bayne, Friction and Wear of Dental Materials, *Friction, Lubrication, and Wear Technology,* Vol 18, *ASM Handbook,* ASM International, 1992, p 665–681

REFERENCES

1. R.G. Craig and J.M. Powers, Ed., *Restorative Dental Materials,* 11th ed., Mosby, Inc., 2002
2. R.G. Craig and J.M. Powers, Wear of Dental Tissues and Materials, *Int. Dent. J.,* Vol 26, 1976, p 121–133
3. M.Z.A.M. Sulong and R.A. Aziz, Wear of Materials Used in Dentistry: A Review of the Literature, *J. Prosthet. Dent.,* Vol 63, 1990, p 342–349
4. J.M. Powers and A. Koran III, The Wear of Hard Dental Tissue—A Review of the Literature, *J. Mich. Dent. Assoc.,* Vol 55, 1973, p 119–126
5. R.W. Leigh, *Dental Pathology of Aboriginal California,* University of California Press, 1928, p 408
6. M. Klatsky, Dental Attrition, *J. Am. Dent. Assoc.,* Vol 26, 1939, p 73–84
7. H.L. Tollens, Atypical Tooth Erosion in a Pygmy Skull, *Dent. Abstr.,* Vol 5, 1960, p 668
8. P.O. Pederson, Investigations into Dental Conditions of about 3000 Ancient and Modern Greenlanders, *Dent. Rec.,* Vol 58, 1938, p 191–198
9. C.E. Snow, Indian Knoll Skeletons of Site Oh 2, Ohio County, Kentucky, *U. Kent. Rep. in Anthrop.,* Vol 4, 1948, p 382–554
10. J.E. Anderson, Human Skeletons of Tehuacan, *Science,* Vol 148, 1965, p 496–497
11. L.H.D. Buxton, The Teeth and Jaws of Savage Man, *Trans. Br. Soc. Study of Orthod.,* Vol 1916–1920, 1920, p 79–88
12. F.St.J. Steadman, Malocclusion in the Tasmanian Aborigines, *Dent. Rec.,* Vol 57, 1937, p 213–249
13. M.S. Goldstein, Dentition of Indian Crania from Texas, *Am. J. Phys. Anthrop.,* Vol 6, 1948, p 63–84
14. A.E. Webster, The Effect of Time and Wear on the Human Teeth, *Dent. Rec.,* Vol 38, 1919, p 331–335
15. G.G. Philippas, Effects of Function on Healthy Teeth: Evidence of Ancient Athenian Remains, *J. Am. Dent. Assoc.,* Vol 45, 1952, p 443–453
16. L. Lysell and R. Filipsson, A Profile Roentgenologic Study of a Series of Medieval Skulls from Northern Sweden, *Dent. Abstr.,* Vol 3, 1958, p 663
17. T. Murphy, Compensatory Mechanisms in Facial Height Adjustment to Function Tooth Attrition, *Aust. Dent. J.,* Vol 4, 1959, p 312–323
18. T. Murphy, Mandibular Adjustment to Functional Tooth Attrition, *Aust. Dent. J.,* Vol 3, 1958, p 171–178
19. D.K. Whittaker, T. Molleson, A.T. Daniel, J.T. Williams, P. Rose, and R. Resteghini, Quantitative Assessment of Tooth Wear, Alveolar-Crest Height and Continuing Eruption in a Romano-British Population, *Archs. Oral Biol.,* Vol 30, 1985, p 493–501

20. A.G. Comuzzie and D.G. Steele, Enlarged Occlusal Surfaces on First Molars Due to Severe Attrition and Hypercementosis: Examples from Prehistoric Coastal Populations of Texas, *Am. J. Phys. Anthropol.,* Vol 78, 1989, p 9–15

21. G.G. Philippas, Influence of Occlusal Wear and Age on Formation of Dentin and Size of Pulp Chamber, *J. Dent. Res.,* Vol 40, 1961, p 1186–1198

22. G.G. Philippas and E. Applebaum, Age Factor in Secondary Dentin Formation, *J. Dent. Res.,* Vol 45, 1966, p 778–789

23. G.G. Philippas and E. Applebaum, Age Changes in the Permanent Upper Lateral Incisor, *J. Dent. Res.,* Vol 46, 1967, p 1002–1009

24. G.G. Philippas and E. Applebaum, Age Change in the Permanent Upper Canine Teeth, *J. Dent. Res.,* Vol 47, 1968, p 411–417

25. M.F. Teaford, A Review of Dental Microwear and Diet in Modern Mammals, *Scanning Microsc.,* Vol 2, 1988, p 1149–1166

26. W. Muller, Xerostomia, *Deut. Zahnarztebl.,* Vol 12, 1958, p 378–380

27. E. Zaus and G.W. Teuscher, Report on Three Cases of Congenital Dysfunction of the Major Salivary Glands, *J. Dent. Res.,* Vol 19, 1940, p 326

28. G.E. Carlsson, A. Hugoson, and G. Persson, Dental Abrasion and Alveolar Bone Loss in the White Rat, Part I: Effect of Ligation of the Major Salivary Gland Ducts, *Odont. Rev.,* Vol 16, 1965, p 308–316

29. M.N. Hatton, M.J. Levine, J.E. Margarone, and A. Aguirre, Lubrication and Viscosity Features of Human Saliva and Commercially Available Saliva Substitutes, *J. Oral. Maxillofac. Surg.,* Vol 45, 1987, p 496–499

30. S.C. Nadler, The Effects of Bruxism, *J. Periodont.,* Vol 37, 1966, p 311–319

31. J. Steel and R.C. Browne, Effect of Abrasion upon the Acid Decalcification of the Teeth, *Br. Dent. J.,* Vol 94, 1953, p 285–288

32. L. Enbom, T. Magnusson, and G. Wall, Occlusal Wear in Miners, *Swed. Dent. J.,* Vol 10, 1986, p 165–170

33. C. Dawes, G.N. Jenkins, and C.H. Tonge, The Nomenclature of the Integuments of the Enamel Surface of Teeth, *Br. Dent. J.,* Vol 115, 1963, p 65–68

34. R.W. Phillips and G. Van Huysen, Dentifrices and the Tooth Surface, *Am. Perf.,* Vol 50, 1948, p 33–41

35. S.D. Gershon, H.H. Pokras, and T.H. Rider, Dentifrices, *Cosmetics, Science and Technology,* E. Saragin, Ed., New York Interscience, 1957, p 296–353

36. American Dental Association, Council on Dental Therapeutics, Abrasivity of Current Dentifrices, *J. Am. Dent. Assoc.,* Vol 81, 1970, p 1177–1178

37. M.S. Putt, C.J. Kleber, and J.C. Muhler, Enamel Polish and Abrasion by Prophylaxis Pastes, *Dent. Hygiene,* Vol 56 (No. 9), 1982, p 38–43

38. J.M. Powers and R.G. Craig, Wear of Fluorapatite Single Crystals, Part I: Method for Quantitative Evaluation of Wear, *J. Dent. Res.,* Vol 51, 1972, p 168–176

39. J.M. Powers and R.G. Craig, Wear of Fluorapatite Single Crystals, Part II: Frictional Behavior, *J. Dent. Res.,* Vol 51, 1972, p 605–610

40. J.M. Powers and R.G. Craig, Wear of Fluorapatite Single Crystals, Part III: Classification of Surface Behavior, *J. Dent. Res.,* Vol 51, 1972, p 611–618

41. J.M. Powers, K.C. Ludema, and R.G. Craig, Wear of Fluorapatite Single Crystals, Part IV: Influence of Sliding Direction on Frictional Behavior and Surface Failure, *J. Dent. Res.,* Vol 52, 1973, p 1019–1025

42. J.M. Powers, K.C. Ludema, and R.G. Craig, Wear of Fluorapatite Single Crystals, Part V: Influence of Environment on Frictional Behavior and Surface Failure, *J. Dent. Res.,* Vol 52, 1973, p 1026–1031

43. J.M. Powers, K.C. Ludema, and R.G. Craig, Wear of Fluorapatite Single Crystals, Part VI: Influence of Multiple-Pass Sliding on Surface Failure, *J. Dent. Res.,* Vol 52, 1973, p 1032–1040

44. J.M. Powers, R.G. Craig, and K.C. Ludema, Frictional Behavior and Surface Failure of Human Enamel, *J. Dent. Res.,* Vol 52, 1973, p 1327–1331

45. K.H.R. Wright, The Abrasive Wear Resistance of Human Dental Tissues, *Wear,* Vol 14, 1969, p 263–284

46. H.M. Rootare, J.M. Powers, and R.G. Craig, Sintered Hydroxyapatite Ceramic for Wear Studies, *J. Dent. Res.,* Vol 57, 1978, p 777–783

47. C.L. Brace and S. Molnar, Experimental Studies in Human Tooth Wear, Part I, *Am. J. Phys. Anthrop.,* Vol 27, 1967, p 213–222

48. R.J. Grabenstetter, R.W. Broge, F.L. Jackson, and A.W. Radike, The Measurement of the Abrasion of Human Teeth by Dentifrice Abrasion: A Test Utilizing Radioactive Teeth, *J. Dent. Res.,* Vol 37, 1958, p 1060–1068

49. K.H.R. Wright and J.I. Stevenson, The Measurement and Interpretation of Dentifrice Abrasiveness, *J. Soc. Cos. Chem.,* Vol 18, 1967, p 387–407

50. G.K. Stookey and J.C. Muhler, Laboratory Studies Concerning the Enamel and Dentin Abrasion Properties of Common Dentifrice Polishing Agents, *J. Dent. Res.,* Vol 47, 1968, p 524–532

51. J.J. Hefferren, A Laboratory Method for Assessment of Dentifrice Abrasivity, *J. Dent. Res.,* Vol 55, 1976, p 563–573

52. H. Ashmore, N.J. Van Abbe, and S.J. Wilson, The Measurement in vitro of Dentin Abrasion by Toothpaste, *Br. Dent. J.,* Vol 133, 1972, p 60–66

53. G.K. Stookey, J.R. Hudson, and J.C. Muhler, Studies Concerning the Polishing Properties of Zirconium Silicate on Enamel, *J. Periodont.,* Vol 37, 1966, p 200–207

54. M.L. Tainter and S. Epstein, A Standard Procedure for Determining Abrasion by Dentifrices, *J. Am. Col. Dent.,* Vol 9, 1942, p 353–379

55. S. Epstein and M.L. Tainter, Abrasion of Teeth by Commercial Dentifrices, *J. Am. Dent. Assoc.,* Vol 30, 1943, p 1036–1045

56. S. Epstein and M.L. Tainter, The Relationship of Particle Size and Other Properties of Dentifrice Ingredients to Toothbrush Abrasion of Enamel, *J. Dent. Res.,* Vol 22, 1943, p 335–344

57. W.H. Bull, R.M. Callender, B.R. Pugh, and G.D. Wood, The Abrasion and Cleaning Properties of Dentifrices, *Br. Dent. J.,* Vol 125, 1968, p 331–337

58. R.S. Manly and D.H. Foster, Importance of Factorial Design in Testing Abrasion by Dentifrices, *J. Dent. Res.,* Vol 46, 1967, p 442–445

59. R.S. Manly, Factors Influencing Tests on the Abrasion of Dentin by Brushing with Dentifrices, *J. Dent. Res.,* Vol 23, 1944, p 59–72

60. R.W. Phillips and M.L. Swartz, Effects of Diameter of Nylon Brushes on Enamel Surface, *J. Am. Dent. Assoc.,* Vol 47, 1953, p 20–26

61. R.S. Manly and F. Brudevold, Relative Abrasiveness of Natural and Synthetic Toothbrush Bristles on Cementum and Dentin, *J. Am. Dent. Assoc.,* Vol 55, 1957, p 779–780

62. F. Mannerberg, Appearance of Tooth Surface as Observed in Shadowed Replicas in Various Age Groups, in Long Term Studies, after Toothbrushing, in Cases of Erosion, and after Exposure to Citrus Fruit Juices, *Odont. Rev. (Malmo),* Vol 11, Supplement 6, 1960, p 1–116

63. J.H. Harrington and I.A. Terry, Automatic and Hand Toothbrushing Studies, *J. Am. Dent. Assoc.,* Vol 68, 1964, p 343–350

64. R.S. Manly, J. Wiren, P.J. Manly, and R.C. Keene, A Method for Measurement of Abrasion by Toothbrush and Dentifrice, *J. Dent. Res.,* Vol 44, 1965, p 533–540

65. D. McConnell and C.W. Conroy, Comparisons of Abrasion Produced by a Simulated Manual Versus a Mechanical Toothbrush, *J. Dent. Res.,* Vol 46, 1967, p 1022–1027

66. V.E. Whitehurst, G.K. Stookey, and J.C. Muhler, Studies Concerning the Cleaning, Polishing, and Therapeutic Properties of Commercial Prophylaxis Pastes, *J. Oral Ther. Pharm.,* Vol 4, 1968, p 181–191

67. G.K. Stookey, In vitro Estimates of Enamel and Dentin Abrasion Associated with a Prophylaxis, *J. Dent. Res.,* Vol 57, 1978, p 36

68. G.K. Stookey and B.R. Schemehorn, A Method for Assessing the Relative

Abrasion of Prophylaxis Materials, *J. Dent. Res.,* Vol 58, 1979, p 588–592

69. Specification 37-1986, American National Standards Institute/American Dental Association, Approved 15 May 1986

70. J.A. von Fraunhofer, C.D. Givens, and T.J. Overmyer, Lubricating Coolants for High-Speed Dental Handpieces, *J. Am. Dent. Assoc.,* Vol 119, 1989, p 291–295

71. G.K. Johnson, F.U. Perry, and G.B. Pelleu, Jr., Effect of Four Anticorrosive Dips on the Cutting Efficiency of Dental Carbide Burs, *J. Am. Dent. Assoc.,* Vol 114, 1987, p 648–650

72. P. Lambrechts, M. Braem, M. Vuylsteke-Wauters, and G. Vanherle, Quantitative in vivo Wear of Human Enamel, *J. Dent. Res.,* Vol 68, 1989, p 1752–1754

73. F. Roulet, P. Mettler, and U. Friedrich, Ein klinischer Vergleich dreier Komposits mit Amalgam für Klasse-II-Füllungen unter besonderer Berücksichtigung der Abrasion, Resultate nach 2 Jähren, *Schweiz. Monatsschr. Zahnkeilkd.,* Vol 90, 1980, p 18–30

74. S. Molnar, J.K. McKee, I.M. Molnar, and T.R. Przybeck, Tooth Wear Rates among Contemporary Australian Aborigines, *J. Dent. Res.,* Vol 62, 1983, p 562–565

75. L. Holmen, A. Thylstrup, and J. Artun, Surface Changes during the Arrest of Active Enamel Carious Lesions in vivo. A Scanning Electron Microscope Study, *Acta Odontol. Scand.,* Vol 45, 1987, p 383–390

76. S.V. Brasch, J. Lazarou, N.J. Van Abbe, and J.O. Forrest, The Assessment of Dentifrice Abrasivity in vivo, *Br. Dent. J.,* Vol 127, 1969, p 119–124

77. A.A. Lugassy and E.H. Greener, An Abrasion Resistance Study of Some Dental Resins, *J. Dent. Res.,* Vol 51, 1972, p 967–972

78. J.M. Powers, L.J. Allen, and R.G. Craig, Two-Body Abrasion of Commercial and Experimental Restorative and Coating Resins and an Amalgam, *J. Am. Dent. Assoc.,* Vol 89, 1974, p 1118–1122

79. J.M. Powell, R.W. Phillips, and R.D. Norman, In vitro Wear Response of Composite Resin, Amalgam and Enamel, *J. Dent. Res.,* Vol 54, 1975, p 1183–1195

80. J.C. Roberts, J.M. Powers, and R.G. Craig, Wear of Dental Amalgam, *J. Biomed. Mater. Res.,* Vol 11, 1977, p 513–523

81. E.W. Tillitson, R.G. Craig, and F.A. Peyton, Friction and Wear of Restorative Dental Materials, *J. Dent. Res.,* Vol 50, 1971, p 149–154

82. J.C. Roberts, J.M. Powers, and R.G. Craig, Fracture Toughness and Critical Strain Energy Release Rate of Dental Amalgam, *J. Mater. Sci.,* Vol 13, 1978, p 965–971

83. J.C. Roberts, J.M. Powers, and R.G. Craig, An Empirical Equation Including Fracture Toughness and Describing Friction of Dental Restorative Materials, *Wear,* Vol 47, 1978, p 139–146

84. G. Johannsen, G. Redmalm, and H. Ryden, Surface Changes on Dental Materials, *Swed. Dent. J.,* Vol 13, 1989, p 267–276

85. J.C. Mitchem and D.G. Gronas, The Continued in vivo Evaluation of the Wear of Restorative Resins, *J. Am. Dent. Assoc.,* Vol 111, 1985, p 961–964

86. P. Lambrechts, G. Vanherle, M. Vuylsteke, and C.L. Davidson, Quantitative Evaluation of the Wear Resistance of Posterior Dental Restorations: A New Three-Dimensional Measuring Technique, *J. Dent. Res.,* Vol 12, 1984, p 252–267

87. American Dental Association, Council on Dental Materials, Instruments, and Equipment, Posterior Composite Resins, *J. Am. Dent. Assoc.,* Vol 112, 1986, p 707–709

88. D.F. Taylor, *Posterior Composites,* D.F. Taylor, 1984, p 360

89. R.A. Draughn, R.L. Bowen, and J.P. Moffa, Composite Restorative Materials, *Restorative Dental Materials,* Vol 1, J.A. Reese and T.M. Valega, Ed., Biddles Ltd., 1985, p 75–107

90. *International State-of-the-Art Conference on Restorative Dental Materials,* Conference Proceedings, National Institute of Health/National Institute of Dental Research, 1986

91. J.F. Roulet, *Degradation of Dental Polymers,* Karger, 1987

92. M. Braem, P. Lambrechts, V. Van Doren, and G. Vanherle, The Impact of Composite Structure on Its Elastic Response, *J. Dent. Res.,* Vol 65, 1986, p 648–653

93. R.A. Draughn, Influence of Filler Parameters on Mechanical Properties of Composite Restorative Materials, *J. Dent. Res.,* Vol 62 (Special Issue), Abstract 187, 1983, p 670

94. K.J. Soderholm, Relationship between Compressive Yield Strength and Filler Fractions in PMMA Composites, *Acta Odontol. Scand.,* Vol 40, 1982, p 145–150

95. J.H. Hembree, W. Fingar, and R.A. Draughn, *South Carolina Dent. J.,* Vol 33, 1975, p 43–47

96. O. Zidan, E. Asmussen, and K.D. Jorgensen, Tensile Strength of Restorative Resins, *Scand. J. Dent. Res.,* Vol 88, 1980, p 285–289

97. H. Oysaed and I.E. Ruyter, Composites for Use in Posterior Teeth: Mechanical Properties Tested under Dry and Wet Conditions, *J. Biomed. Mater. Res.,* Vol 20, 1986, p 261–271

98. A.C. McLundie, C.J.W. Patterson, and D.R. Stirrups, Comparison of the Abrasive Wear in vitro of a Number of Visible-Light-Cured Composite Resins, *Br. Dent. J.,* Vol 159, 1985, p 182–185

99. A. Harrison and T.T. Lewis, The Development of an Abrasion Testing Machine for Dental Materials, *J. Biomed. Mater. Res.,* Vol 9, 1975, p 341–353

100. S.L. Rice, W.F. Bailey, S.F. Wayne, and J.A. Burns, Comparative in vitro Sliding-Wear Study of Conventional Microfilled and Light-Cured Composite Restoratives, *J. Dent. Res.,* Vol 63, 1984, p 1173–1175

101. K.D. Jorgensen, In vitro Wear Tests of Macro-Filled Composite Restorative Materials, *Aust. Dent. J.,* Vol 27, 1982, p 153–158

102. Y. Li, M.L. Swartz, R.W. Phillips, B.K. Moore, and T.A. Roberts, Effect of Filler Content and Size on Properties of Composites, *J. Dent. Res.,* Vol 64, 1985, p 1396–1401

103. R.M. Pilliar, D.C. Smith, and B. Maric, Oscillatory Wear Tests of Dental Composites, *J. Dent. Res.,* Vol 63, 1984, p 1166–1172

104. J.M. Powers, W.H. Douglas, and R.G. Craig, Wear of Dimethacrylate Resins Used in Dental Composites, *Wear,* Vol 54, 1979, p 79–86

105. G.S. Wilson, E.H. Davies, and J.A. von Fraunhofer, Abrasive Wear Characteristics of Anterior Restorative Materials, *Br. Dent. J.,* Vol 151, 1981, p 335–338

106. R.A. Draughn and A. Harrison, Relationship between Abrasive Wear and Microstructure of Composite Resins, *J. Prosthet. Dent.,* Vol 40, 1978, p 220–224

107. G.S. Wilson, E.H. Davies, and J.A. von Fraunhofer, Micro Hardness Characteristics of Anterior Restorative Materials, *Br. Dent. J.,* Vol 148, 1980, p 37–40

108. J.E. McKinney and W. Wu, Relationship between Subsurface Damage and Wear of Dental Restorative Composites, *J. Dent. Res.,* Vol 61, 1982, p 1083–1088

109. L.I. Gallegos and J.I. Nicholls, In vitro Two-Body Wear of Three Veneering Resins, *J. Prosthet. Dent.,* Vol 60, 1988, p 172–178

110. A. Embong, J. Glyn Jones, and A. Harrison, The Wear Effects of Selected Composites on Restorative Materials and Enamel, *Dent. Mater.,* Vol 3, 1987, p 236–240

111. J.M. Powers, J.C. Roberts, and R.G. Craig, Surface Failure of Commercial and Experimental Restorative Resins, *J. Dent. Res.,* Vol 55, 1976, p 432–436

112. J.M. Powers, J.C. Roberts, and R.G. Craig, Wear of Filled and Unfilled Dental Restorative Resins, *Wear,* Vol 39, 1976, p 117–122

113. J.M. Powers and P.L. Fan, Erosion of Composite Resins, *J. Dent. Res.,* Vol 59, 1980, p 815–819

114. J.M. Powers, P.L. Fan, and C.N. Raptis, Color Stability of New Composite Restorative Materials under Accelerated Aging, *J. Dent. Res.,* Vol 59, 1980, p 2071–2074

115. P.L. Fan and J.M. Powers, In vitro Wear of Aged Composite Restorative Materi-

als, *J. Dent. Res.*, Vol 59, 1980, p 2066–2070

116. P.L. Fan and J.M. Powers, Wear of Aged Dental Composites, *Wear,* Vol 68, 1981, p 241–248

117. J.E. McKinney and W. Wu, Chemical Softening and Wear of Dental Composites, *J. Dent. Res.*, Vol 64, 1985, p 1326–1331

118. J.-F. Roulet and C. Walti, Influence of Oral Fluid on Composite Resin and Glass-Ionomer Cement, *J. Prosthet. Dent.*, Vol 52, 1984, p 182–189

119. J.C. Roberts, J.M. Powers, and R.G. Craig, Fracture Toughness of Composite and Unfilled Restorative Resins, *J. Dent. Res.*, Vol 56, 1977, p 748–753

120. A. Harrison and R.A. Draughn, Abrasive Wear, Tensile Strength and Hardness of Dental Composite Resins—Is There a Relationship?, *J. Prosthet. Dent.*, Vol 36, 1976, p 395–398

121. K.D. Jorgensen, Restorative Resins: Abrasion versus Mechanical Properties, *Scand. J. Dent. Res.*, Vol 88, 1980, p 557–568

122. A.J. De Gee, H.C. ten Harkel-Hagenaar, and C.L. Davidson, Structural and Physical Factors Affecting the Brush Wear of Dental Composites, *J. Dent. Res.*, Vol 13, 1985, p 60–70

123. A.J. De Gee, P. Pallav, and C.L. Davidson, Effect of Abrasion Medium on Wear of Stress-Bearing Composites and Amalgams in vitro, *J. Dent. Res.*, Vol 65, 1986, p 654–658

124. K.F. Leinfelder, R.W. Beaudreau, and R.B. Mazer, Device for Determining Wear Mechanisms of Posterior Composite Resins, *J. Dent. Res.*, Vol 68 (Special Issue), Abstract 330, 1989, p 908

125. J.F. Cvar and G. Ryge, "Criteria for the Clinical Evaluation of Dental Restorative Materials," No. 790-244, United States Public Health Service

126. A.J. Goldberg, E. Rydinge, E.A. Santucci, and W.B. Racz, Clinical Evaluation Methods for Posterior Composite Restorations, *J. Dent. Res.*, Vol 63, 1984, p 1387–1391

127. L. Boksman, M. Suzuki, R.E. Jordan, and D.H. Charles, A Visible Light-Cured Posterior Composite Resin: Results of a 3-Year Clinical Evaluation, *J. Am. Dent. Assoc.*, Vol 112, 1986, p 627–631

128. K.F. Leinfelder, A.D. Wilder, and L.C. Teixeira, Wear Rates of Posterior Composite Resins, *J. Am. Dent. Assoc.*, Vol 112, 1986, p 829–833

129. W.F. Vann, W.W. Barkmeier, T.R. Oldenburg, and K.F. Leinfelder, Quantitative Wear Assessments for Composite Restorations in Primary Molars, *Pediatr. Dent.*, Vol 8, 1986, p 7–10

130. K.F. Leinfelder, D.F. Taylor, W.W. Barkmeier, and A.J. Goldberg, Quantitative Wear Measurements of Posterior Composite Resins, *Dent. Mater.*, Vol 2, 1986, p 198–201

131. W.F. Vann, W.W. Barkmeier, and D.B. Mahler, Assessing Composite Resin Wear in Primary Molars: Four-Year Findings, *J. Dent. Res.*, Vol 67, 1988, p 876–879

132. J.P. Moffa and A.A. Lugassy, *The M-L Scale,* Pacific Dental Research Foundation

133. S.C. Bayne, E.D. Rekow, D.F. Taylor, A.D. Wilder, J.R. Sturdevant, H.O. Heymann, T.M. Roberson, and T.B. Sluder, Laser Calibration of Leinfelder Clinical Wear Standards, *J. Dent. Res.*, Vol 69 (Special Issue), Abstract 417, 1990, p 161

134. D.F. Taylor, S.C. Bayne, J.R. Sturdevant, A.D. Wilder, and H.O. Heymann, Vivadent Comparison to M-L, Leinfelder, and USPHS Clinical Wear Scales, *J. Dent. Res.*, Vol 69 (Special Issue), Abstract 416, 1990, p 160

135. D.F. Taylor, J.R. Sturdevant, A.D. Wilder, and S.C. Bayne, Correlation of M-L, Leinfelder, and USPHS Clinical Evaluation Techniques for Wear, *J. Dent. Res.*, Vol 67 (Special Issue), Abstract 1993, 1988, p 362

136. M. Bream, P. Lambrechts, V. Van Doren, and G. Vanherle, In vivo Evaluation of Four Posterior Composites: Quantitative Wear Measurements and Clinical Behavior, *Dent. Mater.*, Vol 2, 1986, p 106–113

137. A.K. Abell, K.F. Leinfelder, and D.T. Turner, Microscopic Observations of

the Wear of a Tooth Restorative Composite in vivo, *J. Biomed. Mater. Res.*, Vol 17, 1983, p 501–507

138. K.D. Jorgensen and E. Asmussen, Occlusal Abrasion of a Composite Restorative Resin with Ultra-Fine Filler—An Initial Study, *Quint. Int.*, Vol 9 (No. 6), 1978, p 73–78

139. J.C. Mitchem and D.G. Gronas, In vivo Evaluation of the Wear of Restorative Resin, *J. Am. Dent. Assoc.*, Vol 104, 1982, p 333–335

140. G.C. McDowell, T.J. Bloem, B.R. Lang, and K. Asgar, In vivo Wear, Part I: The Michigan Computer-Graphic Measuring System, *J. Prosthet. Dent.*, Vol 60, 1988, p 112–120

141. T.J. Bloem, G.C. McDowell, B.R. Lang, and J.M. Powers, In vivo Wear, Part II: Wear and Abrasion of Composite Restorative Materials, *J. Prosthet. Dent.*, Vol 60, 1988, p 242–249

142. H. Xu, T. Wang, and P.A. Vingerling, A Study of Surfaces Developed on Composite Resins in vivo during 4–5 Years; Observations by SEM, *J. Oral Rehabil.*, Vol 16, 1989, p 407–416

143. A.D. Wilder, K.N. May, H.O. Heymann, and K.F. Leinfelder, Three Year Clinical Study of Auto-Cured Composites in Posterior Teeth, *J. Dent. Res.*, Vol 64 (Special Issue), Abstract 1604, 1985, p 353

144. A.D. Wilder, K.N. May, and K.F. Leinfelder, Three-Year Clinical Study of UV-Cured Composite Resins in Posterior Teeth, *J. Prosthet. Dent.*, Vol 50, 1983, p 26–30

145. A.D. Wilder, K.N. May, and K.F. Leinfelder, Eight Year Clinical Study of UV-Polymerized Composites in Posterior Teeth, *J. Dent. Res.*, Vol 66 (Special Issue), Abstract 481, 1987, p 167

146. L. Boksman, R.E. Jordan, M. Suzuki, D.H. Charles, and D.H. Gratton, A Five Year Clinical Evaluation of the Visible Light Cured Posterior Composite Resin Ful-fil, *J. Dent. Res.*, Vol 66 (Special Issue), Abstract 479, 1987, p 166

147. K.F. Leinfelder, Wear Patterns and Rates of Posterior Composite Resins, *Int. Dent. J.*, Vol 37, 1987, p 152–157

148. J.R. Sturdevant, T.F. Lundeen, T.B. Sluder, Jr., A.D. Wilder, and D.F. Taylor, Five-Year Study of Two Light-Cured Posterior Composite Resins, *Dent. Mater.*, Vol 4, 1988, p 105–110

149. P. Lambrechts, M. Bream, and G. Vanherle, Buonocore Memorial Lecture, Evaluation of Clinical Performance for Posterior Composite Resins and Dentin Adhesives, *Oper. Dent.*, Vol 12, 1987, p 53–78

150. F. Lutz, R.W. Phillips, J.F. Roulet, and J.C. Setcos, In vivo and in vitro Wear of Potential Posterior Composites, *J. Dent. Res.*, Vol 63, 1984, p 914–920

151. R.P. Kusy and K.F. Leinfelder, Pattern of Wear in Posterior Composite Restorations, *J. Dent. Res.*, Vol 56, 1977, p 544

152. K.-J. Soderholm, M. Zigan, M. Ragan, W. Fischlschweiger, and M. Bergman, Hydrolytic Degradation of Dental Composites, *J. Dent. Res.*, Vol 63, 1984, p 1248–1254

153. W.D. Brunson, S.C. Bayne, J.R. Sturdevant, T.M. Roberson, A.D. Wilder, and D.F. Taylor, Three-Year Clinical Evaluation of a Self-Cured Posterior Composite Resin, *Dent. Mater.*, Vol 5, 1989, p 127–132

154. K. Ratanapridakul, K.F. Leinfelder, and J. Thomas, Effect of Finishing on the in vivo Wear Rate of a Posterior Composite Resin, *J. Am. Dent. Assoc.*, Vol 118, 1989, p 333–335

155. R. DeLong and W.H. Douglas, A Methodology for the Measurement of Occlusal Wear, Using Computer Graphics, *J. Dent. Res.*, Vol 62, Abstract 456, 1983, p 220

156. R. DeLong, M. Pintado, and W.H. Douglas, Measurement of Change in Surface Contour by Computer Graphics, *Dent. Mater.*, Vol 1, 1985, p 27–30

157. S.C. Bayne, D.F. Taylor, J.R. Sturdevant, A.D. Wilder, H.O. Heymann, W.D. Brunson, and T.M. Roberson, Identification of Clinical Wear Factors, *J. Dent. Res.*, Vol 66 (Special Issue), Abstract 604, 1987, p 182

158. D.F. Taylor, S.C. Bayne, J.R. Sturdevant, A.D. Wilder, W.D. Brunson, and G.G. Koch, General Mathematical

Model for Posterior Composite Wear, *J. Dent. Res.,* Vol 68 (Special Issue), Abstract 332, 1989, p 908

159. S.C. Bayne, H.O. Heymann, J.R. Sturdevant, A.D. Wilder, and T.B. Sluder, Contributing Co-Variables in Clinical Trials, *J. Dent. Res.,* Vol 70 (Special Issue), Abstract 14, 1991, p 267

160. I.E. Ruyter and S.A. Svendsen, Remaining Methacrylate Groups in Composite Restorative Resins, *Acta Odontol. Scand.,* Vol 36, 1978, p 75–82

161. S.I. Stupp and J. Weertman, Characterization of Monomer to Polymer Conversions in Dental Composites, *J. Dent. Res.,* Vol 58 (Special Issue), 1979, p 949

162. E. Asmussen, Restorative Resins: Hardening and Strength versus Quantity of Remaining Double Bonds, *Scand. J. Dent. Res.,* Vol 90, 1982, p 484–489

163. E. Asmussen, Factors Affecting the Quantity of Remaining Double Bonds in Restorative Resin Polymers, *Scand. J. Dent. Res.,* Vol 90, 1982, p 490–496

164. J.L. Ferracane and E.H. Greener, Fourier Transform Infrared Analysis of Degrees of Polymerization in Unfilled Resins—Methods Comparison, *J. Dent. Res.,* Vol 63, 1984, p 1093–1095

165. J.L. Ferracane, J.B. Moser, and E.H. Greener, Ultraviolet Light-Induced Yellowing of Dental Restorative Resins, *J. Prosthet. Dent.,* Vol 54, 1985, p 483–487

166. J.L. Ferracane, Correlation between Hardness and Degree of Conversion during the Setting Reaction of Unfilled Dental Restorative Resins, *Dent. Mater.,* Vol 1, 1985, p 11–14

167. J.L. Ferracane and E.H. Greener, The Effect of Resin Formulation on the Degree of Conversion and Mechanical Properties of Dental Restorative Resins, *J. Biomed. Mater. Res.,* Vol 20, 1986, p 121–131

168. A.K. Abell, K.F. Leinfelder, and D.T. Turner, *Polym. Prepr.,* Vol 20, 1979, p 648–651

169. W.D. Cook, Factors Affecting the Depth of Cure of UV-Polymerized Composites, *J. Dent. Res.,* Vol 59, 1980, p 800–808

170. R. Tirtha, P.L. Fan, J.F. Dennison, and J.M. Powers, In vivo Depth of Cure of Photo-Activated Composites, *J. Dent. Res.,* Vol 61, 1982, p 1184–1187

171. R.L. Leung, P.L. Fan, and W.M. Johnston, Post-Irradiation Polymerization of Visible Light-Activated Composite Resin, *J. Dent. Res.,* Vol 62, 1983, p 363–365

172. E.K. Hansen, After-Polymerization of Visible Light Activated Resins: Surface Hardness versus Light Source, *Scand. J. Dent. Res.,* Vol 91, 1983, p 406–410

173. J.R. Dunn, A.H.L. Tjan, D.L. Morgan, and R.H. Miller, Curing Depths of Composites by Various Light Curing Units, *J. Dent. Res.,* Vol 66 (Special Issue), Abstract 162, 1987, p 127

174. M. Mante, V. Dhuru, and W. Brantley, Relationships between Shade, Thickness, Transmitted Curing Light Intensity and Hardness of a Composite Restorative, *J. Dent. Res.,* Vol 66 (Special Issue), Abstract 163, 1987, p 127

175. T.W. Wilson and D.T. Turner, Characterization of Polydimethacrylates and Their Composites by Dynamic Mechanical Analysis, *J. Dent. Res.,* Vol 66 (Special Issue), Abstract 167, 1987, p 127

176. V.A. Demarest and E.H. Greener, Storage Effects on Dynamic Mechanical Properties of Mica Composites, *J. Dent. Res.,* Vol 66 (Special Issue), Abstract 811, 1987, p 208

177. R.A. Draughn, Compressive Fatigue Limits of Composite Restorative Materials, *J. Dent. Res.,* Vol 58, 1979, p 1093–1096

178. C.N. Raptis, P.L. Fan, and J.M. Powers, Properties of Microfilled and Visible Light-Cured Composite Resins, *J. Am. Dent. Assoc.,* Vol 99, 1979, p 631–633

179. R. Whiting and P.H. Jacobsen, Dynamic Mechanical Properties of Resin-Based Filling Materials, *J. Dent. Res.,* Vol 59, 1980, p 55–60

180. R. Whiting and P.H. Jacobsen, A Non-Destructive Method of Evaluating the Elastic Properties of Anterior Restorative Materials, *J. Dent. Res.,* Vol 59, 1980, p 1978–1984

181. E.H. Greener, C.S. Greener, and J.B. Moser, The Hardness of Composites as a Function of Temperature, *J. Oral Rehabil.,* Vol 11, 1984, p 335–340

182. S.C. Bayne, D.F. Taylor, J.R. Sturdevant, T.M. Roberson, A.D. Wilder, and M.W. Lisk, Protection Theory for Composite Wear Based on 5-Year Clinical Results, *J. Dent. Res.,* Vol 67 (Special Issue), Abstract 60, 1988, p 120

183. J.C. Roberts, J.M. Powers, and R.G. Craig, Wear of Commercial Pit and Fissure Sealants, *J. Dent. Res.,* Vol 56, 1977, p 692

184. M. Houpt, Z. Shey, A. Chosack, E. Eidelman, A. Fuks, and J. Shapira, Occlusal Composite Restorations: 4-Year Results, *J. Am. Dent. Assoc.,* Vol 110, 1985, p 351–353

185. J.M. Powers, J.A. Capp, and R.G. Craig, Abrasion of Temporary Filling Materials, *J. Mich. Dent. Assoc.,* Vol 56, 1974, p 281–283

186. J.M. Powers, P.L. Fan, and R.W. Hostetler, Properties of Class V Restorative Materials, *J. Mich. Dent. Assoc.,* Vol 63, 1981, p 275–278

187. J.E. McKinney, J.M. Antonucci, and N.W. Rupp, Wear and Microhardness of a Silver-Sintered Glass-Ionomer Cement, *J. Dent. Res.,* Vol 67, 1988, p 831–835

188. G.T. Charbeneau and R.R. Bozell III, Clinical Evaluation of a Glass Ionomer Cement for Restoration of Cervical Erosion, *J. Am. Dent. Assoc.,* Vol 98, 1979, p 936–939

189. A. Ekfeldt and G. Oilo, Wear of Prosthodontic Materials—An in vivo Study, *J. Oral Rehabil.,* Vol 17, 1990, p 1–13

190. J.R. Beall, Wear of Acrylic Resin Teeth, *J. Am. Dent. Assoc.,* Vol 30, 1943, p 252–256

191. J.A. Saffir, Further Studies in Evaluating Acrylics for Masticatory Surface Restorations, *J. Am. Dent. Assoc.,* Vol 31, 1944, p 518–523

192. J. Osborne, Abrasion Resistance of Dental Materials, *Br. Dent. J.,* Vol 87, 1949, p 10–12

193. F.A. Slack, A Preliminary Method for Testing Abrasion Hardness, *J. Am. Dent. Assoc.,* Vol 39, 1949, p 47–50

194. G.E. Monasky and D.F. Taylor, Studies on Wear of Porcelain, Enamel, and Gold, *J. Prosthet. Dent.,* Vol 25, 1971, p 299–306

195. C.N. Raptis, J.M. Powers, and P.L. Fan, Frictional Behavior and Surface Failure of Acrylic Denture Teeth, *J. Dent. Res.,* Vol 60, 1981, p 908–913

196. C.N. Raptis, J.M. Powers, and P.L. Fan, Wear Characteristics of Porcelain Denture Teeth, *Wear,* Vol 67, 1981, p 177–185

197. A. Koran, R.G. Craig, and E.W. Tillitson, Coefficient of Friction of Prosthetic Tooth Materials, *J. Prosthet. Dent.,* Vol 27, 1972, p 269–274

198. V.W. Boddicker, Abrasion Tests for Artificial Teeth, *J. Am. Dent. Assoc.,* Vol 35, 1947, p 793–797

199. J.A. Mahalik, F.J. Knap, and E.J. Weiter, Occlusal Wear in Prosthodontics, *J. Am. Dent. Assoc.,* Vol 82, 1971, p 154–159

200. A.R.T. Greenwood, Wear Testing Equipment for Synthetic Resin Teeth, *Abstr. J. Dent. Res.,* Vol 34, 1955, p 741–742

201. J.C. Thompson, Attrition of Acrylic Teeth, *Dent. Pract. (Bristol),* Vol 15, 1965, p 233–236

202. R.E. Myerson, The Use of Porcelain and Plastic Teeth in Opposing Complete Dentures, *J. Prosthet. Dent.,* Vol 7, 1957, p 625–633

203. J.A. Cornell, J.S. Jordan, S. Ellis, and E.E. Rose, A Method of Comparing the Wear Resistance of Various Materials Used for Artificial Teeth, *J. Am. Dent. Assoc.,* Vol 54, 1957, p 608–614

204. J.P. Coffey, R.J. Goodkind, R. DeLong, and W.H. Douglas, In vitro Study of the Wear Characteristics of Natural and Artificial Teeth, *J. Prosthet. Dent.,* Vol 54, 1985, p 273–280

205. W.R. Mann and O.C. Applegate, Acrylic Teeth as a Means of Obtaining Balanced Functional Occlusion in Partial Denture Prosthesis, *J. Am. Dent. Assoc.,* Vol 31, 1944, p 505–514

206. P.G. Lofberg, Pronounced Abrasion of Acrylic Teeth, *Dent. Abstr.,* Vol 2, 1957, p 432–433

207. A.S.T. Franks, Clinical Appraisal of Acrylic Tooth Wear, *Dent. Pract. (Bristol),* Vol 12, 1962, p 149–153

208. V.H. Sears, Occluding Porcelain to Resin Teeth—A Clinical Evaluation, *Dent. Surv.,* Vol 36, 1960, p 1144–1146

209. A. Ekfeldt and G. Oilo, Occlusal Contact Wear of Prosthodontic Materials: An in vivo Study, *Acta Odont. Scand.,* Vol 46, 1988, p 159–169

210. A. Ekfeldt and G. Oilo, Wear Mechanisms of Resin and Porcelain Denture Teeth, *Acta Odont. Scand.,* Vol 47, 1989, p 391–399

211. A. Harrison, Clinical Results of the Measurement of Occlusal Wear of Complete Dentures, *J. Prosthet. Dent.,* Vol 35, 1976, p 504–511

212. R.E. Ogle, L.J. David, and H.R. Ortman, Clinical Wear Study of a New Tooth Material, Part II, *J. Prosthet. Dent.,* Vol 54, 1985, p 67–75

213. L.P. Adams, C.H. Jooste, and C.J. Thomas, An Indirect in vivo Method for Quantification of Wear of Denture Teeth, *Dent. Mater.,* Vol 5, 1989, p 31–34

214. A. Harrison, R. Huggett, and R.W. Handley, A Correlation between Abrasion Resistance and Other Properties of Some Acrylic Resins Used in Dentistry, *J. Biomed. Mater. Res.,* Vol 13, 1979, p 23–34

215. R. Lappalainen, A. Yli-Urpo, and L. Seppa, Wear of Dental Restorative and Prosthetic Materials in vitro, *Dent. Mater.,* Vol 5, 1989, p 35–37

216. G.R. Miller, J.M. Powers, and K.C. Ludema, Frictional Behavior and Surface Failure of Dental Feldspathic Porcelain, *Wear,* Vol 31, 1975, p 307–316

217. R. DeLong, W.H. Douglas, R.L. Sakaguchi, and M.R. Pintado, The Wear of Dental Porcelain in an Artificial Mouth, *Dent. Mater.,* Vol 2, 1986, p 214–219

218. P.L. Fan, J.M. Powers, and B.C. Reid, Surface Mechanical Properties of Stone, Resin, and Metal Dies, *J. Am. Dent. Assoc.,* Vol 103, 1981, p 408–411

219. Y. Shoji, Studies of the Mechanism of the Mechanical Enlargement of Root Canals, *Nihon Univ. Sch. Dent. J.,* Vol 7, 1965, p 71–78

220. H. Ochia, Studies on Dental Hand Reamer, Part I: Automatic Measurement of the Reamer Diameter and Cutting Torque; Part II: Diameter and Cutting Sharpness of Commercial Reamers, *Jpn. J. Conserv. Dent.,* Vol 19, 1976, p 41–73

221. S. Oliet and S.M. Sorin, Cutting Efficiency of Endodontic Reamers, *Oral Surg., Oral Path., Oral Med.,* Vol 36, 1973, p 243–252

222. J. Weber, J.B. Moser, and M.A. Heuer, A Method to Determine the Cutting Efficiency of Root Canal Instruments in Linear Motion, *J. Endodont.,* Vol 6, 1980, p 829–834

223. J.G. Newman, W.A. Brantley, and H. Gerstein, A Study of the Cutting Efficiency of Seven Brands of Endodontic Files in Linear Motion, *J. Endodont.,* Vol 9, 1983, p 316–322

224. R.G. Neal, R.G. Craig, and J.M. Powers, Cutting Ability of K-Type Endodontic Files, *J. Endodont.,* Vol 9, 1983, p 52–57

225. E. Stenman and L.S.W. Spangberg, Machining Efficiency of Endodontic Files: A New Methodology, *J. Endodont.,* Vol 16, 1990, p 151–157

226. R.G. Neal, R.G. Craig, and J.M. Powers, Effect of Sterilization and Irrigants on the Cutting Ability of Stainless Steel Files, *J. Endodont.,* Vol 9, 1983, p 93–96

227. R.A. Felt, J.B. Moser, and M.A. Heuer, Flute Design of Endodontic Instruments: Its Influence on Cutting Efficiency, *J. Endodont.,* Vol 8, 1982, p 253–259

228. L.J. Miserendino, J.B. Moser, M.A. Heuer, and E.M. Osetek, Cutting Efficiency of Endodontic Instruments, Part II: Analysis of Tip Design, *J. Endodont.,* Vol 12, 1986, p 8–12

229. J. Lindhe and L. Jacobson, Evaluation of Periodontal Scalers, Part I: Wear Following Clinical Use, *Odontol. Revy,* Vol 17, 1966, p 1–8

230. J. Lindhe, Evaluation of Periodontal Scalers, Part II: Wear Following Standardized Orthogonal Cutting Tests, *Odontol. Revy,* Vol 17, 1966, p 121–130

231. J. Lindhe, Evaluation of Periodontal Scalers, Part III: Orthogonal Cutting Analyses, *Odontol. Revy,* Vol 17, 1966, p 251–273

232. H. Tal, A. Kozlovsky, E. Green, and M. Gabbay, Scanning Electron Microscope

Evaluation of Wear of Stainless Steel and High Carbon Steel Curettes, *J. Periodontol.,* Vol 60, 1989, p 320–324

233. M.P. Benfenati, M.T. Montesani, S.P. Benfenati, and D. Nathanson, Scanning Electron Microscope: An SEM Study of Periodontally Instrumented Root Surfaces, Comparing Sharp, Dull and Damaged Curettes and Ultrasonic Instruments, *Int. J. Periodont. Rest. Dent.,* Vol 2, 1987, p 51–67

234. H. Tal, J.M. Panno, and T.K. Vaidyanathan, Scanning Electron Microscope Evaluation of Wear of Dental Curettes during Standardized Root Planing, *J. Periodontol.,* Vol 56, 1985, p 532–536

235. D.C. Tidy, Frictional Forces in Fixed Appliances, *Am. J. Orthod. Dentofac. Orthop.,* Vol 96, 1989, p 249–254

236. J. Nicolls, Frictional Forces in Fixed Orthodontic Appliances, *Dent. Prac. Dent. Rec.,* Vol 18, 1967–1968, p 362–366

237. G.F. Andreasen and F.R. Quevedo, Evaluation of Friction Forces in the 0.022 × 0.028 Edgewise Bracket in vitro, *J. Biomech.,* Vol 3, 1970, p 151–160

238. C.A. Frank and R.J. Nikolai, A Comparative Study of Frictional Resistance between Orthodontic Bracket and Arch Wire, *Am. J. Orthod.,* Vol 78, 1980, p 593–609

239. J.G. Stannard, J.M. Gau, and M.A. Hanna, Comparative Friction of Orthodontic Wires under Dry and Wet Conditions, *Am. J. Orthod.,* Vol 89, 1986, p 485–491

240. L.D. Garner, W.W. Allai, and B.K. Moore, A Comparison of Frictional Forces during Simulated Canine Retraction of a Continuous Edgewise Bracket, *Am. J. Orthod. Dentofac. Orthop.,* Vol 90, 1986, p 199–203

241. L. Peterson, R. Spencer, and G. Andreasen, Comparison of Frictional Resistance for Nitinol and Stainless Steel Wire in Edgewise Arch Wire, *Quint. Int.,* Vol 13 (No. 5), 1982, p 563–571

242. D. Drescher, C. Bourauel, and H.-A. Schumacher, Frictional Forces between Bracket and Arch Wire, *Am. J. Orthod. Dentofac. Orthop.,* Vol 96, 1989, p 397–404.

Index